Impact of Psychoendocrine Systems in Cancer and Immunity

Impact
of Psychoendocrine Systems
in Cancer and Immunity

Edited by   **Bernard H. Fox**
Boston University Medical Center

Benjamin H. Newberry
Kent State University

1984
C.J. Hogrefe, Inc.
Lewiston, New York · Toronto

Library of Congress Cataloging in Publication Data
Main entry under title:
Impact of psychoendocrine systems in cancer and immunity.
    Includes bibliographies and indexes.
    1. Cancer–Psychosomatic aspects–Addresses, essays,
lectures. 2. Cancer–Immunological aspects–Addresses,
essays, lectures. 3. Immunity–Endocrine aspects–
Addresses, essays, lectures. 4. Neuroendocrinology–
Addresses, essays, lectures. I. Fox, Bernard H.
II. Newberry, Benjamin H., 1942–   . III. Title:
Psychoendocrine systems in cancer and immunity.
[DNLM: 1. Psychophysiology. 2. Hormones–Physiology.
3. Neoplasms–Psychology. 4. Neoplasms–Immunology.

5. Immunity. 6. Hormones–Immunology. QZ 200 I3458]
RC265.I46 1983   616.99′408   83-18607
ISBN 0-88937-005-2

Canadian Cataloguing in Publication Data
Main entry under title:
Impact of psychoendocrine systems in cancer and
immunity
ISBN 0-88937-005-2

1. Cancer–Psychosomatic aspects–Addresses,
essays, lectures. 2. Stress (Psychology)–
Addresses, essays, lectures. 3. Immune response–
Addresses, essays, lectures. I. Fox, Bernard H.
II. Newberry, Benjamin H.

RC265.I46   616.99′408   C82-094911-6

Copyright © 1984 by C. J. Hogrefe, Inc.

C. J. Hogrefe, Inc.
P. O. Box 51
Lewiston, NY 14092

Canadian Edition published by
C. J. Hogrefe, Inc.
525 Eglinton Avenue East
Toronto, Ontario M4P 1N5

Printed in Canada

Contents

Contributors

David A. Boyle, *Department of Psychology, Kent State University, Kent, Ohio 44242*

Thomas G. Burish, *Department of Psychology, Vanderbilt University, Nashville, Tennessee 37240*

Michael P. Carey, *Department of Psychology, Vanderbilt University, Nashville, Tennessee 37240*

V. M. Dilman, *Professor N. N. Petrov Research Institute of Oncology, Leningrad, USSR*

Dennis G. Dyck, *Department of Psychology, University of Manitoba, Winnipeg, Canada*

Bernard H. Fox, *Department of Biobehavioral Sciences and Hubert Humphrey Cancer Center, Boston University Medical Center, Boston, Massachusetts 02118*

Arnold H. Greenberg, *Department of Pediatrics and Immunology, Manitoba Institute of Cell Biology, University of Manitoba, Winnipeg, Canada*

E. A. Korneva, *Research Institute of Experimental Medicine, USSR Academy of Medical Sciences, Leningrad, USSR*

C. Kubo, *Department of Psychosomatic and Internal Medicine, Faculty of Medicine, Kyushu University, Fukuoka City 812, Japan*

Annabel G. Liebelt, *Northeastern Ohio Universities College of Medicine, Rootstown, Ohio 44272 (Current Address: Registry of Experimental Cancers, National Cancer Institute, Bethesda, Maryland 20205)*

Ruth Lloyd, *Goodwin Institute for Cancer Research, Plantation, Florida 33309 (Current Address: 15 Hereford Street, Boston, Massachusetts 02115)*

Benjamin H. Newberry, *Department of Psychology, Kent State University, Kent, Ohio 44242*

M. N. Ostroumova, *Professor N. N. Petrov Research Institute of Oncology, Leningrad, USSR*

Lorna S. Sandler, *Department of Psychology, University of Manitoba, Winnipeg, Canada*

E. K. Shkhinek, *Research Institute of Experimental Medicine, USSR Academy of Medical Sciences, Leningrad, USSR*

Lydia Temoshok, *Department of Psychiatry, Langley Porter Psychiatric Institute, University of California San Francisco, San Francisco, California 94143*

H. Teshima, *Department of Psychosomatic and Internal Medicine, Faculty of Medicine, Kyushu University, Fukuoka City 812, Japan*

Preface

Recently the belief has been growing that the relationships between psychological processes and disease are of major importance. In this volume two related and central aspects of these relationships, psychological factors in immunity and in cancer, are addressed. Although psychological influences on cancer in animals—both its occurrence and progress—have long been known, the mechanisms have been poorly understood. In man the case is even less clear. Only recently have we been able to isolate some of the bodily intervening processes. Prominent among these are changes in the immune system. But other systems, e. g., the endocrine system, affect and are affected by both psychoneural and immune functions. It is these relationships that have emerged as new concepts in recent years. We no longer merely suspect an impact of neural and endocrine processes on cancer and the immune system; we know it. The task before science now is to explicate how and under what conditions such interactions take place.

If useful applications follow from the area which has come to be called psychoneuroimmunology, they are likely to have a broad impact on health. Any insights into the causes, course, and management of cancer carry immediate impact and capture public as well as scientific attention. In particular, as a reason for considering cancer and immunity together, they are intimately related. And most important, perhaps, the immune system can exercise control over neoplastic diseases.

Realizing this, we selected the book's material primarily to complement rather than merely repeat other recent works in the area. Further, we sought (a) ideas and data from outside the English-speaking scientific community; (b) findings which are too new to have played a large role in shaping recent discussions of the area; (c) inclusion of diverse contexts in which psychological factors and cancer are related; and (d) presentation of new concepts in the field.

Consistent with the third objective, psychological phenomena in the cancer area (personality, feelings of stress, cognitive reactions, various behaviors, etc.) are important as well as the intervening variables mentioned above—the endocrine, neurological and immunological events. We are continually arriving at new inductions, both at the molar and the "black box" (which is not so black these days) levels. It is important to emphasize, as we have done here, that such molar phenomena are elements of the various systems' interactions and are worthy of study in the cancer process as well as more molecular phenomena. Finally, consistent with the fourth objective, authors were invited to be speculative if they wished. Several accepted the invitation, and we trust that their ideas will be stimulating.

We chose to order the chapters roughly in terms of emphasis on review/discussion in their contents, with earlier chapters focusing on discussion and later ones on data. This is a rough classification, however, since most chapters provide both data and general discussion.

Lloyd presents a wide-ranging overview of mechanisms through which psychological processes are involved with immune function. She stresses recent advances in the understanding of relationships among neural and neurohumoral systems as they relate jointly to immunity. She knits together widely diverse topics, portraying a complex system of systems which interact to regulate both normal and pathologic processes.

Dilman and Ostroumova have a slightly more focused view, concentrating on hypothalamic and peripheral metabolic processes as they relate to neoplastic disease and immune function. They suggest a general hyperadaptational syndrome involving a change in the set-point for hypothalamic sensitivity to homeostatic influences. In their view, the neuroendocrine and metabolic components of this syndrome serve to link chronic stress, psychological depression, and normal aging to both immune function and cancer.

In discussing the relation of stress to cancers, Newberry, Liebelt, and Boyle examine the extensive range of environmental and host variables which must be considered in interpreting associations between psychosocial variables and cancer. They apply these in a critical assessment of current views regarding psychobiological factors as modulators of neoplastic processes, concluding that in several respects current research and discussion are too limited.

Burish and Carey review the available research on psychological side effects of cancer chemotherapy, and behavioral interventions in those side effects. They conclude that the side effects can be viewed as the result of classical conditioning, at least to a great degree, and that relaxation is probably a major component of successful interventions.

Shkhinek and Korneva present both discussion and data from their research on immunomodulation by the endocrine system, particularly the effects of corticosteroids on humoral immune function. They present findings in which neuroendocrine or immunological manipulations affect the response of the other system, showing that the effects of hormonal shifts on immune function depend upon both the endocrine pattern and the immune parameter involved.

Greenberg, Dyck, and Sandler report data on the differing response of animals, after acute aversive stimulation, to cancer strains differently resistant to NK cells. Other experiments address repeated vs. acute aversive stimulation, and the effects of hydrocortisone, ACTH, and opiate antagonists. Provocatively, they discuss their findings in terms of a model of conditioned opponent processes.

Teshima and Kubo also present data relevant to animal models of psychological effects on neoplastic disease and immune function. Their experiments examine effects of chronicity on stress-related cytotoxicity, using heterogeneic and EL-4 leukemia cells, macrophage particulate phagocytosis, and transplanted EL-4 tumor growth.

Finally, Temoshok and Fox, in separate series of studies, look at signs and prognosis in melonoma patients, using both medical and psychosocial predictors. Temoshok's group, defining a Type C person, suggest that the medical signs and prognosis of such patients are worse than those of non-C's, and verify their hypotheses. They confirm their hypothesis of earlier relapse among C than non-C patients on the dimension of not expressing dysphoric emotion. However, they did not parallel the earlier data of Rogentine et al., who predicted and found more one-year relapses among those reporting that they were little disturbed by melanoma surgery than among others. Fox follows relapse and mortality experience in Rogentine's samples for two more years, but finds little evidence that can be used to confirm the 1-year data.

We hope that both researchers and practitioners in psychooncology and psychoimmunology will find these chapters interesting and, more importantly, stimulating. A workable understanding of the interrelations among psychosocial factors, immunity, and cancer is still some way off. However, the contributions to this book serve to illustrate both the complexities and the promise of continued research on these problems.

Bernard H. Fox
Benjamin H. Newberry
August, 1983

Mechanisms of Psychoneuroimmunological Response

Ruth Lloyd

> "There is no pure sorrow. Why? It is bedfellow to lungs, lights, bones, guts and gall!"
> –Djuna Barnes, *Nightwood,* 1937

Introduction

The biological principle of homeostasis implies successful psychophysiological adaptation to the vicissitudes of environmental challenge. In man, equilibrium of mind and body describes the healthful state and stress-related processes are seen as the expression of psychological and physiological maladaptation – the psychosomatic relationship gone awry. Maladaptation, in this sense, signifies habitually inappropriate emotional response to perceived stress in association with physiological habit patterns that can predispose the body to tissue damage and organic dysfunction.

Illness, so defined, fits within the biological, psychological and social conceptual framework proposed by G. L. Engel (1973, 1977) to supplant the traditional biochemical model of disease, a model that must be deplored for its narrow emphasis on illness as aberration in the body machine, rather than as human suffering experienced within the social environment. Since it is inclusive rather than exclusive, comprehensive rather than reductive, the biopsychosocial model incorporates an enormous body of research on the symptomatology of various diseases and on the life circumstances that surround disease onset, exacerbation and remission, as well as upon attributes of personality that appear to be associated with physiopathology (Bahnson, 1981; Bakal, 1979; Fox, 1981; Henry & Stephens, 1977; Levy, 1982; Morrison & Paffenbarger, 1981; Weiner, 1977; Weiner, Hofer, & Stunkard, 1980).

The purpose of this review will be to address a central question that is implicit in the published reports on this research: namely, *how* psychogenic stress can modify the internal state to such a degree that normal immunological response to pathogen is either compromised, or altogether undermined (Weiner, 1977). A question of this kind might be approached in any one of several ways. In this present instance, a discussion of the interrelationship among the three regulatory body systems (nervous, endocrine and immune) that are important to healthful functioning and pathologic dysfunction alike will serve as an introduction to the question, and data will later be introduced to illustrate the structural contiguity and functional convergence of these systems. Insofar as necessary, the morphophysiological and genetic substratum underlying disease predisposition will also be described, with particular emphasis being placed upon some of the infinitely small and precise transformations that normally take place between and within somatic cells. Most important of all, given the matter at hand, it will be essential to consider some of the very first links in a so-called "transducer chain" of events (M. Delbrück, cited in Bergman et al., 1969) connecting conscious experience to the endocrine and neurochemical processes that contribute to immunologic competence.

How interpretation between these two realities comes about, how symbol translates into physiological effect, remains, after all, the most basic of all questions in biology (Delbrück, 1970), and although any study of disease must confront the problem of mechanism – the "error in machinery" remaining as much a point of focus as ever – research in medicine and its allied disciplines can only benefit from a theoretical approach that emphasizes the whole person and acknowledges the impelling influence of subjective state on physiologic infrastructure (Rose, 1980; Sperry, 1952, 1976; Weiner, 1972). More to the point, it must be asked whether the immune system is not also sensitive to this same influence. Does it not also contribute to the transductional process and, by implication, to adaptive response and to the protection of internal equilibrium? That is to say, if the phenomenon of psychophysiological encoding is to be defined as the translation of discrete neuronal impulse into highly specific blood-borne hormonal discharge, capable of linking brain and peripheral organ, emotion and endocrine effect (Axelrod, 1974; Scharrer, 1970; Wurtman, 1970, 1971; Wurtman & Anton-Tay, 1969), is it not likely that the generally flawless communication network of immune effector cells fulfills an auxiliary role in this process?

An argument to this effect can be tentatively supported by several observations. It might be remembered, at the outset, that the lymphoid cell membrane incorporates a receptor molecule whose stereoconfiguration permits it to act as a kind of quintessential intermediary between ligand and intracellular transducer (Greaves, 1976), however the latter may be ultimately defined. Furthermore, if it can be assumed that the primary and secondary sites of immune cell genesis and deposition, as well as the interconnected lymphatic vessels that perfuse and drain them, form the representative organ of the immune system (Haurowitz, 1980), it should then follow that communication codes operate within the system, between it and other systems, and that the structural and chemical bases for these apparent codes are decipherable.

Granted that a completely integrated picture of such an intersystem transductional circuitry is not yet in place, the possibility of its existence can hardly be refuted in the light of what is presently known. For example, various immune parameters have been proven to be markedly altered by the experimental manipulation of hypothalamic loci in laboratory animals (Cross et al., 1980; Simon et al., 1980; Solomon & Amkraut, 1981; Spector, 1980); serious compromise of an organism's adaptive resources will be reflected in suppression of immune competence (Locke & Kraus, 1982; Visintainer, Volpicelli, & Seligman, 1982); and perhaps most significantly, the immune response has been shown to be conditionable, a finding that may well have touched upon the underlying psychoimmunological linkage in adaptation (Ader, 1981a; Ader & Cohen, 1981).

In a lighter vein, and as a kind of summing up to these preliminary remarks, various similes can be drawn from the scientific literature that would seem to have bearing on the matter of transduction. It is notable, in the first place, that a terminology exists which could be said to foreshadow the formation of the postulates, comprehensive designs and enduring principles that can eventually bring about the interdisciplinary synthesis that is so needed: terms such as "memory molecule," familiar to immunologist and biochemist alike, or "conformational induction," a term that applies equally to structural alteration in the receptor protein of post-synaptic membranes and to perturbations associated with ligand-receptor binding within the lymphocyte plasma membrane. Nor do other conceptual transliterations seem entirely implausible. A parallel can be drawn, for example, between descriptions of the intracranial circuits of reward, memory and drive as "plastic . . . absorptive . . . ready to pick up programs from the world" (Olds, 1976, p. 48) and the immunological phenomena of surveillance, recognition and memory. Similarly, it is interesting to compare the concept of behavior as dependent variable in a biopsychosocial paradigm (Mason, 1975; Mason et al., 1976; Selye, 1970, 1974) and the definition of the "behavioral code" in operation, whereby behavioral modification, in the broadest sense of that term, becomes mirrored in the tissues, changes in gene expression and synaptic protein becoming the ultimate ultrastructural signs of imprinting, short- and long-term memory retention and associative learning (DeFeudis & DeFeudis, 1977; Kandel & Schwartz, 1982).

General Observations
on the Interaction of Systems

Psychoneuroimmunology has become a newly differentiated field in medical science devoted to the development of new and more inclusive models of brain, mind and behavior in health and illness. Excepting its new energy, some new concepts, increased sophistication in its research tools (Rabkin & Struening, 1976) and remarkable progress in immunology and genetics, the growth of this interdiscipline has taken place in the context of ideas that have contributed to psychosomatic theory over the past thirty years (Murray, 1977). These ideas have been founded upon the presumption that psychosomatic interaction relates, in turn, to genetic predisposition and total life experience, and that these latter influences can incorporate such variables as specific organ susceptibility and perception of self.

This extension of the principle of intrinsic self-governance is a significant departure from previous attempts at synthesis in the biological and behavioral sciences, for it allows a fresh examination of the perturbations in psychoendocrine regulation that jeopardize immunologic protection of the physiological "self." Or, to state the converse, this enlargement of the psychosomatic concept is stimulating basic research on stress-related derangements in intercellular communication which, by either impeding or subverting recognition of pathogen and/or mutagen, threaten the stability of other complementary homeostatic controls.

The three integrative systems of the body differ with respect to the kinds of stimulus induction to which each responds, and salient differences exist between their receptor and effector components. Nevertheless, it is possible to draw analogies between these systems and to describe examples of their complementary, mutually enhancing interaction. The more obvious analogies pertain to the characteristics of systems, *per se*. For in the most general sense, each of the three under consideration behaves as a regulatory unit which monitors the basal metabolic requirements of a discrete population of cells and orchestrates those protective modes of cell interaction that safeguard the internal integrity of the whole organism.

Regulation implies communication, fine-tuned by feedback inhibition, between active elements unique to each system and the receptor proteins, glycoproteins and glycolipids that are integral constituents of target cell membranes. Depending upon its chemical nature, a single efferent molecular "signal" is either acted upon at the cell surface, relayed to the cytoplasm in the form of a ligand-receptor complex enveloped within a receptosome (Pastan & Willingham, 1981), or, once conveyed through the intracellular matrix, introduced into the nucleus of the cell. At the membrane interface and at each conjunction with organelles of the cell, the original chemical mediator is progressively transduced, becoming, at last, the final specific stimulus capable of eliciting an equally specific cellular response.

Specificity of information transfer is common to each of these systems and is a defining characteristic. Hence, in ways that bear similarity to the substrate-specific activity of enzymes (Fersht, 1977; Holloway, 1976), neurotransmitter substances cross the synapse to become selectively bound to specific chemosensitive receptor sites on post-synaptic nerve cell membranes, endocrine hormones traverse the bloodstream to react with specific intramembranous receptor sites on widely dispersed end-organ cells, and microorganisms and other foreign particles succumb to recognition and binding by antigen-specific receptors on the outer surfaces of immunocompetent cells, or lymphocytes.

In an immunological frame of reference, signal specificity is fundamental to lymphoid cell activation and to the lymphocyte's latent capacity for antigen recognition and immunologic memory, capacities encoded in the unique idiotypic configurations of surface receptor molecules, complementary to like spatial arrangements on the surfaces of cognate antigens. In this manner, structural specificity and complementarity act as primary stimuli to lymphoid cell differentiation upon the initial exposure of an organism to antigen and as selective vehicles for the exponential proliferation of lymphocyte clones from lymphoblasts upon subsequent exposure (Katz, 1977; Marchalonis, 1976).

Another obvious parallel between systems can be seen in the transport of glandular secretions, and of immune cells and their assemblage of soluble macromolecules, since, in each instance, the circulating mediums of blood, or of blood and lymph, are essential dynamic principles. It is noteworthy, however, that in contrast to its use in describing the transmission of nerve impulse, or the interlocking of endocrine hormone and tissue cell, "specificity," in the immunologic sense, has a special meaning. Accordingly, in a turn of language appropriate to the phylogenetically ancient guardian role performed by immune cells and their organelles in the evolution of all vertebrate and some invertebrate species, the reactive immune cell is described as possessing specificity "against," or specificity "directed towards," the molecular shape of a particular antigen.

Redundancy, another property of living systems, is also a characteristic of the immune complex. It is no exaggeration to state, for example, that immune response (Ir) genes and their histocompatibility-linked molecular products control a veritable maze of interactions among lymphocytes, phagocytic macrophages and leukocytes and their ancillary soluble products, as well as between these reactive elements and immunogenic stimuli under conditions of acute and inflammatory response and in neoplasia (Cochrum & Hanes, 1980; Dausset, 1981; Nathenson et al., 1980; Sprent & Korngold, 1981; Uehara et al., 1980). Yet, despite their differing capacities and modes of action, the primary immune effector cells, the T and B lymphocytes, demonstrate cooperative and overlapping activities and are part of an armamentarium of immunopotent elements, including closely related cellular subgroups, which collaborate in a complicated and remarkably elaborate interplay.

By means of this interplay, the internal organization of the immune system is expressed and its equilibrium maintained. To be sure, there are provocative, new (and newly resurrected) data to show that this complex organization represents but a subsystem within a systems hierachy and that the "autonomous" immune cell network (Jerne, 1974, 1976) is susceptible to nervous system governance, as well as to inflexible genetic instruction. Nevertheless, through the collective action of its individual regulatory constituents, the immune system unquestionably exhibits many levels of intrinsic stimulatory and inhibitory control (Gershon, 1979; Melchers & Rajewsky, 1976; Loor & Roelants, 1977).

In certain respects, derangements in this kind of control become analogous in different systems and have come to be described in similar terms. Disinhibition in central neurons, for example, is known to result in the "excessive and disorderly" paroxysmal neuronal discharge of epileptic seizure (J. Hughlings Jackson, cited in Taylor, 1958). In like manner, if not in like outcome, a failure in inhibitory feedback in the lymphocyte network can result in excessive proliferation of a single immune cell type, followed by discriminatory disturbance and the production of tissue-damaging autoantibodies – all precursory conditions favoring the development of autoimmune disease (Talal, 1977, 1978).

Beyond serving as an example of profound disturbance in internal organization within a single system, there is an added dimension to the phenomenon of autoimmunity that is particularly relevant to systems interaction. As Heinz Köhler (1980) has recently framed the question: why, in certain disease states, do the "boundary zones" dividing the immune network, the endocrine and nervous systems – zones that are normally strictly delimited – break down? The answer, he suggests, is likely to be found through the interdisciplinary application of hybridoma techniques to one of the focal points of systems convergence: namely, the cell surface receptor and its complementary anti-receptor structure. The significance of this interaction and its converse, the binding of hormonal and neural ligands to their specific receptor sites on primary immune cells, is clear: lymphocyte membrane protein structures comprise the medium of transduction for encoded information from nervous and endocrine tissues to the lymphocytoplasmic matrix (Edelman, Yahara, & Wang, 1973). Consequently, any discussion of effector pathways for psychological influence on immunity must take into account how the psychological status of the organism can influence the complex series of energy transformations that are ultimately resolved at this fundamental, macromolecular level of organization (Rose, 1980).

An appropriate starting point from which to examine this thesis is to describe how the immune system is extrinsically controlled. More specifically, it will be shown how the labyrinthian complex of cells and soluble proteins that comprise the system are affected by neuronal activity in the medial basal hypothalamus, a principal site for the "corebrain control mechanisms" governing emotion, motivation and mood (Pribram, 1980). Inasmuch as the brain and endocrine glands together are thought to form a system equal in importance to the autonomic and somatic nervous systems of the body (Knigge & Silverman, 1972), and the hypothalamus is recognized as a pivotal integrant in autonomic and endocrine activity, certain features of neural and neuroendocrine anatomy and interaction will also be discussed in detail. Revisions in neurological theory that have kept pace with technological advance will also be mentioned, since these new perspectives on cell-to-cell communication have interesting implications for psychoneuroimmunology.

Before introducing this material, it is important to make an additional point: that is to say, it is essential that any argument for brain-mind-immune interconnection be qualified with the realization that the remarkable capacity of the immune system to control the recognition of autologous and foreign molecules, as well as the selective differentiation of lymphocytes, attests to a system of controls that must act at a still more fundamental level. Consequently, a few comments on the genetic control of the immune response are appropriate here, notwithstanding the fact that this subject is tangential to the main thesis to be developed in this chapter.

The Role of
Histocompatibility Genes in Immunity

In the first place, the advent of hybridoma technology (Köhler & Milstein, 1975, 1976) has facilitated the potentially revolutionary clinical procedure of tissue (histo)-compatibility typing (Kennett, McKearn, & Bechtol, 1980; Rose, 1981) and introduced the diagnostic use of monoclonal antibodies to identify genetic predisposition to various chronic diseases, including a number of autoimmune disorders (Benacerraf & McDevitt, 1972; Dausset, 1972; Dausset & Svejgaard, 1977; McDevitt & Bodner, 1972; Ryder, Platz, & Svejgaard, 1980; Sasazuki, Grumet, & McDevitt, 1977). Basic to this work is the discovery of select gene complexes that not only protect self-identity, but also initiate and regulate immune reactions (Cochrum & Hanes, 1980; Dausset, 1981; Nathenson et al., 1980; Sprent & Korngold, 1981; Uehara et al., 1980). Harbored in polymorphic chromosomal loci, these histocompatibility genes encode for glycoprotein molecules expressed as transmembranous cell structures known as HLA histocompatibility antigens in man and as H-2 antigens in the laboratory mouse. These self-determinants comprise two subclasses of the major histocompatibility complex (MHC), or "supergene" (Amos & Kostyu, 1980; Snell, 1980), a division based upon their cellular distribution, some (HLA-A, HLA-B, HLA-C) appearing on most human body cells, others (HLA-D, HLA-DR) appearing only on cells of the human reticuloendothelial system – a selective distribution befitting molecular structures that so profoundly influence the recognitive properties of cells. Still other immune response-associated (Ia) antigens are products of immune response (Ir) genes which map within human D and DR and murine I chromosomal regions of the MHC (Benacerraf & McDevitt, 1972; Gasser & Silvers, 1974; McDevitt et al., 1972). These antigens constitute self-MHC cell-surface markers which mediate many aspects of host response to specific non-MHC-associated (non-self) antigen incursion – not alone response, but appropriateness of response (Dausset, 1980).

In cell-mediated immunity, for example, the macrophage, an ameboid blood monocyte, migrates by pseudopodia and chemotaxis to the site of inflammatory lesion, or potential malignancy, where it processes (chemically alters) and presents antigen to helper T (T_h) cells in the exact genetically (MHC)-restricted orientation that will facilitate T cell induction, recognition, binding and reactivity (Katz & Benacerraf, 1975). In humorally-mediated immunity, a response largely directed against extracellular bacteria and viruses, B lymphocytes undergo differentiation into plasma cells, each plasma cell and its B cell precursor being capable of producing one or more surface glycoprotein antibody molecules from amongst five possible classes (M, G, A, D, E). Each such molecule shares an identical specificity according to its idiotype, i.e., an array of surface antigenic determinants associated with precisely those genetically-encoded hypervariable (V) regions on the amino terminal portions of the polypeptide chains of which the antibody molecule is comprised (Brack et al., 1978; Cooper et al., 1979; Seidman et al., 1978).

In further illustration of histocompatibility-linked Ir gene control of humoral and cell-mediated immunity, the binding of the Ia receptor molecule and its attached antigen to the macrophage surface is an essential prerequisite to T_h cell proliferation: that is, helper, suppressor and cytotoxic T lymphocyte (CTL) specializations are elaborated during differentiation in an histocompatibility "context," T cell commitment to autologous MHC antigens during differentiation pointing, therefore, to a kind of immune cell imprinting that must have inevitable salutary consequences to the immunologic defense and adaptive endowment of the host (Benacerraf, 1981).

Moreover, the histocompatibility context has a potent effect on the discriminative capability of T lymphocyte subpopulations. Helper and suppressor/cytotoxic T cells (each of the two subsets distinguished by a different surface antigen) have been found to respond to different protein products of the major histocompatibility complex, the helper T cells alone responding selectively and vigorously to HLA-DR antigens associated with immune response genes of the MHC (Engleman et al., 1981). It has also been shown that cytotoxic T lymphocyte precursor cells from congenitally athymic mice are developmentally restricted by the particular specificity of engrafted semi- and fully-allogeneic neonatal thymic H-2 complex, strongly indicating that it is "the MHC phenotype of the intrathymic environment that dictates which MHC determinants the CTL precursors differentiating within it will specifically recognize as self-determinants" (Kruisbeek et al., 1981, p. 2175).

It is hoped that this very brief condensation of a complex topic should at least have suggested that no matter how complicated a web of data might be spun to illustrate the extrinsic control of immune reactivity, there are immutable forces within the system itself that remain untouched by these influences. Also, it is obvious that arguments for the compelling effects of attitudinal, behavioral and environmental variables on disease susceptibility must be countered with irrefutable evidence that this susceptibility is to some extent genetically pre-programmed in particular individuals.

The Central Regulation of the Immune Response

Neurophysiological Determinants of Immune Function

The main thrust of immunological theory and experimentation has tended to dwell, not without reason, on the seeming autonomy of immune effector mechanisms. This idea of autonomy persists, to be expressed most recently in an essay by Köhler, Levitt and Bach (1981), which describes the system as a "minicosmos," a self-contained, self-directing complementary network with a seemingly boundless capacity to "create a mirror image for all structures in the universe" (p. 58). In fairness, however, this bias in contemporary immunological research should be placed in historical context by noting that nearly a century and a half of achievements in the study of immune mechanisms had passed before S. Metal'nikov was to insist, on the basis of his own research at the Pasteur Institute, that the very complexity of immunologic responses made "l'intervention du système nerveux" an essential requisite to their regulation (Metal'nikov [1934], quoted in Spector, 1980).

A number of recent publications indicate that Metal'nikov's ideas are shared by a growing cadre of investigators (Ader, 1980, 1981b; Riley, 1981; Rogers, Dubey, & Reich, 1979; Solomon & Amkraut, 1981; Stoll, 1979; Weiss, Herd, & Fox, 1981) and that traditionally divided research interests are coming to view the immune system in its proper context, in an "intermediate position," as Herbert Weiner has said, "between the self-regulatory function of an organ and its superordinate regulation by the brain" (Weiner, 1977, p. 604). The investigations that have helped to bring about this more propitious research climate began in the early 1940's and continue to this day.

Broadly speaking, lesions, ablation and electrical stimulation of hypothalamic nuclei can both activate (see, e.g., Dann, Wachtel, & Rubin, 1979) and suppress the immune system, a suppressive effect being the more commonly reported result (Cross et al., 1980; Simon et al., 1980; Solomon & Amkraut, 1981; Spector, 1980; Spector & Korneva, 1981; Stein, Keller, & Schleifer, 1979, 1981; Stein, Schleifer, & Keller, 1981). Varying with choice of antigen and experimental species, immunosuppression has been shown to take the form of anaphylaxis inhibition, depressed delayed hypersensitivity response, thymic involution, reduced circulating antibody titer, lymphocyte depletion and impaired mitogen-induced lymphocyte blastogenesis.

How electrolytic ablation influences plasma transmitter levels, cytotropic antibodies and the receptivity of autonomic receptor subunits on tissue-fixed mast cells and target shock organs remains unclear, as do the mediator pathways between the brain, inflammation loci in peripheral tissue, and recognition sites on lymphoid organs and activated lymphoid cells. Direct experimental evidence has been either slim or lacking in this regard (Devoino, 1979; Fessel & Forsyth, 1963). However, indirect support, confirming earlier Soviet investigations into this question (Klimenko, 1972, 1975; Korneva & Klimenko, 1976), comes from a study by Besedovsky et al. (1977), which has demonstrated *afferent* linkages between immunoregulatory factors and the central nervous system; i.e., the firing frequency of individual nerve cells in the ventromedial nucleus of the hypothalamus in preimmunized rats will increase following systemic administration of sheep red blood cells (SRBC) and trinitrophenylated-hemacyanin (TNP-Hae).

In spite of the present paucity of data relating to this matter, inductive reasoning, exemplified by such arguments as those developed in a 1973 paper by Janković and Isaković, would dictate that incursion into subcortical tissue, by whatever means, must markedly influence neurotransmitter outflow, neuropeptide secretion and the activity levels of peripheral corticosteroid hormones. It will be seen that diencephalic structures are densely reticulated by the "dorsal norepinephrine bundle" (Ungerstedt, 1971), as well as by other transmitter systems that exert strong influence on the pituitary-adrenal axis (Renaud, Pittman, & Blume, 1979; Záborsky, 1982). Bearing in mind that steroid hormones are generally immunosuppressive (Claman, 1972, 1975; Ignarro, 1977; Parillo & Fauci, 1979), three of the more striking immunologic reactions to plasma glucocorticoid elevation brought about by the activation of this axis (Lang et al., 1976) include (1) the hormone-induced sequestering of effector (helper) T lymphocytes by their redistribution to sites of origin, i. e., the bone marrow and spleen (Fauci, 1978; Haynes & Fauci, 1978); (2) the inhibition of mast cell agranulation and histamine release (Schmutzler & Freundt, 1975); and (3) the inhibition of lymphokine synthesis (Wahl, Altman, & Rosenstreich, 1975, (the term, "lymphokine," denoting a host of biologically active mediator substances acting upon lymphocytes and their accessory cells [Cohen, Pick, & Oppenheim, 1979; Pick, 1981a, 1981b]). Logically enough, it follows from these observations that the immunosuppressive effects of anterior hypothalamic lesions can be abrogated by adrenalectomy, hypophysectomy (Tyrey & Nalbandov, 1972) and the metopirone (metyrapone)-induced paralysis of adrenocortical secretion (Gainer, Peng-Loy, & Sarne, 1977).

Experimental evidence leaves no doubt that this cascade of effects does in fact occur under particular conditions of stress in the intact organism. Some of these effects will be examined in considerable detail, discussed as separate threads of evidence, before their reassembly into a clearer, if more complicated, picture of neuroimmunological response. Still, it should be noted that, straightforward as the above sequence might seem, the immunosuppression that follows anterior hypothalamic lesioning is not invariably correlated with increased steroid production and release (Cross et al., 1980). As R.J. Cross and his colleagues have pointed out (Brooks et al., 1982), there may be other, non-steroid neuroendocrine hormones responsible for the immunosuppression that follows destructive lesions. They have shown, furthermore, that preoptic and anterior hypothalamic lesions in rats will induce an increase in the activity of splenic, macrophage-like suppressor cells (Roszman et al., 1982).

There is little question that patterns of activation in various transmitter and hormonal systems under conditions of immune suppression and potentiation will eventually be fully analyzed and defined. By comparison, a more complete understanding of the relationship between changes in immunologic parameters as these are induced by both psychosocial influence and experimentally-manipulated conditioning procedures may be closer at hand. Apart from their intrinsic interest, the studies that have illustrated these phenomena will surely help to provide a larger perspective on behavioral adaptation and its relevance to immune status. For the purposes of this review, they can, in addition, provide an appropriate *psychological* background for the detailed physiological descriptions that are to follow in the later sections of this chapter.

Psychological Determinants of Immune Function

At the outset, it is fair to say that behavioral research has proceeded with reasonable confidence on the premise that adaptation is an expression of learning: an organism learns contingencies between its behavior and environmental outcome, and to the degree to which its innumerable and continuous acts of self-reference and experiential validation succeed (Cullen, 1980), it can be said to have learned to cope, to adapt. Once confined to the more straightforward tenets of causality, to strict emphasis upon the response-reinforcer bond, the principles of learning that have evolved from this research are now shown to be equally pertinent to the ambiguities of perception and cognition. As a consequence, attention has come to be focused not alone on how an organism perceives surrounding events – are these predictable? controllable? – but also on its ability to resolve conflict and so make the instrumental choices that will assure its well-being and survival (Miller, 1980a, 1980b; Overmier, Patterson, & Wielkiewicz, 1980). This final point has been illustrated in a series of recent psychoimmunological studies, of which the following few are but selected examples.

Locke and Kraus (1982) have observed significant diminution in natural killer (NK) cell activity in young adults who are inadequately adjusted to high levels of "life change stress." In a second such example taken from animal research, Reite, Harbeck, and Hoffman (1981) have found cellular immunity to be depressed in infant monkeys during and immediately following peer separation.

There is still other evidence to show that immune function can be impaired under circumstances in which adaptive, coping strategies are patently futile. Thus, Keller et al. (1981) have shown that unavoidable aversive stimulation administered to rats in the form of a graded series of electric shocks, paired with restraint, will be directly reflected in T lymphocyte activity–increasing levels of shock and decreasing cellular response to the mitogen, phytohemagglutinin (PHA), having been found to describe a continuum.

There are related studies that have more directly addressed the issue of psychological state as it may bear upon immune competence by evaluating the relationship between coping and tumor susceptibility (Sklar & Anisman, 1981). Thus, in the "yoked" testing procedure (random, inescapable shock *vs* control over shock delivery, both animals receiving identical shocks), adult male rats have been found to have a much-reduced capacity to reject tumor cell implantation (Visintainer, Volpicelli, & Seligman, 1982) and to show more rapid and exaggerated tumor development and reduced survival rate (Sklar & Anisman, 1979).

The classical conditioning of the immune response has added still another facet to the study of central influence on immune function. It has proven to be a replicable, generalizable phenomenon in both adrenalectomized and intact animals (Ader, Cohen, & Grota, 1979), one that holds true for both humoral, antibody-mediated immunity (Ader & Cohen, 1981; Cohen et al., 1979; Rogers et al., 1976; Wayner, Flannery, & Singer, 1978) and cellular, T cell-mediated immunity (Ader & Cohen, 1981; Bovbjerg, Ader, & Cohen, 1982; Gorczynski, Macrae, & Kennedy, 1982). In this work, conditioned immunosuppression is initially established by the *single* pairing of an innocuous gustatory stimulus with illness-induced taste aversion: i.e., presentation of sodium saccharin, acting as conditioned stimulus (CS), is temporally associated with the intraperitoneal injection of an aversive, immunosuppressive drug (e.g., cyclophosphamide [Cupps, Edgar, & Fauci, 1982]), acting as unconditioned stimulus (US). The acquisition of conditioned immunosuppression is then demonstrated by a depressed hemagglutinin antibody titer serving as the measure of conditioned response (CR) to antigen (i.p. injection of sheep red blood cells SRBC) presented in association with the once-innocuous, now behaviorally significant, conditioned stimulus (saccharin).

Not to be described as an original discovery in itself, inasmuch as pioneering efforts to relate immunologic enhancement to the conditioned reflex were undertaken by Metal'nikov and Chorine at the Pasteur Institute as early as 1926, and later diligently pursued in the Soviet Union (Ader, 1981a), these more recent demonstrations of the phenomenon have a special significance, for they come at a time that is ripe for interdisciplinary cohesion. Obviously, too, the implications of this work are far-reaching. Given the fact that the significant pairing in the conditioning paradigm (i.e., the pairing of a neutral stimulus with an unconditioned response) operates in both immunosuppression and immunopotentiation, the potential for the therapeutic application of these behavioral procedures becomes immediately apparent.

It has been shown, for example, that onset of proteinuria and subsequent lethal glomerulonephritis in systemic lupus erythematosis (SLE) can be significantly delayed by the application of this same taste aversion conditioning paradigm to female, New Zealand hybrid mice, a standard experimental model for the study of this autoimmune disease (Ader & Cohen, 1982). By contrast, in CBA mice, the pairing of a neutral stimulus (sham skin graft) (CS) with either inoculation of foreign alloantigenic (C57BL/6) lymphoid cells (US), or skin allograft (CS + US), has been shown to elicit the classically conditioned enhancement of an antigen-specific cellular immune response—in this case, the proliferation of cytotoxic T lymphocyte precursors (CTLp) in peripheral blood. This particular study by Gorcznski, Macrae and Kennedy (1982) went a step further in illustrating the extent to which immune response parameters can be manipulated, by showing both positive reinforcement of the conditioned response (i.e., increased frequency of CTLp following the reintroduction of the CS and US) and extinction of the response (following the reintroduction of the CS alone) in a pre-selected subgroup of "responder" animals.

Overall, these experiments on the behavioral conditioning of immune reactions suggest, as Ader and Cohen (1975) have stated, "an intimate and virtually unexplored relationship between the central nervous system and immunologic processes . . . a mechanism that may be involved in the complex pathogenesis of psychosomatic disease" (pp. 338–9). In a word, it is no longer enough to describe putative mechanisms for the neuroendocrine modulation of the immune response in a strictly mechanistic fashion. The following detailed, if less than comprehensive, over-view of these and other central mechanisms will seem a barren scaffold indeed if the dynamics of intrapsychic perceptual process were not to be borne in mind.

Neural and Neuroendocrine Pathways in Pituitary Regulation

It is now well established that the pituitary gland, i.e., adenohypophysis, receives indirect stimulation from afferent fiber systems that converge on the medial hypothalamus from the neocortex, thalamus, limbic structures, preoptic area, midbrain and brainstem (Anschel, Alexander, & Perachio, 1982; Renaud et al., 1979; Záborsky, 1982). Understandably, its strategic position within this neuroaxis renders this "master gland" exquisitely sensitive to both intraorganismic and environmental influence (Hennessy & Levine, 1979). It is with good reason, therefore, that the tropic endocrine hormones of the pituitary have been described as the biologic transformation of sensory inflow, and that their area of origin, the hypothalamic-hypophyseal region of the brain, is generally considered to be a primary site of neuroendocrine transduction.

Present knowledge of this critical interface would not be possible were it not for the remarkable evolution of investigative technique in brain research, dating from the early axon-degeneration studies of Nauta and Gygax (1954) and the histochemical fluorometric and elec-tromicroscopic work carried out by Fuxe and his colleagues in the 1960's (Andén et al., 1966; Falck & Hillarp, 1959; Fuxe, 1965; Hillarp, Fuxe, & Dahlström, 1966). Now in common use are: (1) specific anti-sera raised against peptides as fixable antigens; (2) histochemical stain-ing with unlabeled antibody peroxidase-antiperoxidase (PAP) for light and electron microscopic analysis (immunohistochemistry); (3) the se-quential immunoprecipitation of radioactively-labeled cellular proteins from culture medium (radioimmunoassay; gel electrophoretic and fil-tration analysis); (4) gel permeation chromatography; (5) the mapping of neurotransmitter and neuropeptide receptor distribution in the brain by means of autoradiographic tracing of anterograde axonal transport following *in vivo* and *in vitro* labeling with radioactive ligands; and (6) the autoradiographic measurement of glucose utilization in neuronal systems.

The fine structure and pharmacology of central neurons is being illu-minated to such a degree by procedures of this kind that previously un-suspected varieties of anatomical, bioelectric and biochemical relation-ship between and within neurons have become evident. The most fun-damental contribution of this technology has been to bring about the essentially complete characterization of a number of brain transmitter systems, each with its own distinct morphology. The following descrip-tion of these several systems is an encapsulation of an extensive litera-ture representing this prodigious effort. It does not by any means pre-sent an exhaustive listing of either all possible neurotransmitter, nor of all possible neuropeptide, candidates.

Neurotransmitter Systems

A diffuse noradrenergic (NE) fiber system has been shown to inner-vate the cerebral cortex, the hippocampal formation, the cerebellum, the hypothalamus, the medial forebrain bundle and the median eminence (infundibulum) (Amoral & Sinnamon, 1977; Lindvall & Björklund,

1978; Moore & Bloom, 1979; Savaki et al., 1982; Ungerstedt, 1971), this last structure serving as a neurohemal end-organ for the entire hypothalamic-hypophysiotropic system (Brawer & Walsh, 1982; Knigge, Scott, & Weindl, 1972). The noradrenergic network originates in cell groups within the brainstem reticular formation and the nucleus locus coeruleus (Dahlström & Fuxe, 1965; Moore, 1980).

Epinergic (epinephrine) nerve terminals, derived from cell bodies in the lateral reticular nucleus of the medulla (Hökfelt et al., 1974), have been traced to the median eminence and to the ventromedial and arcuate nuclei of the hypothalamus (Hökfelt et al., 1978; Moore & Bloom, 1979; Palkovits et al., 1980; Van der Gugten et al., 1976). Somata of a dopaminergic (DA) system, situated in the arcuate, dorsomedial and periventricular nuclei of the hypothalamus, in the caudate thalamus, and in the pars compacta of the midbrain substantia nigra (Jacobowitz, 1978), have been shown to give rise to terminal fibers which not only lie in close proximity to the infundibular capillary plexi of the anterior pituitary (Fuxe, 1965; Fuxe & Hökfelt, 1969; Moore & Kromer, 1978; Ungerstedt, 1971), but extend as well to the posterior pituitary (Björklund & Nobin, 1973) and basal ganglia (Andén et al., 1966; Carpenter & Peter, 1972; Dahlström & Fuxe, 1964; Ungerstedt, 1971).

The raphe cell groupings of the midbrain have been identified as the source of a serotoninergic (5-HT) axonal system which innervates the median eminence (Andén et al., 1966; Belenky, Chetverukhin, & Polenov, 1979) and hypothalamus (Azmitia & Segal, 1978; Belenky et al., 1979; Moore, Halaris, & Jones, 1978; Parent, Descarries, & Beaudet, 1981), including the preoptic area (Saavedra et al., 1974; Van der Kar & Lorens, 1979). 5-HT neurons have also been identified within the hypothalamus itself (Kent & Sladek, 1978).

The release of the inhibitory amino acid neurotransmitter, γ-aminobutyric acid (GABA), has been shown to be mediated by axonal fibers in the median eminence and the pars reticulata of the substantia nigra— projections which originate in the arcuate nucleus (Tappaz & Brownstein, 1977; Walaas & Fronnum, 1978) and basal ganglia (caudate nucleus of the neostriatum [Bak et al., 1975; Kim et al., 1971]), respectively. Finally, ascending acetylcholine-containing (cholinergic) axons have been traced in the cortex, striatum, medial forebrain bundle and median eminence from their locus of origin in the septum (Carson et al., 1978; Moroni, Cheney, & Costa, 1977; Shute & Lewis, 1966).

Neurosecretory Systems

Another—and as will be seen, not entirely disassociated—transmitter network (Barker, 1977) originates in the parvicellular tuberoinfundibular, paraventricular and supraoptic nuclei of the hypothalamus. The first of these neurosecretory systems synthesizes a number of small peptide hormones (e. g., somatostatin [growth hormone release-inhibiting hormone], thyrotropin-releasing hormone [TRH], luteinizing hormone-releasing hormone [LHRH], substance P and neurotensin) which are secreted into a sinusoidal capillary plexus in an area of the hypothalamus situated directly above the neurovascular infundibular stem (Elde et al., 1976; Johansson et al., 1978; Kobayashi, Matsui, & Ishii, 1970; McCann & Porter, 1969). Drained downward from this plexus through large capillaries to a secondary plexus in the anterior pituitary lobe, these releasing hormones either selectively stimulate, or inhibit, the secretion of the pituitary tropic hormones, prolactin (PRL), growth hormone (GH), luteinizing hormone (LH), follicle-stimulating hormone (FSH) and thyroid-stimulating hormone (TSH).

The paraventricular and supraoptic nuclei of the hypothalamus form a magnocellular neurosecretory system, or supraoptic-hypophyseal tract, which crosses the median eminence and extends the entire length of the pituitary stalk (Brownstein, Russell, & Gainer, 1980; Defendini & Zimmerman, 1978; Joseph & Knigge, 1978; Renaud et al., 1979). In common with tuberoinfundibular neurons, these cells also mediate an exchange between neural elements and the blood stream, although in this case, the mechanisms for exchange are both direct and indirect.

In the first instance, the two nonapeptide neurohormones, oxytocin and vasopressin, and their carrier proteins, estrogen-stimulated neurophysin (ESN) and nicotine-stimulated neurophysin (NSN), are independently secreted from separate groups of cells (Seif & Robinson, 1978) into capillaries that discharge into the systemic venous system from the posterior lobe terminus (Bargmann & Scharrer, 1951; Bisset, 1976; Scharrer & Scharrer, 1954). In the second instance, vasopressin behaves as a regulatory hormone that is secreted into the anterior lobe circulation, either by way of a neurosecretory pathway from the magnocellular paraventricular nucleus (Antunes, Carmel, & Zimmerman, 1977; Zimmerman & Robinson, 1976), or through a vascular connection that has been found to join the two pituitary lobes and the median eminence (Baertshi et al., 1980). There is also new evidence to show that vasopressin and oxytocin secretion may be facilitated by electrotonic coupling (local circuitry) between cells in both the paraventricular and supraoptic hypothalamic nuclei (Andrew et al., 1981) and that these two nuclei are innervated by ascending noradrenergic fibers (Sawchenko & Swanson, 1981). The many axonal collaterals that have been shown to project from the paraventricular nucleus to both intra- and extra-hypothalamic sites (cortex, striatum, olfactory tract, pons and cerebellum) (Eiden & Brownstein, 1981; Krieger, 1980; Pittman, Blume, & Renaud, 1981) further suggest a local, integrative activity.

Adrenocorticotropin (ACTH), melanocyte-stimulating hormone (MSH), methionine [Met]-enkephalin and the biologically inactive prohormone of the endorphins, β-lipotropin (β-LPH), have all have been found to be synthesized *de novo* from pro-opiomelanocortin (POMC), or pro-opiocortin (Chrétien et al., 1979; Cohen et al., 1980; Eipper & Mains, 1980; Mains, Eipper, & Ling, 1977; Roberts & Herbert, 1977a, 1977b), a macromolecular glycoprotein found in anterior pituitary endocrine cells (Eipper & Mains, 1978; Pelletier et al., 1977; Roberts & Herbert, 1977a, 1977b; Rubinstein, Stein, & Udenfriend, 1978) and in nerve cell bodies in the arcuate nucleus of the hypothalamus (Liotta et al., 1979; Pelletier, 1980). This second, endogenous CNS source of pro-opiocortin forms two fiber systems: a tuberoinfundibular peptidergic tract which terminates at the median eminence capillary bed; and a second, more restricted system which appears to synapse with other non-peptidergic infundibular neurons (Bugnon et al., 1979). A recent immunohistochemical study undertaken by Schwartzberg and Nakane (1982) has determined that the appearance of antigenic determinants of ACTH-related peptides (e. g., ACTH, γ-lipotropin, β-endorphin and a 16K opiocortin fragment) in the median eminence of the fetal rat precedes their appearance in the pituitary gland (day 12 *vs* day 16).

Immunocytochemical staining of rat brain sections has shown that ACTH-immunoreactive fibers of the opiocortin system originate from the basal hypothalamus, to converge in high concentration on the paraventricular nucleus, with extensions to the limbic system and brainstem (Knigge & Joseph, 1982; Krieger, 1980). In addition, radioimmunoassay, gel exclusion chromatography and immunochemical staining have revealed dense concentrations of β-endorphin in both anterior and posterior pituitary lobes and a much reduced, but strategic, localization in the brain, notably in the arcuate nucleus and median eminence (Sofroniew, 1979; Wilkes et al., 1980).

The distribution of another group of opioid peptides, the methionine [Met]- and leucine [Leu]-enkephalins, is characterized by cell bodies in the paraventricular nucleus of the hypothalamus, with projections to the posterior pituitary (Chavkin, James, & Goldstein, 1982, Rossier et al., 1980b) and a widespread distribution to other areas of the brain (Watson et al., 1982). The heptadecapeptide, dynorphin (Goldstein et al., 1979), forms still a third endogenous opioid system, with anatomic and biosynthetic features resembling those of the enkephalin system

(Kakidani et al., 1982; Watson et al., 1982), but nonetheless distinct (Goldstein & Ghazarossian, 1980). The exact relationship between the distribution patterns of these two peptides remains to be elucidated (Watson et al., 1981). The paraventricular nucleus, however, has been found to be the site of origin of corticotropin-releasing hormone (corticoliberin) (CRH) (Gibbs & Vale, 1982; Rivier et al., 1982; Spiess et al., 1981; Vale et al., 1981), α-Neo-endorphin, vasopressin, and two fragments of the dynorphin molecule, dynorphin-(1–17) and dynorphin-(1–8), and immunoreactivity by CRH and dynorphin-(1–8) has been observed in some of the same paraventricular neurons (see Roth et al. [1983] for a discussion of the close, and perhaps "synergistic," relationship between peptidergic paraventricular cells).

As a class, neurosecretory cells are derived from the neural crest, neuroectoderm and ectoblast (Said, 1980). Consequently, they share certain structural and chemical features, and so have been accorded the acronym descriptor, APUD (amine precursor uptake and decarboxylation) (Pearse, 1981). For example, in contrast to the enzymatically controlled synthesis of conventional neurotransmitters from amino acids and monoamines, peptide synthesis comes about through the selective proteolytic cleavage of a larger, genetically-encoded parent molecule, or pro-hormone (e.g., pro-opiocortin), a ribosomal-dependent process which takes place on RNA template within the nucleus of the peptidergic cell (Acher, 1976; Gainer et al., 1977; McKelvy & Epelbaum, 1978; Sachs et al., 1969).

Additionally, neurosecretory cells are electrically active and therefore capable of impulse generation and propagation from axonal bouton terminals (Cooke, 1977; Maddrell & Nordmann, 1979). They are also indisputably "endocrine," precisely as their dual properties were first conceptualized by Ernst and Bertha Scharrer forty years ago (Scharrer & Scharrer, 1940). Hence, unlike other "first messengers" involved in neurotransmission, neurosecretory cells have been found to be more sensitive to hormonal and metabolic signals and to exert more potent and relatively longer-lasting effects upon target tissues (Brownstein, 1978; Emson, 1977; Knowles & Howard, 1966).

Aside from their localization in both brain and pituitary gland (Elde & Hökfelt, 1979; Krieger, 1980; Krieger & Martin, 1981a, 1981b; Shepherd, 1974; de Wied & Jolles, 1982), the distribution of peptidergic neurosecretory cells has been found to be extraordinarily diffuse. To date, they have been found in the urogenital and gastrointestinal tracts, pancreas, thyroid gland and lung (Ghatei et al., 1982; Hökfelt et al., 1979a; Kendall & Orwoll, 1980; Larsson, 1978; Said, 1980). In the brain, but outside the blood-brain barrier (in the ventral median eminence), neurohemal contacts exist (Halász, Kosaras, & Lengvari, 1972) which presumably allow hormonal flow to take place between the axonal projections of peptidergic cells and portal vessel fenestrae (Carlisle & Knowles, 1953; Monroe & Holmes, 1982; Renaud et al., 1979). Although anastomosis has been demonstrated in other circumventricular organs of the brain that lack the blood-brain barrier (van Breeman & Clemente, 1955; Duvernoy & Koritke, 1964; Hofer, 1958, 1965; Weindl & Joynt, 1972), these particular linkages are presumed to delineate a final common pathway in neuroendocrine regulation (Knigge, 1967; Scharrer, 1965). Therefore, in view of its probable importance in terms of psychoendocrine and immune regulation, it would be well, at this point, to describe aspects of the morphology and integrative capacities of this infundibular pathway in greater detail.

The Ventricular System and Median Eminence

In certain respects, the median eminence is a unique hypothalamic tissue. Characterized by an extremely high rate of metabolic activity (Knigge & Silverman, 1972; Silverman, Knigge, & Peck, 1972), it has been described as a "pulsatile system" with relatively few true synapses, an interstitial space in which enzymes, transmitters and neurohormones mingle in high concentration (Joseph & Knigge, 1978; Kobayashi et al., 1970; Kordon et al., 1979). In addition, the median eminence has been shown to be densely populated by short capillary loops and by tanycytes, or specialized ependymocytes, cells with pleomorphic characteristics and apparently phagocytic capacity (Brawer & Walsh, 1982). Tanycytes are presumed to provide both a vehicle for the selective transport of biologically active materials between hypothalamus, cerebrospinal fluid and the adenohypophyseal circulatory network (Bleier, 1972; Pilgrim, 1978; Porter et al., 1975; Rodriguez, 1969), and a channel for their retrograde passage along this same corridor (Dorsa et al., 1981). Intercellular tight junctions in the ependymal covering of the median eminence, and between ependyma on the infundibular floor, may also serve as differentially permeable barriers to the movement of hormonal substances (Brightman, Prescott, & Reese, 1975; Monroe & Holmes, 1982; Richards, 1978). On the other hand, the role of gap junctions between ependyma found in this area, and at the ventrolateral wall of the third ventricle, is still imperfectly understood (Monroe & Holmes, 1982), although it is known that they, too, permit the intercellular flux of ions and small molecules (e.g., negatively-charged polypeptides) (Bennett, Spray, & Harris, 1981).

In a general sense, this ventricular transport mechanism fits the model of brain-endocrine interaction along a "glial-vascular chain" first proposed by Folke Löfgren in 1959 – although, understandably, the model has been undergoing considerable modification. For one thing, three-dimensional electron-microscopic examination of circulatory patterns in the infundibulum, infundibular process, pituitary gland and third ventricle, as seen in vascular casts of these structures (Page, Munger, & Bergland, 1970), has so altered the traditional concept of their function that a "new paradigm" for neuroendocrine integration is now emerging (Bergland & Page, 1979). Hence, when viewed posteriorly, from above, and as one with the anastomotic arteries of the neurohypophysis and the fenestrated capillaries on the infundibular surface, the capillary circuitry common to both pituitary lobes suggests a diversified pattern of hormonal flow, not alone within the gland itself, but also between it, the carotid circulation, the third ventricle and the cerebrospinal fluid.

With respect to the importance of the median eminence and the ubiquitous neuropolypeptides in complex behavior, an observation by Mayeri and Rothman (1981) deserves special mention. From their study of "selective and specific" *nonsynaptic* peptidergic transmission in the abdominal ganglion of the marine mollusk, *Aplysia,* these investigators surmised that a mode of information processing in which the extracellular space acts as a medium for transmitter-specific, rather than synapse-specific, interneuronal communication might well characterize the activity of peptide neurons in the vertebrate brain. Although they did not suggest a likely CNS locus for this form of neuronal connection, several lines of evidence would seem to implicate the infundibular zone.

Selective
Observations on the Interaction of Systems

Hormones and the Brain

The possibility exists that hormones synthesized within the pituitary gland may gain access to the brain and so influence its function (Dunn & Gispen, 1977), and that they may do so by more than one route. The central effects of corticotropin (ACTH), for example, had originally been understood to be indirect and to be limited to the dynamics of its own release: namely, to the long-loop negative feedback inhibition of its hypothalamic "releasor," corticotropin-releasing hormone (CRH), by circulating plasma levels of ACTH and the adrenal corticosteroids, cortisol and corticosterone (de Kloet, Veldhuis, & Bohus, 1980; McEwen et al., 1979; Smelik & Papaikonomou, 1973; Yates & Maran,

1974). It is now known that CRH secretion is not only modified by feedback of its own peripheral end-products, but that it is also influenced by a short-loop feedback circuit within the hypothalamic-hypophyseal neurosecretory unit itself, an inhibitory control system that is entirely independent of the adrenal cortex (Bergland et al., 1980; Krieger & Liotta, 1979; Motta, Fraschini, & Martini, 1969). Both of these reflex systems, short and long, have been found to be affected by patterns of sleep and wakefulness, darkness and light (Krieger, Kreuzer, & Rizzo, 1971; Orth & Island, 1969); circadian variation in hormone secretion entrained to patterns of food intake (Holloway et al., 1979; Krieger, 1974; Wilkinson, Shiusako, & Dallman, 1979); elevations in corticosteroids and ACTH in response to physical stressors (Hennessy & Levine, 1979; Yuwiler, 1976); and by even so subtle a psychological stressor as failed expectancy (Levine, Goldman, & Coover, 1972).

The exact sites at which these modulatory actions take place *in vivo*, whether at the level of the hypothalamus or the hypophysis, remain unclear. However, recent CRH bioassays, carried out *in vivo* by Catherine Rivier and colleagues (Rivier et al., 1982), "confirm the fact that the pituitary represents an important inhibitory feedback site" (p. 277). (It will be remembered that the hypothalamus and pituitary gland are independent sites of origin for ACTH peptidergic cells [Schwartzberg & Nakane, 1982].) There is, in addition, a report by Schachter et al. (1982) showing that glucocorticoids will inhibit *de novo* synthesis of pro-opiocortin (POMC) (the precursor to ACTH and β-endorphin) in rat anterior pituitary tissue in culture by selectively decreasing POMC mRNA levels. Glucocorticoid feedback on central structures is evidently mediated by a steroid receptor system within pituitary, hypothalamic and extra-hypothalamic sites, particularly dense receptor concentrations having been found in the hippocampus (Bohus, de Kloet, & Veldhuis, 1982).

These demonstrations of endocrine hormone influence on the brain take on added significance in the light of research that has shown associations between ACTH and the morphinomimetic opioid pentapeptides, the endorphins; between β-endorphin and the pituitary tropic hormone, prolactin; between the endorphins, the enkephalins and lymphoid cells; and between ACTH and the potent T lymphocyte mediator products, the lymphokines. Furthermore, there is recent work indicating that immunopotent factors may themselves perform an endocrine role.

At risk of introducing an ostensibly random collection of facts, evidence for each of the foregoing observations will be listed, in turn. Perhaps, in being presented in this way, these diverse data will appear less as heterogeneous elements than as characteristics of a more or less integral system, joined by common properties and by a kind of architectural logic, form closely relating to function. What is more, certain of these studies would appear to add support to the long-held belief that the hypothalamus, brainstem and vagus nerve are involved in anaphylactic shock (Karczewski, 1964; Mills & Widdicombe, 1970) and bronchial allergy (Gold, Kessler, & Yu, 1972; Szentivanyi, 1968). Still other studies suggest the presence of a lymphoid-pituitary-adrenal axis (Blalock & Smith, 1981) and/or hypothalamic-infundibular-thymic axis, although a cautionary note is in order in this regard, given the preliminary nature of the data.

The Interrelatedness of Neuropeptides

Although their degree of coexistence is not invariably balanced, indicating either a differential processing from the glycoprotein precursor, pro-opiocortin, or, in some instances, the likelihood of different precursors, ACTH and β-endorphin have been found to be localized within the same nerve cell bodies, to occupy the same pituitary cell, and to be released stoichiometrically from the same secretory granules (Agnati et al., 1982; Guillemin et al., 1978). This particular pairing is not unlike others of its kind, and may reflect a general, rather than exceptional, condition in the infundibular hypothalamus (Hökfelt et al., 1979a, 1979b, 1980a, 1980b). Similar relationships have been discovered, for example, between β-endorphin and α-MSH (Watson & Akil, 1981); between the cholinergic neurotransmitter, acetylcholine, and central monoamines (Hökfelt et al., 1978); between acetylcholine and vasoactive intestinal peptide (VIP) (Johansson & Lundberg, 1981; Lundberg et al., 1981); between the polypeptide transmitter, substance P, and serotonin (Björklund et al., 1979; Chan-Paly, Jonsson, & Paly, 1978); and between substance P and the neuropeptide, cholecystokinin (CCK) (Hökfelt et al., 1980b).

In certain cases, these proximal relationships have proven functional as well. Thus, ACTH, β-lipotropin and β-endorphin are each released in response to serotoninergic mediation (Bruni, Hawkins, & Yen, 1982) and stressful stimuli (Rossier et al., 1980a). So, too, is the pituitary tropic hormone, prolactin (Nicoll, Talwalker, & Meites, 1960). Moreover, under conditions of stress, β-endorphin seems to act as an endogenous agonist in regulating the secretion of prolactin, perhaps exerting its control "by a local endocrine mechanism" (Rossier et al., 1980a, p. 373), or, as de Wied and Jolles (1982) have suggested, β-endorphin may be a "second-order precursor molecule for neuropeptides with neuroleptic and psychostimulant effects" (p. 1040).

The Psychoactive Role of Neuropeptides
and Adrenocortical Hormones

Of interest in this connection are the extensive investigations that
have been carried out on the psychological and behavioral effects of
the neuropeptides, their proteolytically-cleaved molecular fragments
(Bohus & de Wied, 1981; Herman & Goldstein, 1981; Herman, Leslie,
& Goldstein, 1980; de Wied & Jolles, 1982; Wiegant & de Wied, 1981;
Witter, Gispen, & de Wied, 1981), and the adrenal corticosteroids (Bohus et al., 1982). Research into this intriguing biobehavioral domain
has shown that intraventricular and intracerebral administration of
these neuro- and adrenal hormones exerts significant effects upon numerous behavioral components of adaptation. They have been found,
for example, to enhance memory consolidation, vigilance and concentration, and to be implicated in the maintenance, facilitation and/or inhibition of a broad range of species- and self-preservative behaviors:
e. g., self-stimulatory behavior in the experimental response-contingent
reward paradigm, conditioned approach, avoidance and extinction behavior, locomotor activity and sexual and agonistic behavior. (It should
be noted here that the behavioral and endocrinologic [feedback] regulatory actions of the adrenal steroids seem to be disassociated [Bohus et
al., 1982].)

The significance of these findings comes into full focus with the realization that peptide and other central transmitter systems together occupy cortical and limbic structures that control the viscero-motor, som-
ato-motor and sensory processes involved in selective attention, learning (Roberts, 1981), emotionally-motivated behavior (Roberts, 1970)
and stress responding (Palkovits, 1979). Existing data on the interaction of these two brain systems have lately been characterized as confusing and contradictory (de Wied & Jolles, 1982). Nevertheless, the
potential importance of this avenue of research is obvious, in view of
the specificity and likely interdependence of these systems in psychopathology, neuropathy and normal brain function. Recent studies have,
for example, implicated the brain monoamine, epinephrine, in the tonic
inhibition of adrenal steroid hormone release, i. e., in a neuroendocrine
role (Ganong, 1980; Roth et al., 1981). In like manner, the neurotransmitter, dopamine, has been shown to inhibit the synthesis and release of
β-endorphin (Farah, Malcolm, & Mueller, 1982) (evidently by inhibiting the synthesis of the precursor, pro-opiocortin [Höllt et al., 1982]),
as well as that of prolactin (Farah et al., 1982) and [Met]enkephalin
(Hong et al., 1979).

Opioid Peptides and Lymphoid Cells

Judging from initial reports, the association between the opioid peptides and immune effector cells promises to be complex. By way of illustration: (1) β-endorphin has been shown to induce a two- to fourfold increase in T cell proliferation in the presence of the mitogen, Concanavalin A (Con A) (Gilman et al., 1981); (2) high molarities of [Met]enkephalin and low [Leu]enkephalin concentrations will enhance lymphocyte blastogenesis in the presence of the mitogen, phytohemagglutinin (PHA) (Plotnikoff, 1982); (3) [Met] and [Leu]enkephalins have been found to enhance the chemiluminescence of neutrophils from cancer patients, in contrast to cells from healthy subjects (Miller, Murgo, & Plotnikoff, 1982); (4) [Met]enkephalin will also increase active rosette formation in normal human blood T lymphocytes (Wybran et al., 1979); and (5), as *in vivo* corroboration to these *in vitro* studies, the survival rate of leukemia-inoculated mice has been found to be prolonged by injections of [Met] and [Leu]enkephalin (Plotnikoff, Miller, & Murgo, 1982).

Adding a new dimension to this line of investigation is the recent discovery that lymphocytes are themselves a source of ACTH, the β-endorphin fragment, γ-endorphin, and a sub-class of human interferon, human leukocyte interferon (HuIFN-α). Antigenic and structural similarities among HuIFN-α, ACTH and γ-endorphin had indicated that the lymphokine might be a precursor to the peptide hormones (Blalock & Smith, 1980), an hypothesis that seemed confirmed by subsequent pepsin-digestion and acid treatment of the molecule, and an *in vivo* demonstration of analgesic and behavioral effects far exceeding those for β-endorphin (Smith & Blalock, 1981).

It is evidently premature, however, to suggest a "pivotal" role for interferon in psychoneuroendocrine regulation on the basis of these data. For in direct contradiction to these findings, Epstein et al. (1982) were unable to find significant structural and functional homology between ACTH and β-endorphin, and either natural IFN-α or human IFN-α prepared by recombinant DNA technique. Comparisons between lymphokine and peptide molecules were made on the basis of antiviral protective activity, in addition to radioimmunoassay, whereby a ^{125}I-human β-endorphin probe failed to detect peptide-like material in either form of interferon, a result that would seem to preclude a precursor role for the molecule.

A later study by Smith, Meyer and Blalock (1982) has helped to resolve this particular issue (suggesting that ACTH and interferon may in fact be the products of different genes) and has uncovered still other neurohormonal-endocrine-lymphoid interrelationships. They have reported a coordinated, but evidently dissociated, production of IFN and an ACTH-like substance in female, hypophysectomized mice in response to Newcastle disease virus (NDV) injection. The use of the synthetic steroid, dexamethasone, served to illustrate both the dissociation and the likely source of the ACTH-like material: i. e., prior drug treatment in hypophysectomized animals suppressed production of the peptide-like substance and corticosterone release, but did not affect interferon production; and in contrast to those from control and dexamethasone-treated animals, spleen cells from NDV-infected, hypophysectomized mice showed positive immunofluorescence when stained with antiserum to ACTH-(1-13 amide). If, as the investigators propose, the lymphocyte–or, by inference, the immune system–performs a "sensory function" by way of a lymphoid-adrenal axis, the findings from this study offer yet one more piece of evidence to uphold the notion that the system is, in at least certain important respects, autonomous. (Contributing a final footnote to these findings as a whole is evidence showing that T cell production of γ-interferon can be modulated both by the neurohypophyseal hormone, vasopressin [Johnson, Farrer, & Torres, 1982], and by a desacetylated recombinant DNA-derivation of the thymic hormone, thymosin α_1, or N^α-desacetylthymosin α [DTα_1] [Svedersky et al., 1982].)

A Neuroendocrine Role for Thymic Hormones: Preliminary Evidence

The thymus gland is essential to the development of a viable immune system, to the development of a thymic "imprint," or characteristic surface antigens (idiotypes) on regulatory T-cell subpopulations (Douglas, 1980; Reinherz & Schlossman, 1980; Waldmann & Broder, 1977), and to the balanced output of these differentiated populations during an immune response. Its epithelial cells are the source of a number of thymic hormones, or factors (Bach et al., 1979; Goldstein et al., 1981; Low et al., 1979), that are directly instrumental in regulating the system.

With regard to a presumptive neuroendocrine role for the immune system, the polypeptide thymic hormone, thymosin β_4 (Low, Hu, & Goldstein, 1981), has not only shown a peripheral distribution in lung, liver and kidney, but has been shown to be present in the brain, with relatively high concentrations in the olfactory bulb (Hannappel et al., 1982). It is of interest that thymosin β_4 has also been shown to be synthesized by peritoneal macrophages and adherent spleen cells (Xu et al., 1982), as well as by the structural epithelial cells of the thymus gland.

Thymosin β_4 will elicit the release of luteinizing hormone-releasing hormone (LHRH) from medial basal hypothalamic tissue and from pituitary tissue superfused with hypothalamic tissue, *in vitro* (Rebar et al., 1981), and the intraventricular injection of thymosin β_4 will bring about a significant increase in serum luteinizing hormone (LH) levels, *in vivo* (Hall et al., 1982). Furthermore, extensive thymosin α_1-like immunoreactivity (Goldstein et al., 1977; Low et al., 1979) has been demonstrated in guinea pig brain tissue, with highest concentrations detected in the tuberal region of the hypothalamus, i.e., the arcuate nucleus and the median eminence (Hall et al., 1981).

If indeed thymic peptide infiltration into the brain and pituitary gland takes place, the precise route remains unknown. However, by use of the horseradish peroxidase (HRP)-retrograde transport technique for thymic injection in mice and rats, Bulloch and Moore (1981) have postulated the existence of a preganglionic cholinergic pathway to the thymus gland from brainstem nuclei (retrofacial nucleus and nucleus ambiguus) and spinal cord neurons (three separate groups located medially to the ventral horn).

By way of summary, the activities of β-endorphin might serve as a sort of axial principle around which to summarize the preceding material – bearing in mind that the endogenous neuropeptide has been implicated as "a circulating immunosuppressive agent in ... situations of stress-related immune deficiency" (McCain et al., 1982, p.1622). This orientation is of course arbitrary and an undoubted over-simplification of neuro-endocrine-immune interconnection. Yet, it might nonetheless suggest additional cross-linkages that may exist between systems:

(1) It warrants repeating, at the start, that β-endorphin has been shown to be a product of the brain, the pituitary gland (Schwartzberg & Nakane, 1982) and of at least some peripheral organs (Tsong et al., 1982); (2) β-endorphin shows familial features in common with another neuropeptide (ACTH), but its reputed similarities to an immunoregulatory lymphokine (interferon) are presently open to debate; (3) in its capacity to bind to non-opiate receptors (Hazum, Chang, & Cuatrecasas, 1979) and to modulate the activities of both a neurotransmitter (acetylcholine) and a tropic hormone (prolactin), β-endorphin gives evidence of acting as a rather generalized effector substance in the brain, if not also in the body periphery; (4) in thus acting as a releasing hormone to prolactin, β-endorphin holds a characteristic in common with the thymic peptide hormone, thymosin β_4, given the capacity of the latter to release the tropic hormone, luteinizing hormone, *in vivo;* (5) β-endorphin production is itself stimulated by the very same neurohormone (vasopressin) that is found to modulate T cell production of the lymphokine (interferon) with which it appears to be "familially" re-

lated, the activity of the latter peptide (vasopressin) thus resembling that of a lymphokine; and lastly (6), both opiate neuropeptides (β-endorphin, the enkephalins) are able to evoke a proliferative response in lymphoid cells.

Neuroimmunomodulation

This brief, rather circumvoluted summary can only hint at how great a challenge it will be to discover the ways in which brain chemistry, the secretory products of endocrine glands, and the activated constituents of the immune system complement and counteract one another in the behaving, adapting organism. As though it were not challenge enough, the task is made considerably more difficult when things are not what they seem. For these data illustrate an intriguing, yet confounding, phenomenon in neurobiology (and now apparently in immunology, as well). It is one that was first observed in the behavior of neurosecretory neurons, but has since been found to characterize an ever-increasing number of effector agents involved in processes which may themselves require redefinition. It has in fact undermined established definitions of nervous pathway, synapse and "private" interneuronal message.

The process in question has been defined as "neuromodulation," and terms such as "cybernin," "parahormone" (Guillemin, 1977) and "paraneurone" (Fujita et al., 1981) have been used as descriptors for mediator substances "which serve to optimize nervous system function without themselves being involved in specific information transmittal" (Guillemin quoted in Roberts, 1978, p. 235) – quite as a catalyst might do in expediting a chemical reaction. There is now a wealth of experimental evidence to indicate that a given "classical" neurotransmitter can behave as neurohormone, a neurohormone as neurotransmitter, and either as neuromodulator (Siggins, 1979), depending upon such factors as the intrinsic spontaneous activity and environmental matrix of the effector cell, the locus, speed and duration of its biologic action, and the stable and dynamic characteristics of receptor sites (Barchas et al., 1978; Barker, 1977; Barker et al., 1978; Bloom, 1979; Kordon et al., 1979; Roberts, 1978; Rotsztejn, 1980; Weight, 1973). Hence, there would appear to be circumstances in which the neuronal signal, in a manner similar to that of the neuropeptide, fulfills only an indirect facilitative role by either amplifying or dampening synaptic events. Moreover, it has been determined that pre- and post-synaptic nerve cell membranes possess varieties of voltage-sensitive ion channels, or currents, that can subtly modify neuronal function, providing neurotransmitters "with a rich lexicon for communication" (Nicoll, 1982, p. 374).

It is likewise possible that indirect mediation and direct signal transmission are not solely attributable to the secretory cells of the APUD group, but are interchangeable properties common to all neurons. The statement by Defendini and Zimmerman (1978) to the effect that "a particular peptide may exercise different effects at different sites by different mechanisms, doubtless in response to different stimuli" (p. 138), suggests that the phenomenon is by no means simple. When the potential neuroendocrine modulatory capacity of the immune system is introduced into the picture, as the foregoing research reports ostensibly warrant, the phenomenon is indeed by no means simple.

Local Circuit Neurons

There are discoveries in neuroanatomical research that hint at mechanisms that may at least partially explain these "mediating," or "modulatory" effects in the intercommunication of cells. For example, one of the most important revelations stemming from this research has been the wholly new representation of the dendrite as an active, rather than purely receptive, neuronal element. Accordingly, in contrast to the rapid, regenerative spike-wave conduction of nerve impulse through extended axon, terminal bouton and synapse, dendrites have been shown to exhibit relatively slow transmittal of graded, low voltage electrotonic potentials across cell membranes (Brightman & Reese, 1969; Gilula, 1974; Schmitt, Dev, & Smith, 1976; Sotelo, 1977). In addition, the dendrite is seen to have a number of different affiliations with other dendrites and with axons, such as dendrodendritic, somatosomatic and somatodendritic couplings (desmosomes), serial and reciprocal synapses, unidirectional and bidirectional gap junctions (nexi), etc. (Rakic, 1975; Schmitt et al., 1976; Sotelo, 1977).

Many years ago, Ramón y Cajal (1852–1934) vehemently defended the view, founded upon his own voluminous research, that "all three parts of the neuron, the cell body, the dendrites and the axon, conduct nervous impulses equally" (Cajal, 1909, p. 110), and that the "prodigious abundance and unaccustomed wealth of forms of the so-called neurons with short axons ('les cellules à cylindre-axe court')" probably represented the morphological basis for the "functional superiority of the human brain" (Cajal, 1937, p. 480). Recent research on local circuit neurons (LCNs) has vindicated Cajal's vision, healed the breach in neuroanatomical theory, and opened up a new perspective on the biology of the central nervous system (Rakic, 1975; Roberts & Bush, 1981; Schmitt & Worden, 1979; Schmitt et al., 1976; Sheperd, 1974). Described as "multiple terminal networks" (Guillemin, 1977), or as "small

computational units or modules" (Schmitt et al., 1976), local circuit
neurons have seemingly limitless ramifications, allowing a degree of
cell-to-cell communication and an intricacy and variety of electrochem-
ical exchange that is commensurate with the known modifiability of
neurons. They have been observed in the sensory cortex (Sloper, 1972),
between the specialized ependymocytes that line an area of the third
ventricle immediately adjacent to the paraventricular nucleus, and
within delimited cell groupings in the supraoptic region of the hypothalamus (Andrew et al., 1981).

To further illustrate the point, the dendritic membrane has been
shown to be permeable to such small molecules as transmitters, enzymes, nucleotides, amino acids and glycoproteins (Gilula, 1974;
Griepp & Revel, 1977; Kreutzberg et al., 1973; Peracchia, 1977). In
view of research showing the peptidergic neuronal system to be capable
of at least partial utilization of this alternative mode of information exchange (Barker et al., 1978), it might be asked whether these various
properties, expressed in a single structural entity of the neuron, might
not provide a basis for neuronal membrane permeation by immune
products (e.g., lymphokines). Furthermore, given the proven junctional
permeability of the lymphocyte (Oliveira-Castro & Dos Reis, 1977;
Resch, 1976), is it not reasonable to suppose that these same properties
might contribute to the neuroendocrine mediation of immune function?

The Cyclic Nucleotides

If there are still more fundamental levels of cellular activity that can
help to explain the neuroendocrine modulation of immune function under conditions of psychological stress, these may lie in the transmembranous and intracellular mechanisms for stimulus transduction, cell
metabolism and proliferation mediated by the cyclic nucleotides, cyclic
AMP (3', 5'-adenosine monophosphate) and cyclic GMP (3', 5'-guano-
sine monophosphate) (Amkraut & Solomon, 1975). By acting as vital,
virtually ubiquitous intermediates in these processes (Cramer &
Schultz, 1977; Greengard & Robison, 1980), these two molecules exercise control over what A. A. Monjan (1981) has defined as "the final
common site of action for the varied stress-induced humors" (p. 217).
Their behavior has a special significance with respect to cell membrane
and membrane receptor physiology, areas currently under intense investigation (Baxter & Funder, 1979). But more relevant to this present thesis is research that has designated the cyclic AMP cascade as the essential mediating element in the phosphorylation of pre-synaptic protein;

or, to state the case more broadly, of particular interest is research that is succeeding in isolating the structural, biochemical and genetic transformations within neurons through which sensitization, learning and memory become manifest (Kandel & Schwartz, 1982).

Hormones, neurotransmitters and immunoglobulins depend upon cyclic AMP and cyclic GMP for their biological efficacy, even as the activities of the nucleotides within the cell membrane and cytoplasm depend, in turn, upon the external hormonal environment of the cell and upon the direct stimulatory action of a regulatory ligand-receptor complex (Baxter & Funder, 1979; Hirata & Axelrod, 1980; Iyengar et al., 1980). The actions of the nucleotides are maintained by their differing responses to this environment, and their mediatorial roles have been shown to be differentially expressed according to cell type (Goldberg et al., 1975). Cytoplasmic levels of cyclic AMP are increased by a number of pituitary tropic hormones, including ACTH (Schimmer, 1980), as well as by epinephrine, dopamine, histamine, the enkephalins and the prostaglandins, PGE_1 and PGE_2, whereas intramembranous levels of cyclic GMP are augmented by norepinephrine, serotonin, acetylcholine, thymosin, thymopoietin and insulin (Bartfai, 1978; Hadden, Coffey, & Spreafico, 1977; Hadden et al., 1975).

The adrenal glucocorticoids also interact with the cyclic nucleotides, but their behavior differs in certain respects from that of other agonists. For example, corticosterone enhances the phosphorylation of proteins by cyclic AMP-dependent kinase enzymes (Liu, Walter, & Greengard, 1981), both within the fluid matrix of the cell membrane, where modifications of ion channels are thought to take place in the lipoprotein bilayer, and within the nucleus itself, where the combined effects of (1) a translocated catalytic subunit of cytosolic protein kinase and (2) an interaction between the receptor-hormonal unit and nuclear chromatin alter ribonucleic acid (RNA)-mediated synthesis of specific proteins and gene expression (Nathanson & Greengard, 1977).

In contrast to all other cells of the body, increased levels of both cyclic AMP and the humoral and hormonal ligands which induce its elevation *inhibit*, rather than stimulate, the metabolic, proliferative, cytotoxic and secretory activity of virtually all reticuloendothelial cells derived from hemopoietic lineage, whereas cyclic GMP does precisely the opposite (Braun, Lichtenstein, & Parker, 1974; Hadden et al., 1975; Parker, 1979; Strom, Lundin, & Carpenter, 1977). It has been suggested that this anomaly in the behavior of the nucleotides in hemopoietic cells may make an important contribution to homeostasis by protecting the host "from the dangerous consequences of an unregulated immune response" (Bourne et al., 1974, p. 19). The point is well taken, particularly in view of the stimulatory (i.e., immunodepressant) effects of

ACTH and the adrenocortical hormones. (It will be recalled that ACTH increases intracellular levels of cyclic AMP.) It may also be possible that the inversed behavior of nucleotides in lymphocytes and accessory cells counterbalances the usual stimulatory influence of these hormones on body cells, and so protects *immune* homeostasis by providing a kind of buffer against the lability of the neuroendocrine axis.

Contrary to the original interpretation of nucleotide effects proposed by Goldberg and colleagues (Goldberg et al., 1975), which presumed their balanced, oppositional ("Yin Yang") coupling in the plasma membrane and in intracellular signal transduction, later research has placed this hypothesis in doubt and the precise role of cyclic GMP remains a controversial issue (Goldberg & Haddox, 1977; Hardman, 1982). Nevertheless, there are interesting facets to the nucleotide regulation of immune cell systems which reflect just such a reciprocal influence. For example, chemotaxis in non-lymphoid immune cells (i.e., polymorphonuclear leukocytes [PMNs], monocytes and macrophages), a process that is characterized by the development of a motile configuration (polarization) and by sustained, directed movement, has been shown to be moderated by cGMP, but inhibited by cAMP. The differential response evidently results from the ligand-mediated inhibition of the catalytic enzyme molecule, adenylate cyclase (Stephens & Snyderman, 1982), and/or the stimulation of guanylate cyclase (Coffey, Hadden, & Hadden, 1981). There are also studies to show that early and late phases of cell-mediated immune responsivity are mediated, first by cholinergic-, then by epinergic-specific ligand-receptor binding on the surfaces of activated T lymphocytes (Strom & Carpenter, 1980; Strom, George, & Lane, 1979), their activation "dramatically altering the distribution and concentration of receptor units" (Strom & Carpenter, 1980, p. 309).

Conclusions

Perhaps inevitably, the attempt to integrate what is presently known regarding the interaction of complex systems only serves to underscore their complexity. Accordingly, rather than to further belabor this particular aspect of the subject under review, it might be well, in summary, to reexamine more directly two premises that can lend cohesion to the material presented thus far.

In this review, as elsewhere, it has been argued that the central nervous system exercises a modulating influence on immunologic function. This fact alone provides a unifying theme, a framework for research findings in immunology which might otherwise appear unrelated or incongruous. To frame the argument another way: if the immune system is influenced by the brain, and this influence were to be ignored, the system would then indeed seem to act in overly-complicated, strange and mysterious ways. Its "autonomy" would continue to fascinate, but this very fascination would act as an impediment to the full understanding of disease susceptibility, and to a more informed appreciation of what Aaron Antonovsky (1981) has called "salutogenesis," or genesis of health. The considerable extent to which these latter two processes are affected by the social milieu, by the *symbolic* climate of everyday life (Amkraut & Solomon, 1975; Mason, 1968), would be overlooked, depriving immunological research of an important theoretical dimension.

A second organizing principle is embedded within this first premise. In view of evidence suggesting a direct CNS axis to the thymus gland (Bulloch & Moore, 1981), ample documentation of autonomic innervation to it, the lymph nodes and spleen (Crotti, 1918; Engel et al., 1977; Felten et al., 1981; Fillenz, 1970; Galindo & Imaeda, 1962; Giron, Crutcher, & Davis, 1980; Hammar, 1935; Reilly et al., 1979; Sergeeva, 1974; Williams & Felten, 1981; Williams et al., 1981), as well as mounting evidence for the presence of transmitter- and peptide-specific binding sites on lymphocytes and accessory phagocytic leukocytes (Lopker et al., 1980; Maslinski, Grabczewska, & Ryzewski, 1980; Pochet et al., 1979; Shapiro & Strom, 1980; Stepien et al., 1981; Strom, Lane, & George, 1981; Wybran et al., 1979), it would be reasonable to expect thymic hormone synthesis to be modulated by "target" organ hormone inhibitory feedback on the sources of that synthesis. In other words, is there not a long-loop feedback connection between the brain and the primary and secondary tissues of immunity? Established concepts of efferent tropism and end-organ feedback may not pertain here in the strictest sense, yet there is speculation that primary, secondary and even tertiary levels of feedback most probably exist (Besedovsky & Sorkin, 1981; Blalock & Smith, 1981; Hall & Goldstein, 1981; Smith & Blalock, 1981).

One such internal regulatory circuit has been recently demonstrated by Besedovsky, Del Rey and Sorkin (1981), who have shown that injections of lymphokine-containing supernatants from mitogen (Con A)-activated human peripheral blood leukocytes and rat spleen cells will elicit significant (2-3-fold) increases in circulating (immunosuppressive) corticosterone levels in rats. Two previous observations bear repeating in this context: first of all, this same investigative group has demonstrated an afferent link between peripheral sites of humorally-mediated acute inflammatory response and specific hypothalamic nuclei (Besedovsky et al., 1977); and secondly, lymphocytes are evidently a source of "tropic" stimulation to corticosterone production (Smith et al.,

1982). Taken together, these studies indicate that immunological signals are not only transmitted to the adrenal gland and brain from distant tissue sites, but show that they are also capable of eliciting CNS activity, perhaps even capable of initiating a condition of positive feedback.

To further pursue the idea of feedback: what might the presence of thymosin α_1 in the brain signify, given the demonstrably neuroendocrine-like characteristics of thymic hormones? what is its source? its role in brain function and its relationship to other brain peptides and transmitters? Does its presence in the median eminence and mediobasal hypothalamus not implicate the brain itself as an organ of feedback, as has been postulated to be the case with respect to the central activity of the tropic hormone, prolactin (Thompson, 1982)? In other words, is it not possible that thymosin α_1, like prolactin, might be "acting as an agent to regulate its own secretion" (p. 88)? And again, like prolactin (Landas et al., 1981), does hormonal flow not take place between cerebrospinal fluid, brain and pituitary, its extent and direction largely determined by ependymocytes?

If these kinds of feedback modes should prove to be in operation in varying degree in the modulation of all systems – nervous, endocrine and immune – this review chapter will have revealed nothing if not that the pertinent circuits for these modes are probably oblique and multichanneled, as well as direct. Hence, it would seem only realistic to suppose that each primary signal is continuously transmuted by excitatory and inhibitory input, by internuncial effects and a sort of inter-signal mix, or "cross-talk," all of which are presumably elaborated, in part, through the superimposition of dendritic fields. Obviously, too, there are many biosynthetic, as well as anatomic, relationships in this local circuitry that have yet to be explored.

Potentially intriguing parallels and contrasts also remain to be defined between feedback as an underlying process in psychoneuroimmunological regulation, and feedforward, as the latter has been discussed in the context of classically conditioned immunological response (Bovbjerg, Cohen, & Ader, 1982). Beyond question, the conditioning paradigm itself offers one of the most promising experimental strategies for illustrating the integration of systems and for analyzing their interlocking segments. Notwithstanding the manifest difficulties to be encountered along this avenue of research, there will surely be some compensation in the realization that, of all physiological systems, the nervous and immune systems alone have the capacity to learn and to remember.

References

Acher, R. Molecular evolution of the polypeptide hormones. In *Polypeptide hormones: Molecular and cellular aspects.* Ciba Foundation Symposium 41 (new series). New York: Elsevier Excerpta Medica, North-Holland, 1976.

Ader, R. Presidential address: Psychosomatic and psychoimmunological research. *Psychosom. Med.,* 1980, *42,* 307–321.

Ader, R. An historical account of conditioned immunologic responses. In R. Ader (Ed.), *Psychoneuroimmunology.* New York: Academic Press, 1981 a.

Ader, R. (Ed.), *Psychoneuroimmunology.* New York: Academic Press, 1981 b.

Ader, R., & Cohen, N. Behaviorally conditioned immunosuppression. *Psychosom. Med.,* 1975, *37,* 333–340.

Ader, R., & Cohen, N. Conditioned immunopharmacological responses. In R. Ader (Ed.), *Psychoneuroimmunology.* New York: Academic Press, 1981.

Ader, R., & Cohen, N. Behaviorally conditioned immunosuppression and murine systemic lupus erythematosus. *Science,* 1982, *215,* 1523–1536.

Ader, R., Cohen, N., & Grota, L. J. Adrenal involvement in conditioned immunosuppression. *Int. J. Immunopharmacol.,* 1979, *1,* 141–145.

Agnati, L. F., Fuxe, K., Locatelli, V., Benfenati, F., Zini, I., Panerai, A. E., El Etreby, M. F., & Hökfelt, T. Neuroanatomical methods for the quantitative evaluation of coexistence of transmitters in nerve cells. Analysis of the ACTH- and β-endorphin immunoreactive nerve cell bodies of the mediobasal hypothalamus of the rat. *J. Neurosci. Meth.,* 1982, *5,* 203–214.

Amkraut, A. A., & Solomon, G. F. From symbolic stimulus to the pathophysiologic response: Immune mechanisms. *Int. J. Psychiat. Med.,* 1975, *5,* 541–563.

Amoral, D. G., & Sinnamon, H. M. The locus coeruleus: Neurobiology of a central noradrenergic nucleus. *Prog. Neurobiol.,* 1977, *9,* 147–196.

Amos, D. B., & Kostyu D. D. HLA: A central immunological agency of man. In H. Harris & K. Hirschhorn (Ed.), *Advances in human genetics* (Vol. 10). New York: Plenum Press, 1980.

Andén, N. N., Dahlström, A., Fuxe, K., Larsson, K., & Olson, L. Ascending monoamine neurons to the telencephalon and diencephalon. *Acta. Physiol. Scand.,* 1966, *67,* 313–326.

Andrew, R. D., MacVicar, B. A., Dudek, F. E., & Hatton, G. L. Dye transfer through gap junctions between neuroendocrine cells of rat hypothalamus. *Science,* 1981, *211,* 1187–1189.

Anschel, S., Alexander, M., & Perachio, A. A. Multiple connections of medial hypothalamic neurons in the rat. *Exp. Brain Res.,* 1982, *46,* 383–392.

Antonovsky, A. *Health, stress and coping.* San Francisco: Jossey-Bass Publishers, 1981.

Antunes, J. L., Carmel, P. W., & Zimmerman, E. A. Projections from the paraventricular nucleus to the zona externa of the median eminence of the rhesus monkey: An immunohistochemical study. *Brain Res.,* 1977, *137,* 1–10.

Axelrod, J. The pineal gland: A neurochemical transducer. *Science,* 1974, *184,* 1341–1348.

Azmitia, E. C., & Segal, M. An autoradiographic analysis of the differential ascending projections of the dorsal and median raphe nuclei in rat. *J. Comp. Neurol.,* 1978, *179,* 641–668.

Bach, J.-F., Bach, M.-A., Charrière, J., & Dardenne, M. The mode of action of thymic hormones. *Ann. N. Y. Acad. Sci.,* 1979, *332,* 23–32.

Baertschi, A. J., Vallet, P., Baumann, J. B., & Girard, J. Neural lobe of pituitary modulates corticotropin release in the rat. *Endocrinology,* 1980, *106,* 878–882.

Bahnson, C. B. Stress and cancer: The state of the art, (Part 2). *Psychosomatics,* 1981, *22,* 207–230.

Bak, I. J., Choi, W. B., Hassler, R., Usunoff, K. G., & Wagner, A. Fine structural organization of the corpus striatum and substantia nigra in rat and cat. In D. Calne, T. N. Chase, & A. Barbeau (Eds.), *Advances in neurology (Vol. 9): Dopaminergic mechanisms.* New York: Raven Press, 1975.

Bakal, D. A. *Psychology and medicine: Psychobiological dimensions of health and illness.* New York: Springer Publishing Co., 1979.

Barchas, J. D., Akil, H., Elliot, G. R., Holman, R. Bruce, & Watson, S. J. Behavioral neurochemistry: Neuroregulators and behavioral states. *Science,* 1978, *200,* 964–973.

Bargmann, W., & Scharrer, E. The site of origin of the hormones of the posterior pituitary. *Amer. Scientist,* 1951, *39,* 255–259.

Barker, J. L. Physiological roles of peptides in the nervous system. In H. Gainer (Ed.), *Peptides in neurobiology.* New York: Plenum Press, 1977.

Barker, J. L., Neale, J. H., Smith, T. J., & McDonald, R. L. Opiate peptide modulation in amino acids: Rsponses suggest novel form of neuronal communication. *Science,* 1978, *199,* 1451–1453.

Bartfai, T. Cyclic nucleotides in the nervous system. *Trends Biochem. Sci.,* 1978, *3,* 121–124.

Baxter, J. D., & Funder, J. W. Hormone receptors. *New Engl. J. Med.,* 1979, *301,* 1149–1161.

Belenky, M. A., Chetverukhin, V. K., & Polenov, A. L. Quantitative radiographic light and electron microscopic analysis of the localization of monoamines in the median eminence of the rat. II. Serotonin. *Cell Tissue Res.,* 1979, *204,* 305–317.

Benacerraf, B. Role of MHC gene products in immune regulation. *Science,* 1981, *212,* 1229–1238.

Benacerraf, B., & McDevitt, H. O. Histocompatibility-linked immune response genes. *Science,* 1972, *175,* 273–279.

Bennett, M. V. L., Spray, D. C., & Harris, A. L. Gap junctions and development. *Trends Neurosci.,* 1981, *4,* 159–163.

Bergland, R. M., & Page, R. B. Pituitary-brain vascular relations: A new paradigm. *Science,* 1979, *204,* 18–24.

Bergland, R. M., Blume, H., Hamilton, A., Monica, P., & Patterson, R. Adrenocorticotropic hormone may be transported directly from the pituitary to the brain. *Science,* 1980, *210,* 541–543.

Bergmann, K., Burke, P. V., Cerda-Olmedo, E., David, C. N., Delbrück, M., Foster, K. W., Goodell, E. W., Heisenberg, M., Meissner, G., Zalokar, M., Dennison, D. S., & Shropshire, W. Phycomyces. *Bacteriol. Rev.,* 1969, *33,* 99–157.

Besedovsky, H. O., & Sorkin, E. Immunologic-neuroendocrine circuits: Physiologic approaches. In R. Ader (Ed.), *Psychoneuroimmunology.* New York: Academic Press, 1981.

Besedovsky, H. O., Del Rey, A., & Sorkin, E. Lymphokine-containing supernatants from Con A-stimulated cells increase corticosterone blood levels *J. Immunol.,* 1981, *126,* 385–387.

Besedovsky, H. O., Sorkin, E., Felix, D., & Haas, H. Hypothalamic changes during the immune response. *Eur. J. Immunol.,* 1977, *7,* 325–328.

Bisset, G. W., Neurohypophyseal hormones. In J. A. Parsons (Ed.), *Peptide hormones.* University Park Press, 1976.

Björklund, A., & Nobin, A. Fluorescence histochemical and microspectrofluorometric mapping of dopamine and noradrenaline cell groups in the rat diencephalon. *Brain Res.,* 1973, *51,* 193–205.

Björklund, A., Emson, P. C., Gilbert, R. F. T., & Skagerberg, G. Further evidence for the possible co-existence of 5-hydroxytryptamine and substance P in medullary raphe neurons of rat brain. *Brit. J. Pharmacol.,* 1979, *66,* 112–113.

Blalock, J. E., & Smith, E. M. Human leukocyte interferon: Structural and biological relatedness to adrenocorticotropic hormone and endorphins. *Proc. Natl. Acad. Sci. USA.,* 1980, *77,* 5972–5974.

Blalock, J. E., & Smith, E. M. Human leukocyte interferon (HuIFN-α): Potent endorphin-like opioid activity. *Biochem. Biophys. Res. Commun.,* 1981, *101,* 472–478.

Bleier, R. Structural relationship of ependymal cells and their processes within the hypothalamus. In K. M. Knigge, D. E. Scott, & A. Weindl (Eds.), *Brain-endocrine interaction: Median eminence: Structure and function.* Basel: S. Karger, 1972.

Bloom, F. E. Contrasting principles of synaptic physiology: Peptidergic and non-peptidergic neurons. In K. Fuxe, T. Hökfelt, & R. Luft (Eds.), *Central regulation of the endocrine system.* New York: Plenum Press, 1979.

Bohus, B., & de Wied, D. Actions of ACTH- and MSH-like peptides on learning, performance and retention. In J. L. Martinez, Jr., R. A. Jensen, R. N. Messing, H. Rigter, & J. L. McGaugh (Eds.), *Endogenous peptides and learning and memory processes.* New York: Academic Press, 1981.

Bohus, B., de Kloet, E. R., & Veldhuis, H. D. Adrenal steroids and behavioral adaptation: Relationship to brain corticoid receptors. In D. Ganten, & D. Pfaff (Eds.), *Adrenal actions on the brain. Current topics in neuroendocrinology* (Vol. 2). New York: Springer-Verlag, 1982.

Bourne, H. R., Lichtenstein, L. M., Melmon, K. L., Henney, C. S., Weinstein, Y., & Shearer, G. M. Modulation of inflammation and immunity by cyclic AMP. *Science,* 1974, *184,* 19–28.

Bovbjerg, D., Ader, R., & Cohen, N. Behaviorally conditioned suppression of a graft-*vs*-host response. *Proc. Natl. Acad. Sci. USA,* 1982, *79,* 583–585.

Bovbjerg, D., Cohen, N., & Ader, R. The central nervous system and learning: A strategy for immune regulation. *Immunol. Today,* 1982, *3,* 287–291.

Brack, C., Hirama, M., Lenhard-Schiller, R., & Tonegawa, S. A complete immunoglobulin gene is created by somatic recombination. *Cell,* 1978, *15,* 1–14.

Braun, W., Lichtenstein, L. M., & Parker, C. W. (Eds.), *Cyclic AMP, cell growth, and the immune response.* New York: Springer-Verlag, 1974.

Brawer, J. R., & Walsh, R. J. Response of tanycytes to aging in the median eminence of the rat. *Amer. J. Anat.,* 1982, *163,* 247–256.

van Breeman, V. L., & Clemente, C. D. Silver deposition in central nervous system and hematoencephalic barrier studies with the electron microscope. *J. Biophys. Biochem. Cytol.,* 1955, *1,* 161–166.

Brightman, M. W., & Reese, T. S. Junctions between intimately apposed cell membranes in the vertebrate brain. *J. Cell Biol.,* 1969, *40,* 648–677.

Brightman, M. W., Prescott, L., & Reese, T. S. Intercellular junctions of special ependyma. In K. M. Knigge, D. E. Scott, H. Kobayashi, & S. Ishii (Eds.), *Brain-endocrine interaction. II. The ventricular system in neuroendocrine mechanisms.* Basel: S. Karger, 1975.

Brooks, W. H., Cross, R. J., Roszman, T. L., & Markesbery, W. R. Neuroimmunomodulation: Neural anatomical basis for impairment and facilitation. *Ann. Neurol.,* 1982, *12,* 56–61.

Brownstein, M. J. Biologically active peptides in the brain. In A. Karlin, V. M. Tennyson, & H. J. Vogel (Eds.), *Neuronal information transfer.* New York: Academic Press, 1978.

Brownstein, M. J., Russell, J. T., & Gainer, H. Synthesis, transport, and release of posterior pituitary hormones. *Science,* 1980, *207,* 373–378.

Bruni, J. F., Hawkins, R. L., & Yen, S. S. C. Serotonergic mechanism in the control of beta-endorphin and ACTH release in male rats. *Life Sci.,* 1982, *30,* 1247–1254.

Bugnon, C., Bloch, B., Lenys, D., & Fellman, D. Cyto-immunological study of infundibular neurons of the human hypothalamus simultaneously reactive with antisera against endorphins, ACTH, MSH, and beta-LPH. *Cell Tissue Res.,* 1979, *199,* 177–196.

Bulloch, K., & Moore, R. Y. Thymus gland innervation by brainstem and spinal cord in mouse and rat. *Amer. J. Anat.,* 1981, *162,* 157–166.

Carlisle, D. B., & Knowles, F. G. W. Neurohaemal organs in crustaceans. *Nature (Lond.),* 1953, *172,* 404–405.

Carpenter, M. B., & Peter, P. Nigrostriatal and nigrothalamic fibers in the rhesus monkey. *J. Comp. Neurol.,* 1972, *144,* 93–116.

Carson, K. A., Nemeroff, C. B., Rone, M. S., Nicholson, G. F., Kizer, J. S., & Hanker, J. S. Experimental studies on the ultrastructural localization of acetylcholinesterase in the mediobasal hypothalamus of the rat. *J. Comp. Neurol.,* 1978, *182,* 201–220.

Chan-Paly, V., Jonsson, G., & Paly, S. L. On the co-existence of serotonin and substance P in neurons of the rat central nervous system. *Proc. Natl. Acad. Sci. USA.,* 1978, *75,* 1582–1586.

Chavkin, C., James, I. F., & Goldstein, A. Dynorphin is a specific endogenous ligand of the K opioid receptor. *Science,* 1982, *215,* 413–415.

Chrétien, M., Benjannet, S., Gossard, F., Gianoulakis, C., Crine, P., Lis, M., & Seidah, N. G. From beta-lipotropin to beta-endorphin and 'pro-opiomelanocortin.' *Can. J. Biochem.,* 1979, *57,* 1111–1121.

Claman, H. N. Corticosteroids and lymphoid cells. *New Engl. J. Med.,* 1972, *287,* 388–397.

Claman, H. N. How corticosteroids work. *J. Allergy Clin. Immunol.,* 1975, *55,* 145–151.

Cochrum, K. C., & Hanes, D. M. The role of histocompatibility antigens in clinical transplantation. In R. A. Reisfeld, & S. Ferrone (Eds.), *Current trends in histocompatibility* (Vol. 2). New York: Plenum Press, 1980.

Coffey, R. G., Hadden, E. M., & Hadden, J. W. Phytohemagglutinin stimulation of guanylate cyclase in human lymphocytes. *J. Biol. Chem.,* 1981, *256,* 4418–4424.

Cohen, N., Ader, R., Green, N., & Bovbjerg, D. Conditioned suppression of a thymus-independent antibody response. *Psychosom. Med.,* 1979, *41,* 487–491.

Cohen, S., Pick, E., & Oppenheim, J. J. (Eds.). *The biology of the lymphokines.* New York: Academic Press, 1979.

Cohen, S. N., Chang, A. C., Nakanishi, S., Inoue, A., & Numa, S. Studies of clone DNA encoding for the structure for the bovine corticotropin beta-lipotropin precursor protein. *Ann. NY Acad, Sci.,* 1980, *343,* 415–424.

Cooke, I. M. Electrical activity of neurosecretory terminals and control of peptide hormone release. In H. Gainer (Ed.), *Peptides in neurobiology.* New York: Plenum Press, 1977.

Cooper, M., Mosier, D. E., Scher, I., & Vitetta, E. S. (Eds.), *B lymphocytes in the immune response.* New York: Elsevier North-Holland, Inc., 1979.

Cramer, H., & Schultz, J. (Eds.), *Cyclic 3', 5'-nucleotides: Mechanisms of action.* New York: John Wiley & Sons, 1977.

Cross, R. J., Markesbery, W. R., Brooks, W. H., & Roszman, T. L. Hypothalamic-immune interactions. I. The acute effect of anterior hypothalamic lesions on the immune response. *Brain Res.,* 1980, *196, 79*–87.

Crotti, A. *Thyroid and thymus.* Philadelphia: Lea & Febiger, Publishers, 1918.

Cullen, J. Coping and health: A clinician's perspective. In S. Levine & H. Ursin (Eds.), *Coping and health.* New York: Plenum Press, 1980.

Cupps, T. R., Edgar, L. C., & Fauci, A. S. Suppression of human B lymphocyte function by cyclophosphamide. *J. Immunol.,* 1982, *128,* 2453–2457.

Dahlström, A., & Fuxe, K. Evidence for the existence of monoamine-containing neurons in the central nervous system. I. Demonstration of monoamines in the cell bodies of brainstem neurons. *Acta Physiol. Scand.,* 1964, *62 (Suppl. 232),* 1–55.

Dann, J. A., Wachtel, S. S., & Rubin, A. L. Possible involvement of the central nervous system in graft rejection. *Transplantation,* 1979, *27,* 223–226.

Dausset, J. Correlation between histocompatibility antigens and susceptibility to illness. *Progr. Clin. Immunol.,* 1972, *1,* 183–210.

Dausset, J. Are D and DR two distinct entities? In R. A. Reisfeld & S. Ferrone (Eds.), *Current trends in histocompatibility* (Vol. 1). New York: Plenum Press, 1980.

Dausset, J. The major histocompatibility complex in man: Past, present and future concepts. *Science,* 1981, *213,* 1469–1474.

Dausset, J., & Svejgaard, A. (Eds.), *HLA and disease.* Copenhagen: Munksgaard, 1977.

Defendini, R., & Zimmerman, E. A. The magnocellular neurosecretory system of the mammalian hypothalamus. In S. Reichlin, R. J. Baldessarini, & J. B. Martin (Eds.), *The hypothalamus. Research publications: Association for research in nervous and mental diseases* (Vol. 56). New York: Raven Press, 1978.

DeFeudis, F. V., & DeFeudis, P. A. *Elements of the behavioral code.* New York: Academic Press, 1977.

Delbrück, M. A physicist's renewed look at biology: Twenty years later. *Science,* 1970, *168,* 1312–1315.

Devoino, L. V. Serotoninergic system of raphe nucleus of the midbrain in immune reaction regulation. *Vyssch. Funkzii. Mozga. Norme. Pathol.,* 1979.

Dorsa, D. M., de Kloet, E. R., van Dijk, A. M. J., & Mezey, É. Retrograde transport of neuropeptides as a pituitary-brain communication system. In D. S. Farner & K. Lederis (Eds.), *Neurosecretion: Molecules, cells, systems.* New York: Plenum Press, 1981.

Douglas, S. Cells involved in immune responses. In H. H. Fudenberg, D. P. Stites, J. L. Caldwell, & J. V. Wells (Eds.), *Basic & clinical immunology.* Los Altos, Cal.: Lange Medical Publications, 1980.

Dunn, A. J., & Gispen W. H. How ACTH acts on the brain. *Biobehav. Rev.,* 1977, *1,* 15–23.

Duvernoy, H., & Koritke, J. G. Contribution à l'étude de l'angioarchitectonie des organes circumventriculaires. *Arch. Biol.,* 1964, *75 (Suppl.),* 693–748.

Edelman, G. M., Yahara, I., & Wang, J. L. Receptor mobility and receptor-cytoplasmic interactions in lymphocytes. *Proc. Natl. Acad. Sci. USA,* 1973, *70,* 1442–1446.

Eiden, L. E., & Brownstein, M. J. Extrahypothalamic distributions and functions of hypothalamic peptide hormones. *Fed. Proc.,* 1981, *40,* 2553–2559.

Eipper, B. A., & Mains, R. E. Existence of a common precursor to ACTH and endorphin in the anterior and intermediate lobe of the rat pituitary. *J. Supramol. Struct.,* 1978, *8,* 247–262.

Eipper, B. A., & Mains, R. E. Structure and biosynthesis of pro-adrenocorticotropin/endorphin and related peptides. *Endocr. Rev.,* 1980, *1,* 1–27.

Elde, R. P., & Hökfelt, T. Localization of hypophysiotropic peptides and other biologically active peptides within the brain. *Ann. Rev. Physiol.,* 1979, *41,* 587–602.

Elde, R. P., Hökfelt, T., Johansson, O., Efendic, S., & Luft, R. Immunohistochemical studies using antibodies to leucine enkephalin: Observations on nervous system of the rat. *Neurosci. Abstr.,* 1976, *1,* 759.

Emson, P. C. Peptides as neurotransmitter candidates in the mammalian CNS. *Progr. Neurobiol.,* 1977, *13,* 61–116.

Engel, G. L. Enduring attributes of medicine relevant for the education of the physician. *Ann. Int. Med.,* 1973, *78,* 587–593.

Engel, G. L. The need for a new medical model: A challenge for biomedicine. *Science,* 1977, *196,* 129–136.

Engel, W. K., Trotter, J. L., McFarlin, D. E., & McIntosh, C. L. Thymic epithelial cell contains acetylcholine receptor. *Lancet,* 1977, *1,* 1310.

Engleman, E. G., Benike, C. J., Grumet, F. C., & Evans, R. L. Activation of human T lymphocyte subsets: Helper and suppressor/cytotoxic T cells recognize and respond to distinct histocompatibility antigens. *J. Immunol.,* 1981, *127,* 2124–2129.

Epstein, L. B., Rose, M. E., McManus, N. H., & Choh Hao, L. Absence of functional and structural homology of natural and recombinant human leukocyte interferon (IFN-α) with human α-ACTH and β-endorphin. *Biochem. Biophys. Res. Commun.,* 1982, *104,* 341–346.

Falck, B., & Hillarp, N. Å. On the cellular localization of catecholamines in the brain. *Acta Anat. (Basel),* 1959, *38,* 277–279.

Farah, J. M., Jr., Malcolm, D. S., & Mueller, G. P. Dopaminergic inhibition of pituitary β-endorphin-like immunoreactivity secretion in the rat. *Endocrinology,* 1982, *110,* 657–659.

Fauci, A. S. Mechanisms of corticosteroid action on lymphocyte subpopulations. I. Redistribution of circulating T and B lymphocytes to the bone marrow. *Immunology,* 1978, *28,* 669–680.

Felten, D. L., Overhage, J. M., Felten, S. Y., & Schmedtje, J. F. Noradrenergic sympathetic innervation of lymphoid tissue in the rabbit appendix: Further evidence for a link between the nervous and immune systems. *Brain Res. Bull.,* 1981, *7,* 595–612.

Fersht, A. *Enzymes: Structure and mechanism.* San Francisco: W. H. Freeman & Co., Publishers, 1977.

Fessel, W. J., & Forsyth, R. P. Hypothalamic role in control of gamma globulin levels. *Arthr. Rheum.,* 1963, *6,* 771–772.

Fillenz, M. The innervation of the cat spleen. *Proc. Roy. Soc. Lond. [Biol.],* 1970, *174,* 459–468.

Fox, B. H. Psychosocial factors and the immune system in human cancer. In R. Ader (Ed.), *Psychoneuroimmunology.* New York: Academic Press, 1981.

Fujita, T., Iwanaga, T., Kusumoto, Y., & Yoshie, S. Paraneurons and neurosecretion. In D. S. Farner & K. Lederis (Eds.), *Neurosecretion: Molecules, cells, systems.* New York: Plenum Press, 1981.

Fuxe, K. Evidence for the existence of monoamine neurons in the central nervous system. IV. Distribution of monoamine nerve terminals in the central nervous system. *Acta Physiol. Scand.,* 1965, *65 (Suppl. 247),* 37–85.

Fuxe, K., & Hökfelt, T. Catecholamines in the hypothalamus and the pituitary gland. In W. F. Ganong & L. Martini (Eds.), *Frontiers in endocrinology, 1969.* New York: Oxford University Press, 1969.

Gainer, H., Peng-Loy, Y., & Sarne, Y. Biosynthesis of neuronal peptides. In H. Gainer (Ed.), *Peptides in neurobiology.* New York: Plenum Press, 1977.

Galindo, B., & Imaeda, T. Electron microscope study of the white pulp of the mouse spleen. *Anat. Rec.,* 1962, *143,* 399–415.

Ganong, W. F. Neurophysiologic basis of instinctual behavior and emotions. In W. F. Ganong (Ed.), *Review of medical physiology.* Los Altos, CA.: Lange Medical Publications, 1971.

Ganong, W. F. Neurotransmitters and pituitary function: Regulation of ACTH secretion. *Fed. Proc.,* 1980, *39,* 2923–2930.

Gasser, D. L., & Silvers, W. K. Genetic determinants of immunological responsiveness. *Adv. Immunol.,* 1974, *18,* 1–66.

Gershon, R. K. Immune regulation. *Fed. Proc.,* 1979, *38,* 2051–2077.

Ghatei, M. A., Sheppard, M. N., O'Shaughnessy, D. J., Adrian, T. E., McGregor, G. P., Polak, J. M., & Bloom, S. R. Regulatory peptides in the mammalian respiratory tract. *Endocrinology,* 1982, *111,* 1248–1254.

Gibbs, D. M., & Vale, W. Presence of corticotropin releasing factor-like immunoreactivity in hypophysial portal blood. *Endocrinology,* 1982, *111,* 1418–1420.

Gilman, S. C., Schwartz, J. M., Milner, R. J., Bloom, F. E., & Feldman, J. D. Enhancement of lymphocyte proliferative responses by β-endorphin, *Soc. Neurosci.,* 1981, *7,* 880. (Abstract)

Gilula, N. B. Junctions between cells. In R. P. Cox (Ed.), *Cell communications.* New York: John Wiley & Sons, 1974.

Giron, L. T., Crutcher, K. A., & Davis, J. N. Lymph nodes: A possible site for sympathetic neuronal regulation of immune responses. *Ann. Neurol.,* 1980, *8,* 520–525.

Gold, W. M., Kessler, G. F., & Yu, D. Y. C. Role of the vagus nerves in experimental asthma in allergic dogs. *J. Appl. Physiol.,* 1972, *33,* 719–725.

Goldberg, N. D., & Haddox, M. K. Cyclic GMP metabolism and involvement in biological regulation. *Ann. Rev. Biochem.,* 1977, *46,* 823–896.

Goldberg, N. D., Haddox, M. K., Nicol, S. E., Glass, D. B., Sanford, C. H., Kuehl, F. A., & Estensen, R. Biologic regulation through opposing influences of cyclic GMP and cyclic AMP: The Yin Yang hypothesis. *Adv. Cyclic Nucl. Res.,* 1975, *5,* 307–330.

Goldstein, A., & Ghazarossian, V. E. Immunoreactive dynorphin in pituitary and brain. *Proc. Natl. Acad. Sci. USA,* 1980, *77,* 6207–6210.

Goldstein, A., Tachibana, S., Lowney, L. I., Hunkapiller, M., & Hood, L. Dynorphin-(1-13), an extraordinarily potent opioid peptide. *Proc. Natl. Acad. Sci. USA,* 1979, *76,* 6666–6670.

Goldstein, A. L., Low, T. L. K., McAdoo, M., McClure, J., Thurman, G. B., Rossio, J., Lai, C. Y., Chang, D., Wang, S. S., Harvey, C., Ramel, A. H., & Meienhofer, J. Thymosin alpha 1: Isolation and sequence analysis of an immunologically active thymic polypeptide. *Proc. Natl. Acad. Sci. USA,* 1977, *74,* 725–729.

Goldstein, A. L., Low, T. L., Thurman, G. B., Zata, M. M., Hall, N. R., Chen, J., Hu, S. K., Naylor, P. B., & McClure, J. E. Current status of thymosin and other hormones of the thymus gland. *Recent Progr. Horm. Res.,* 1981, *37,* 369–415.

Gorczynski, R. M., Macrae, S., & Kennedy, M. Conditioned immune response associated with allogeneic skin grafts in mice. *J. Immunol.,* 1982, *129,* 704–709.

Greaves, M. F. Cell surface receptors: A biological perspective. In P. Cuatrecasas & M. F. Greaves (Eds.), *Receptors and recognition.* London: Chapman and Hall, 1976.

Greengard, P., & Robison, G. A. (Eds.), *Advances in cyclic nucleotide research* (Vol. 13). New York: Raven Press, 1980.

Griepp, E. B., & Revel, J. P. Gap junctions in development. In W. E. de Mello (Ed.), *Intracellular communication.* New York: Plenum Press, 1977.

Guillemin, R. The expanding significance of hypothalamic peptides; or, endocrinology as a branch of neuroendocrinology. *Recent Progr. Horm. Res.,* 1977, *33,* 1–28.

Guillemin, R. The endocrinology of the neuron and the neural origin of endocrine cells. In J. C. Porter (Ed.), *Hypothalamic peptide hormones and pituitary regulation. Advances in experimental medicine and biology* (Vol. 87). New York: Plenum Press, 1977.

Guillemin, R., Vargo, T., Rossier, J., Minick, S., Ling, N., Rivier, C., Vale, W., & Bloom, F. E. β-endorphin and adrenocorticotrophin are secreted concomitantly by the pituitary gland. *Science,* 1978, *197,* 1367–1369.

Hadden, J. W., Coffey, R. G., & Spreafico, F. (Eds.), *Immunopharmacology. Comprehensive immunology.* New York: Plenum Press, 1977.

Hadden, J. W., Johnson, E. M., Hadden, E. M., Coffey, R. G., & Johnson, L. D. Cyclic GMP and lymphocyte activation. In A. S. Rosenthal (Ed.), *Immune recognition.* New York: Academic Press, 1975.

Halász, B., Kosaras, B., & Lengvari, I. Ontogenesis of the neurovascular link between the hypothalamus and the anterior pituitary in the rat. In K. M. Knigge, D. E. Scott & A. Weindl (Eds.), *Brain-endocrine interaction. I. Median eminence: Structure and function.* Basel: S. Karger, 1972.

Hall, N. R., & Goldstein, A. L. Neurotransmitters and the immune system. In R. Ader (Ed.), *Psychoneuroimmunology.* New York: Academic Press, 1981.

Hall, N. R., McGillis, J. P., Spangelo, B. L., & Goldstein, A. L. Evidence for an interaction between thymosin peptides and the pituitary-gonadal axis. *Fed. Proc.,* 1981, *41,* 1267. (Abstract)

Hall, N. R., McGillis, J. P., Spangelo, B. L., Palaszynski, E., Moody, T., & Goldstein, A. L. Evidence for a neuroendocrine-thymus axis mediated by thymosin polypeptide. In B. Serrou, C. Rosenfeld, J. C. Daniels, & J. P. Saunders (Eds.), *Current concepts in human immunology and cancer immunomodulation* (Vol. 17). *Developments in immunology.* New York: Elsevier North-Holland, Inc., 1981.

Hammar, J. A. Konstitutionsanatomische Studien über die Neurotisierung des Menschenembryos. IV. Über die Innervationsverhältnisse der Inkretorgane und der Thymus bis in den 4 Fetalmonat. *Zeit. Mikrosk. Forsch.,* 1935, *38,* 253–293.

Hannappel, E., Xu, G., Morgan, J., Hempstead, J., & Horecker, B. L. Thymosin β4: A ubiquitous peptide in raι and mouse tissues. *Proc. Natl. Acad. Sci. USA,* 1982, *79,* 2172–2175.

Hardman, J. G. Guanylate cyclase: Properties and regulation. In S. Swillens & J. E. Dumont (Eds.), *Cell regulation by intracellular signals.* New York: Plenum Press, 1982.

Haurowitz, F. The foundations of immunology. In H. H. Fudenberg, D. P. Stites, J. L. Caldwell, & J. V. Wells (Eds.), *Basic & clinical immunology.* Los Altos, CA: Lange Medical Publications, 1980.

Haynes, B. F., & Fauci, A. S. The differential effect of in vivo hydrocortisone on the kinetics of subpopulations of human peripheral blood thymus-derived lymphocytes. *J. Clin. Invest.,* 1978, *61,* 703–707.

Hazum E., Chang, K.-J., & Cuatrecasas, P. Specific nonopiate receptors for beta-endorphin. *Science,* 1979, *205,* 1033–1035.

Hennessy, J. W., & Levine, S. Stress arousal and the pituitary adrenal system: A psychoendocrine hypothesis. *Progr. Psychobiol. Physiol. Psychol.,* 1979, *8,* 133–178.

Henry, J. P., & Stephens, P. M. *Stress, health, and the social environment.* New York: Springer-Verlag, 1977.

Herman, B. H., Leslie, F., & Goldstein, A. Behavioral effects and *in vivo* degradation of intraventricularly administered dynorphin-(1-13) and D-ALA^2-dynorphin-(1-11) in rats. *Life Sci.,* 1980, *27,* 883–892.

Herman, B. H., & Goldstein, A. Cataleptic effects of dynorphin-(1-13) in rats made tolerant to a *Mu* opiate receptor agonist. *Neuropeptides,* 1981, *2,* 13–22.

Hillarp, N. Å., Fuxe, K., & Dahlström, A. Demonstration and mapping of central neurons containing dopamine, noradrenaline, and 5-hydroxytryptamine and their reactions to psychopharmaca. *Pharmac. Rev.,* 1966, *18,* 727–741.

Hirata, F., & Axelrod, J. Phospholipid methylation and biological signal transmission. *Science,* 1980, *209,* 1082–1090.

Hofer, H. Zur Morphologie der circumventrikulären Organe des Zwischenhirns der Säugetiere. *Verh. Deutsch. Zool. Ges.,* 1958, *24,* 202–251.

Hofer, H. Circumventrikulären Organe des Zwischenhirns. *Primatologia* (Vol. 2, pt. 2). Basel: S. Karger, 1965.

Hökfelt, T., Fuxe, K., Goldstein, M., & Johansson, O. Immunohistochemical evidence for the existence of adrenaline neurons in the rat brain. *Brain Res.,* 1974, *66,* 235–252.

Hökfelt, T., Johansson, O., Ljungdahl, A., Lundberg, J., Schultzberg, M., Fuxe, K., Pernow, B., & Goldstein, M. Peptide neurons. In A. M. Gotto, E. J. Peck, & A. E. Boyd (Eds.), *Brain peptides: A new endocrinology.* New York: Elsevier North-Holland Biomedical Press, 1979 a.

Hökfelt, T., Johansson, O., Ljungdahl, A., Lundberg, J., Schultzberg, M., Fuxe, K., Goldstein, M., Steinbusch, H., Verofstad, A., & Elde, R. Neurotransmitters and neuropeptides: Distribution patterns and cellular localization as revealed by immunocytochemistry. In K. Fuxe, T. Hökfelt, & R. Luft (Eds.), *Central regulation of the endocrine system.* New York: Plenum Press, 1979 b.

Hökfelt, T., Johansson, O., Ljungdahl, A., Lundberg, J. M., & Schultzberg, M. Peptidergic neurons. *Nature (Lond.),* 1980 a, *284,* 515–521.

Hökfelt, T., Lundberg, J. M., Schultzberg, M., Johansson, O., Skirboll, L., Änggard, A., Fredholm, B., Hamberger, B., Pernow, B., Rehfeld, J., & Goldstein, M. Cellular localization of peptides in neural structures. *Proc. Roy. Soc. [Biol.],* 1980 b, *210,* 63–77.

Hökfelt, T., Elde, R., Fuxe, K., Johansson, O., Ljungdahl, A., Goldstein, M., Luft, R., Efendic, S., Nilsson, G., Terenius, L., Ganten, D., Jeffcoate, S.L., Rehfeld, J., Said, S., Perez de la Mora, M., Possani, L., Tapia, R., Teran, L., & Palacios, R. Aminergic and peptidergic pathways in the nervous system with special reference to the hypothalamus. In S. Reichlin, R.J. Baldessarini, & J.B. Martin (Eds.), *The hypothalamus.* New York: Raven Press, 1978.

Holloway, W.R. The mechanism of enzyme action. *Oxford biology reader* (Vol. 45). Oxford: Oxford University Press, 1976.

Holloway, W.R., Tsui, H.W., Grota, L.J., & Brown, G.M. Melatonin and corticosterone regulation: Feeding time or daylight, dark cycle? *Life Sci.,* 1979, *25,* 1837–1842.

Höllt, W., Haarmann, I., Seizinger, B.R., & Herz, A. Chronic haloperidol treatment increases the level of *in vitro* translatable messenger ribonucleic acid coding for the β-endorphin/adrenocorticotropin precursor proopiomelanocortin in the pars intermedia of the rat pituitary. *Endocrinology,* 1982, *110,* 1885–1891.

Hong, J.S., Yang, H.Y., Gillin, J.C., di Guilio, A.M., Fratta, W., & Costa, E. Chronic treatment with haloperidol accelerates the biosynthesis of enkephalins in rat striatum. *Brain Res.,* 1979, *160,* 192–195.

Ignarro, L.J. Regulation of polymorphonuclear leukocyte, macrophage and platelet formation. In J.W. Hadden, R.G. Coffey, & F. Spreafico (Eds.), *Immunopharmacology. Comprehensive immunology* (Vol. 3). New York: Plenum Press, 1977.

Iyengar, R., Birnbaumer, L., Schulster, D., Houslay, M., & Michell, R.H. Modes of membrane receptor signal coupling. In D. Schulster & A. Levitzki (Eds.), *Cellular receptors for hormones and neurotransmitters.* New York: John Wiley & Sons, 1980.

Jackson, J.H. In Taylor J. (Ed.), *The collected works of John Hughlings Jackson.* London: Staples Press, 1958. *(q. v.)*

Jacobowitz, D.M. Monoaminergic pathways in the central nervous system. In M.A. Lipton, A. DiMascio, & K.F. Killam (Eds.), *Psychopharmacology: A generation of progress.* New York: Raven Press, 1978.

Janković, B.D., & Isaković, K. Neuroendocrine correlates of immune response. I. Effects of brain lesions on antibody production, Arthus reactivity and delayed hypersensitivity in the rat. *Int. Arch. Allergy Appl. Immunol.,* 1973, *45,* 360–372.

Jerne, N.K. Towards a network theory of the immune system. *Ann. Immunol. (Paris),* 1974, *125,* 373–389.

Jerne, N.K. The immune system: A web of V-domains. *Harvey Lect.,* 1976, *70,* 93–110.

Johansson, O., & Lundberg, J.M. Ultrastructural localization of VIP-like immunoreactivity in large dense-core vesicles of "cholinergic-type" nerve terminals in cat exocrine glands. *Neuroscience,* 1981, *6,* 847–862.

Johansson, O., Hökfelt, T., Elde, R.P., Jeffcoate, S.L., & White, N. Thyrotropin-releasing hormone (TRH) and somatostatin: Immunocytochemical distribution in the central nervous system. *Neurosci. Lett.,* 1978, *220 (Suppl. 1).*

Johnson, H.M., Farrer, W.L., & Torres, B.A. Vasopressin replacement of interleukin II requirement in gamma-interferon production: Lymphokine activity of a neuroendocrine hormone. *J. Immunol.,* 1982, *129,* 983–986.

Joseph, S.A., & Knigge, K.M. The endocrine hypothalamus: Recent anatomical studies. In S. Reichlin, R.J. Baldessarini, & J.B. Martin (Eds.), *The hypothalamus. Research publications: Association for research in nervous and mental diseases* (Vol. 56). New York: Raven Press, 1978.

Kakidani, H., Furutani, Y., Takahashi, H., Noda, M., Morimoto, Y., Hirose, T., Asai, M., Inayama, S., Nakanishi, S., & Numa, S. Cloning and sequence analysis of cDNA for porcine β-Neo-endorphin/dynorphin precursor. *Nature (Lond.),* 1982, *298,* 245–249.

Kandel, E. R., & Schwartz, J. H. Molecular biology of learning: Modulation of transmitter release. *Science,* 1982, *218,* 433–443.

Karczewski, W. The electrical activity of the vagus nerve after an "anti-anaphylactic" stimulation of the brain. *Acta Allerg.,* 1964, *19,* 229–235.

Katz, D. H. *Lymphocyte differentiation, recognition, and regulation.* New York: Academic Press, 1977.

Katz, D. H., & Benacerraf, B. The function and interrelationships of T-cell receptors, Ir genes and other histocompatibility gene products. *Transpl. Rev.,* 1975, *22,* 175–195.

Keller, S. E., Weiss, J. M., Schleifer, S. J., Miller, N. E., & Stein, M. Suppression of immunity by stress: Effects of a graded series of stressors on lymphocyte stimulation in the rat. *Science,* 1981, *213,* 1397–1400.

Kendall, J. W., & Orwoll, E. Anterior pituitary hormones in the brain and other extrapituitary sites. In L. Martini & W. F. Ganong (Eds.), *Frontiers in neuroendocrinology* (Vol. 6). New York: Raven Press, 1980.

Kennett, R. H., McKearn, T. J., & Bechtol, K. B. (Eds.), *Monoclonal antibodies: A new dimension in biological analyses.* New York: Plenum Press, 1980.

Kent, D. L., & Sladek, S. R., Jr. Histochemical, pharmacological and microspectrofluorometric analysis of new sites of serotonin localization in the rat hypothalamus. *J. Comp. Neurol.,* 1978, *180,* 221–236.

Kim, J.-S., Bak, I. J., Hassler, R., & Okada, Y. The role of γ-aminobutyric acid (GABA) in the extrapyramidal motor system. 2. Some evidence of a type of GABA-rich strio-nigral neuron. *Exp. Brain Res.,* 1971, *14,* 95–104.

Klimenko, V. M. *The study of some neuronal mechanisms of hypothalamic regulation of immune reactions in rabbits.* Avtoref., kand. diss. Inst. Expt. Med., Acad. Med. Sci. USSR, Leningrad, 1972.

Klimenko, V. M. *The dynamics of neuronal activity-reconstruction during the last periods of immunogenesis.* Tesisy Dokl., Leningrad 1975.

de Kloet, E. R., Veldhuis, D., & Bohus, B. Significance of neuropeptides in the control of corticosterone-receptor activity in rat brain. In G. C. Pepeu, M. J. Kuhar, & S. J. Enna (Eds.), *Receptors for neurotransmitters and peptide hormones. Advances in biochemical psychopharmacology* (Vol. 21). New York: Raven Press, 1980.

Knigge, K. M. Brain and endocrine function. *Amer. Zool.,* 1967, *7,* 135–144.

Knigge, K. M., & Joseph, S. A. Relationship of the central ACTH-immunoreactive opiocortin system to the supraoptic and paraventricular nuclei of the hypothalamus of the rat. *Brain Res.,* 1982, *239,* 655–658.

Knigge, K. M., & Silverman, A. J. Transport capacity of the median eminence. In K. M. Knigge, D. E. Scott, and A. Weindl (Eds.), *Brain-endocrine interaction: Median eminence: Structure and function.* Basel: S. Karger, 1972.

Knigge, K. M., Scott, D. E., & Weindl, A. (Eds.), *Brain-endocrine interaction: Median eminence: Structure and function.* Basel: S. Karger, 1972.

Knowles, F. G. W., & Howard, A. B. The function of neurosecretion in endocrine regulation. *Nature (Lond.),* 1966, *210,* 271–272.

Kobayashi, H., Matsui, T., & Ishii, S. Functional electron microscopy of the hypothalamic median eminence. *Int. Rev. Cytol.,* 1970, *29,* 281–381.

Köhler, G., & Milstein, C. Continuous cultures of fused cells secreting antibody of prede-fined specificity. *Nature (Lond.),* 1975, *256,* 495–497.

Köhler, G., & Milstein, C. Derivation of specific antibody-producing tissue culture and tumor lines of cell fusion. *Eur. J. Immunol.,* 1976, *6,* 511–519.

Köhler, H. Idiotypic network interactions. *Immunol. Today,* 1980, *1,* 18–21.

Köhler, H., Levitt, D., & Bach, M. A non-galilean view of the immune network. *Immunol. Today,* 1981, *2,* 58–60.

Kordon, C., Enjalbert, A., Epelbaum, J., & Rotsztejn. W. Neurotransmitter interactions with adenohypophysial regulation. In A. M. Gotto, E. J. Peck, & A. E. Boyd (Eds.), *Brain peptides: A new endocrinology.* New York: Elsevier North-Holland Biomedical Press, 1979.

Korneva, E. A., & Klimenko, V. M. Neuronale Hypothalamusaktivität und homöosta-tische Reaktionen. *Ergebn. exp. Med.,* 1976, *23,* 373–382.

Kreutzberg, G. W., Schubert, P., Toth, L., & Rieske, E. Intradendritic transport to post-synaptic sites. *Brain Res.,* 1973, *62,* 399–404.

Krieger, D. T. Food and water restriction shifts corticosterone, temperature, activity and brain amine periodicity. *Endocrinology,* 1974, *95,* 1195–1201.

Krieger, D. T. Pituitary hormones in the brain. What is their function? *Fed. Proc.,* 1980, *39,* 2937–2941

Krieger, D. T., & Liotta, A. S. Pituitary hormones in brain: Where, how and why? *Science,* 1979, *205,* 366–372.

Krieger, D. T., & Martin, J. B. Brain peptides (first of two parts). *New Engl. J. Med.,* 1981 a, *304,* 876–885.

Krieger, D. T., & Martin, J. B. Brain peptides (second of two parts). *New Engl. J. Med.,* 1981 b, *304,* 944–951.

Krieger, D. T., Kreuzer, J., & Rizzo, F. A. Constant light: Effect on circadian pattern and phase reversal of steroid and electrolyte levels in man. *J. Clin. Endocrin. Metab.,* 1971, *32,* 266–284.

Kruisbeek, A. M., Sharrow, S. O., Mathieson, B. J., & Singer, A. The H-2 phenotype of the thymus dictates the self-specificity expressed by thymic but not splenic cytotoxic T lymphocyte precursors in thymus-engrafted mice. *J. Immunol.,* 1981, *127,* 2168–2176.

Landas, S., Thompson, S., Lewis, R., Stamler, G., Raizada, M., & Phillips, M. Uptake of prolactin from cerebrospinal fluid in rat brain. *The Physiologist,* 1981, *24,* 33. (Abstract)

Lang, R. W., Voight, K. H., Fehm, H. L., & Pfeiffer, E. F. Localization of corticotropin re-leasing activity in the rat hypothalamus. *Neurosci. Lett.,* 1976, *2,* 19–22.

Larsson, L. I. Distribution of ACTH-like immunoreactivity in rat brain and gastrointesti-nal tract. *Histochemistry,* 1978, *55,* 225–233.

Levine, S., Goldman, L., & Coover, G. D. Expectancy and the pituitary-adrenal system. In *Physiology, emotion, and psychosomatic illness.* Ciba Foundation Symposium (new series). New York: Elsevier Excerpta Medica North-Holland, 1972.

Levy, S. M. (Ed.), *Biological mediators of behavior and disease: Neoplasia.* New York: Else-vier Biomedical, 1982.

Lindvall, O., & Björklund, A. Organization of CA neurons in the rat CNS. In L. Iversen, S. Iversen, & S. Snyder (Eds.), *Handbook of psychopharmacology.* New York: Plenum Press, 1978.

Liotta, A. S., Gildersleeve, D., Brownstein, M. J. & Krieger, D. T. Biosynthesis *in vitro* of immunoreactive 31,000 dalton corticotropin/β-endorphin-like material by bovine hypothalamus. *Proc. Natl. Acad. Sci. USA,* 1979, *76,* 1448–1452.

Liu, A. Y. C., Walter, U., & Greengard, P. Steroid hormones may regulate autophosphorylation of cyclic adenosine 3′, 5′-monophosphate-dependent protein kinase in target tissue. *Eur. J. Biochem.,* 1981, *144,* 539–548.

Locke, S. E., & Kraus, L. Modulation of natural killer cell activity by life stress and coping ability. In S. M. Levy (Ed.), *Biological mediators of behavior and disease: Neoplasia.* New York: Elsevier Biomedical, 1982.

Löfgren, F. New aspects of the hypothalamic control of the adenohypophysis. *Acta Morph. Neerl. Scand.,* 1959 a, *2,* 220–229.

Löfgren, F. The infundibular recess: A component of the hypothalamo-adreno-hypophyseal system. *Acta Morph. Neerl. Scand.,*1959 b, *3,* 55–78.

Loor, F., & Roelants, G. E. *B- and T-cells in immune recognition.* New York: John Wiley & Sons, 1977.

Lopker, A., Abood, G., Hoss, W., & Lionetti, F. J. Stereospecific muscarinic acetylcholine and opiate receptors in human phagocytic leukocytes. *Biochem. Pharmacol.,* 1980, *29,* 1361–1365.

Low, T. L. K., Hu, S. K., & Goldstein, A. L. Complete amino acid sequence of bovine thymosin β_4: A thymic hormone that induces terminal deoxynucleotidyl transferase activity in thymocyte populations. *Proc. Natl. Acad. Sci. USA,* 1981, *78,* 1162–1166.

Low, T. L. K., Thurman, G. B., Chincarini, C., McClure, J. E., Marshall, G. D., Hu, S. K., & Goldstein, A. L. Current status of thymosin research: Evidence for the existence of a family of thymic factors that control T-cell maturation. *Ann. NY Acad. Sci.,* 1979, *332,* 33–48.

Low, T. L. K., Thurman, G. B., McAdoo, M., McClure, J. E. Rossio, J. L., Naylor, P. H., & Goldstein, A. L. The chemistry and biology of thymosin. I. Isolation, characterization, and biological activities of thymosin α_1 and polypeptide β_1 from calf thymus. *J. Biol. Chem.,* 1979, *254,* 981–986.

Lundberg, J. M., Fried, G., Fahrenkrug, J., Hoomstedt, B., Hökfelt, T., Lagercrantz, H., Lundgren, G., & Änggard, A. Subcellular fractionation of cat submandibular gland: Comparative studies on the distribution of acetylcholine and vasoactive intestinal polypeptide (VIP). *Neuroscience,* 1981, *6,* 1001–1010.

Maddrell, S. H. P., & Nordmann, J. J. *Neurosecretion.* New York: John Wiley & Sons, 1979.

Mains, R. E., Eipper, B. A., & Ling, N. Common precursor to corticotropin and endorphins. *Proc. Natl. Acad. Sci. USA,* 1977, *74,* 3014–3018.

Marchalonis, J. J. Surface immunoglobulins of B and T lymphocytes: Molecular properties, association with the cell membrane, and a unified model of antigen recognition. *Contemp. Topics Mol. Immunol.,* 1976, *5,* 125–160.

Maslinski, W., Grabczewska, E., & Ryzewski, J. Acetylcholine receptors of rat lymphocytes. *Biochim. Biophys. Acta,* 1980, *633,* 269–273.

Mason, J. W. A review of psychoendocrine research on the pituitary-adrenal cortical system. *Psychosom. Med.,* 1968, *30,* 576–607.

Mason, J. W. Emotion as reflected in patterns of endocrine integration. In L. Levi (Ed.), *Emotions: Their parameters and measurement.* New York: Raven Press, 1975.

Mason, J. W., Maher, J. T., Hartley, L. H., Mougey, E. H., Perlow, M. J., & Jones, L. G. Selectivity of corticosteroid and catecholamine responses to various natural stimuli. In G. Serban (Ed.), *Psychopathology of human adaptation.* New York: Plenum Press, 1976.

Mayeri, E., & Rothman, B. S. Nonsynaptic peptidergic neurotransmission in the abdominal ganglion of *Aplysia.* In D. S. Farner & K. Lederis (Eds.), *Neurosecretion: Molecules, cells, systems.* New York: Plenum Press, 1981.

McCain, H. W., Lamster, I. B., Bozzone, J. M., & Grbic, J. T. β-endorphin modulates human immune activity via non-opiate receptor mechanisms. *Life Sci.,* 1982, *31,* 1619–1624.

McCann, S. M., & Porter, J. C. Hypothalamic pituitary-stimulating and inhibiting hormones. *Physiol. Rev.,* 1969, *49,* 240–284.

McDevitt, H. O., & Bodner, W. F. Histocompatibility antigens, immune responsiveness and susceptibility to disease. *Amer. J. Med.,* 1972, *52,* 1–8.

McDevitt, H. O., Deak, B. D., Schreffler, D. C., Klein, J., Stimpfling, J. H., & Snell, G. D. Genetic control of the immune response: Mapping of the Ir-1 locus. *J. Exp. Med.,* 1972, *135,* 1259–1278.

McEwen, B. S., Davis, P. G., Parsons, B., & Pfaff, D. W. The brain as a target for steroid hormone action. *Ann. Rev. Neurosci.,* 1979, *2,* 65–112.

McKelvy, J. F., & Epelbaum, J. Biosynthesis, packaging, transport and release of brain peptides. In S. Reichlin, R. J Baldessarini, & J. B. Martin (Eds.), *The hypothalamus. Research publications: Association for research in nervous and mental diseases* (Vol. 56). New York: Raven Press, 1978.

Melchers, F., & Rajewsky, D. *The immune system.* New York: Springer-Verlag, 1976.

Metal'nikov, S. *Rôle du système nerveux et des facteurs biologiques et psychiques dans l'immunité.* Paris: Masson, 1934.

Metal'nikov, S., & Chorine, V. Rôle des réflexes conditionnels dans l'immunité. *Ann. Inst. Pasteur (Paris),* 1926, *40,* 893–900.

Miller, N. E. A perspective on the effects of stress and coping on disease and health. In S. Levine & H. Ursin (Eds.), *Coping and health.* New York: Plenum Press, 1980 a.

Miller, N. E. Effects of learning on physical symptoms produced by psychological stress. In H. Selye (Ed.), *Selye's guide to stress research.* New York: Van Nostrand Reinhold Co., 1980 b.

Miller, G. C., Murgo, A. J., & Plotnikoff, N. P. The influence of leucine and methionine enkephalin on immune mechanisms. *Int. J. Immunopharmac.,* 1982, *4,* 366–367.

Mills, J. E., & Widdicombe, J. G. Role of vagus nerve in anaphylaxis and histamine-induced bronchial constrictions by guinea pigs. *Brit. J. Pharmac.,* 1970, *39,* 724–731.

Monjan, A. A. Stress and immunologic competence: Studies in animals. In R. Ader (Ed.), *Psychoneuroimmunology.* New York: Academic Press, 1981.

Monroe, B. G., & Holmes, E. M. The freeze-fractured median eminence. I. Development of intercellular junctions in the ependyma of the 3rd ventricle of the rat. *Cell Tissue Res.,* 1982, *222,* 389–408.

Moore, R. Y. The reticular formation: Monoamine neuron system. In J. A. Hobson & M. A. B. Brazier (Eds.), *The reticular formation revisited: Specifying functions for a nonspecific system.* (IBRO Monograph Ser., Vol. 6). New York: Raven Press, 1980.

Moore, R. Y., & Bloom, F. E. Central catecholamine neuron systems: Anatomy and physiology of the norepinephrine and epinephrine systems. *Ann. Rev. Neurosci.,* 1979, *2,* 113–168.

Moore, R. Y., & Kromer, L. F. The organization of central catecholamine neuron systems. In B. Haber & M. H. Aprison (Eds.), *Neuropharmacology and behavior.* New York: Plenum Press, 1978.

Moore, R. Y., Halaris, A. E., & Jones, B. E. Serotonin neurons of the midbrain raphe: Ascending projections. *J. Comp. Neurol.,* 1978, *180,* 417–438.

Moroni, F., Cheney, D. L., & Costa, E. Inhibition of acetylcholine turnover in rat hippocampus by intraseptal injection of β-endorphin and morphine. *Naunyn-Schmiedeberg's Arch. Pharmac.,* 1977, *299,* 149–153.

Morrison, F. R., & Paffenbarger, R. A. Epidemiological aspects of biobehavior in the etiology of cancer: A critical review. In S. M. Weiss, J. A. Herd, & B. H. Fox (Eds.), *Perspectives in behavioral medicine.* New York: Academic Press, 1981.

Motta, M., Fraschini, F., & Martini, L. Short feedback mechanisms in the control of anterior pituitary function. In W. F. Ganong & L. Martini (Eds.), *Frontiers in neuroendocrinology, 1969.* New York: Oxford University Press, 1969.

Murray, J. B. New trends in psychosomatic research. *Genetic Psychol. Monogr.,* 1977, *96,* 3–74.

Nathanson, J. A., & Greengard, P. "Second messengers" in the brain. *Sci. Amer.,* 1977, *237,* 109–119.

Nathenson, S. G., Ewenstein, B. M., Uehara, H., Martinko, J. M., Coligan, J. E., & Kindt, T. J. Structure of H-2 major histocompatibility complex products: Recent studies on the H-2K^b glycoprotein and on the H-2K^b MHC mutants. In R. A. Reisfeld & S. Ferrone (Eds.), *Current trends in histocompatibility* (Vol. 1). New York: Plenum Press, 1980.

Nauta, W. J. H., & Gygax, P. A. Silver impregnation of degenerating axons in the central nervous system. *Stain Tech.,* 1954, *29,* 91–93.

Nicoll, R. A. Neurotransmitters can say more than just 'yes' or 'no'. *Trends Neurosci.,* 1982, *5,* 369–371, 374.

Nicoll, C. S., Talwalker, P. K., & Meites, J. Initiation of lactation in rats by nonspecific stresses. *Amer. J. Physiol.,* 1960, *198,* 1103–1106.

Olds, J. Do reward and drive neurons exist? In G. Serban (Ed.), *Psychopathology of human adaptation.* New York: Plenum Press, 1976.

Oliveira-Castro, G. M., & Dos Reis, G. A. Cell communication in the immune response. In W. C. de Mello (Ed.), *Intercellular communication in the immune response.* New York: Plenum Press, 1977.

Orth, D. W., & Island, D. P. Light synchronization of the circadian rhythm in plasma cortisol (17-OHCS) concentration in man. *J. Clin. Endocrin. Metab.,* 1969, *29,* 479–486.

Overmier, J. B., Patterson, J., & Wielkiewicz, R. M. Environmental contingencies as sources of stress in animals. In S. Levine & H. Ursin (Eds.), *Coping and health.* New York: Plenum Press, 1980.

Page, R. B., Munger, B. L., & Bergland, R. M. Scanning microscopy of pituitary vascular casts. *Amer. J. Anat.,* 1970, *146,* 273–301.

Palkovits, M. Changes in brain amines during stress. In M. T. Jones, B. Gillham, M. F. Dallman, & S. Chattopadhyay (Eds.), *Interactions within the brain-pituitary adrenocortical system.* New York: Academic Press, 1979.

Palkovits, M., Mezey, É., Záborszky, L., Feminger, A., Versteeg, D. H. G., Wijnen, H. L. J. M., DeJong, W., Fekete, M. I. K., Herman, J. P., & Kanyicska, B. Adrenergic innervation of the rat hypothalamus. *Neurosci. Lett.,* 1980, *18,* 237–243.

Parent, A., Descarries, L., & Beaudet, A. Organization of ascending serotonin system in the adult rat brain. A radioautographic study after intraventricular administration of [^{3}H] 5-hydroxytryptamine. *Neurosciences,* 1981, *6,* 115–138.

Parillo, J. E., & Fauci, A. S. Mechanisms of glucocorticoid action on immune processes. *Ann. Rev. Pharmacol. Toxicol.,* 1979, *19,* 179–201.

Parker, C. W. The role of intracellular mediators in the immune response. In S. Cohen, E. Pick, & J. J. Oppenheim (Eds.), *Biology of the lymphokines.* New York: Academic Press, 1979.

Pastan, I. H., & Willingham, M. C. Journey to the center of the cell: Role of the receptosome. *Science,* 1981, *214,* 504–509.

Pearse, A. G. E. Molecular markers and the APUD concept. In D. S. Farner & K. Lederis (Eds.), *Neurosecretion: Molecules, cells, systems.* New York: Plenum Press, 1981.

Pelletier, G. Ultrastructural localization of a fragment (16K) of the common precursor for adrenocorticotropin (ACTH) and β-lipotropin (β-LPH) in the rat hypothalamus. *Neurosci. Lett.,* 1980, *16,* 85–90.

Pelletier, G., Leclerc, R., Labrie, F., Côté, J., Chrétien, M., & Li, M. Immunohistochemical localization of β-lipotropic hormone in the pituitary gland. *Endocrinology,* 1977, *100,* 700–776.

Peracchia, C. Gap junction structure and function. *Trends Biochem.,* 1977, *2,* 26–31.

Pick, E. (Ed.), *Lymphokine reports: Lymphokines in macrophage activation* (Vol. 3). New York: Academic Press, 1981 a.

Pick, E. (Ed.), *Lymphokine reports: A forum of immune immunoregulatory cell products* (Vol. 4). New York: Academic Press, 1981 b.

Pilgrim, C. Commentary: Transport function of hypothalamic tanycyte ependyma: How good is the evidence? *Neurosci.,* 1978, *3,* 277–283.

Pittman, Q. J., Blume, H. W., & Renaud, L. P. Connections of the hypothalamic paraventricular nucleus with the neurohypophysis, median eminence, amygdala, lateral septum and midbrain periaqueductal gray: An electrophysiological study in the rat. *Brain Res.,* 1981, *215,* 15–28.

Plotnikoff, N. P. The central nervous system control of the immune system: Enkephalins: Antitumor activites. *Psychopharmacol. Bull.,* 1982, *18,* 148.

Plotnikoff, N. P., Miller, G. C., & Murgo, A. J. Enkephalins-endorphins: Immunomodulations in mice. *Int. J. Immunopharmacol.,* 1982, *4,* 366–367.

Pochet, R., Delespesse, G., Gausset, P. W., & Collet, H. Distribution of beta-adrenergic receptors on human lymphocyte subpopulations. *Clin. Exp. Immunol.,* 1979, *38,* 578–584.

Porter, J. C., Ben-Jonathan, N., Oliver, C., & Eskay, R. L. Secretion of releasing hormones and their transport from CSF to hypophysial portal blood. In K. M. Knigge, D. E. Scott, H. Kobayashi, & S. Ishii (Eds.), *Brain-endocrine interaction. II. The ventricular system in neuroendocrine mechanisms.* Basel: S. Karger, 1975.

Pribram, K. H. The biology of the emotions and other feelings. In R. Plutchnik & H. Kellerman (Eds.), *Emotion: Theory, research and experience.* New York: Academic Press, 1980.

Rabkin, J. G., & Struening, E. L. Life events, stress and illness. *Science,* 1976, *194,* 1013–1020.

Rakic, P. Local circuit neurons. *Neurosci. Res. Progr. Bull.,* 1975, *13,* 291–346.

Ramón y Cajal, S. *Recollections of my life.* (E. Horne Craigie, transl.). Philadelphia: The American Philosophical Society, 1937.

Ramón y Cajal, S. Histologie du système nerveux de l'homme et des vertébrés. Madrid: Instituto Ramón y Cajal, 1952. (Orig. Publ., 1909).

Rebar, R.W., Miyake, A., Low, T.L.K., & Goldstein, A.L. Thymosin stimulates secretion of luteinizing hormone-releasing factor. *Science,* 1981, *213,* 669–671.

Reilly, F.D., McCuskey, P.A., Miller, M.L., McCuskey, R.S., & Meineke, H.A. Innervation of the periarteriolar lymphatic sheath of the spleen. *Tissue Cell,* 1979, *11,* 121–126.

Reinherz, E.L., & Schlossman, S.F. Regulation of the immune response: Inducer and suppressor T-lymphocyte subsets in human beings. *New Engl. J. Med.,* 1980, *303,* 370–373.

Reite, M., Harbeck, R., & Hoffman, A. Altered cellular immune response following peer separation. *Life Sci.,* 1981, *29,* 1133–1136.

Renaud, L.P., Pittman, Q.J., & Blume, H.W. Neurophysiology of hypothalamic peptidergic neurons. In K. Fuxe, T. Hökfelt, & R. Luft (Eds.), *Central regulation of the endocrine system.* New York: Plenum Press, 1979.

Resch, K. Membrane-associated events in lymphocyte activation. In P. Cuatrecasas & M.F. Greaves (Eds.), *Receptors and recognition.* London: Chapman and Hall, 1976.

Richards, J.G. Permeability of intercellular junctions in brain epithelia and endothelia to exogenous amine: Cytochemical localization of extracellular 5-hydroxydopamine. *J. Neurocytol.,* 1978, *7,* 61–70.

Riley, V. Psychoneuroendocrine influences on immunocompetence and neoplasia. *Science,* 1981, *212,* 1100–1109.

Rivier, C., Brownstein, M., Spiess, J., Rivier, J., & Vale, W. *In vivo* corticotropin-releasing factor-induced secretion of adrenocorticotropin, beta-endorphin, and corticosterone. *Endocrinology,* 1982, *110,* 272–278.

Roberts, A., & Bush, B.M.H. (Eds.), *Neurons without impulses: Their significance for vertebrate and invertebrate nervous systems.* Cambridge: Cambridge University Press, 1981.

Roberts, D.C.S. An evaluation of the role of noradrenaline in learning. In S.J. Cooper (Ed.), *Theory in psychopharmacology* (Vol. 1). New York: Academic Press, 1981.

Roberts, E. Role of GABA in neurons in information processing in the vertebrate CNS. In A. Karlin, V.M. Tennyson, & H.L. Vogel (Eds.), *Neuronal information transfer.* New York: Academic Press, 1978.

Roberts, J.L., & Herbert, E. Characterization of a common precursor to corticotropin and β-lipotropin: Cell-free synthesis of the precursor and identification of corticotropin peptides in the molecule. *Proc. Natl. Acad. Sci. USA,* 1977a, *74,* 4826–4830.

Roberts, J.L., & Herbert, E. Characterization of a common precursor to corticotropin and β-lipotropin: Identification of β-lipotropin peptides and their arrangement relative to corticotropin in the precursor synthesized in a cell-free system. *Proc. Natl. Acad. Sci. USA,* 1977b, *74,* 5300–5304.

Roberts, W.W. The hypothalamic mechanisms for motivational and species-typical behavior. In R.E. Whalen, R.F. Thompson, J. Verzeano, & N.W. Weinberger (Eds.), *The neural control of behavior.* New York: Academic Press, 1970.

Rodriguez, E.M. Ependymal specializations. I. Fine structure of the neural (internal) region of the toad median eminence, with particular reference to the connections between ependymal cells and the subependymal capillary loops. *Zeit. Zellforsch. Mikrosk. Anat.,* 1969, *102,* 153–171.

Rogers, M.P., Dubey, D., & Reich, P. The influence of the psyche and the brain on immunity and disease susceptibility: A critical review. *Psychosom. Med.,* 1979, *41,* 147–164.

Rogers, M. P., Reich, P., Strom, T. B., & Carpenter, C. B. Behaviorally conditioned immunosuppression: Replication of a recent study. *Psychosom. Med.,* 1976, *38,* 447–452.

Rose, N. R. Autoimmune diseases. *Sci. Amer.,* 1981, *244,* 80–103.

Rose, R. M. Endocrine responses to stressful psychological events. *Psychiat. Clin. N. Amer.,* 1980, *3,* 251–276.

Rossier, J., French, E., Guillemin, R., & Bloom, F. E. On the mechanisms of the simultaneous release of immunoreactive β-endorphin, ACTH, and prolactin by stress. *Adv. Biochem. Psychopharmacol.,* 1980a, *22,* 363–375.

Rossier, J., Pittman, Q., Bloom, F. E., & Guillemin, R. Distribution of opioid peptides in the pituitary: A new hypothalamic-pars nervosa enkephalinergic pathway. *Fed. Proc.,* 1980b, *39,* 2555–2560.

Roszman, T. L., Cross, R. J., Brooks, W. H., & Markesbery, W. R. Hypothalamiç-immune interactions. II. The effect of hypothalamic lesions on the ability of adherent spleen cells to limit lymphocyte blastogenesis. *Immunology,* 1982, *45,* 737–742.

Roth, K. A., Katz, F. J., Sibel, M., Mefford, I. N., Barchas, J. D., & Carroll, B. J. Central epinergic inhibition of corticosterone release in the rat. *Life Sci.,* 1981, *28,* 2389–2394.

Roth, K. A., Weber, E., Barchas, J. D., Chang, D., & Chang, J.-K. Immunoreactive dynorphin-(1-8) and corticotropin-releasing factor in subpopulation of hypothalamic neurons. *Science,* 1983, *291,* 189–190.

Rotsztejn, N. H. Neuromodulation in neuroendocrinology. *Trends Neurosci.,* 1980, *3,* 67–70.

Rubinstein, M., Stein, S., & Udenfriend, S. Characterization of pro-opiocortin, a precursor of opioid peptides and corticotropin. *Proc. Natl. Acad. Sci. USA,* 1978, *75,* 669–671.

Ryder, L. P., Platz, P., & Svejgaard, A. Histocompatibility antigens and susceptibility to disease: Genetic considerations. In R. A. Reisfeld & S. Ferrone (Eds.), *Current trends in histocompatibility* (Vol. 2). New York: Plenum Press, 1980.

Saavedra, J. M., Palkovits, M., Brownstein, M., & Axelrod, J. Serotonin distribution in the nuclei of the rat hypothalamus preoptic region. *Brain Res.,* 1974, *77,* 157–165.

Sachs, H., Faucett, P., Takabatake, Y., & Portanova, R. Biosynthesis and release of vasopressin and neurophysin. *Recent Progr. Horm. Res.* 1969, *25,* 447–491.

Said, S. I. Peptides common to the nervous system and the gastrointestinal tract. In L. Martini & W. F. Ganong (Eds.), *Frontiers in neuroendocrinology.* New York: Raven Press, 1980.

Sasazuki, T., Grumet, F. C., & McDevitt, H. O. The association of genes in the major histocompatibility complex and disease susceptibility. *Ann. Rev. Med.,* 1977, *28,* 425–452.

Savaki, H. E., Kadekaro, M., McCulloch, J., & Sokoloff, L. The central noradrenergic system in the rat: Metabolic mapping with α-adrenergic blocking agents. *Brain Res.,* 1982, *234,* 65–79.

Sawchenko, P. E., & Swanson, L. W. Central noradrenergic pathways for the integration of hypothalamic, neuroendocrine and autonomic responses. *Science,* 1981, *214,* 685–687.

Schachter, B. S., Johnson, L. K., Baxter, J. D., & Roberts, J. L. Differential regulation by glucocorticoids of pro-opiomelanocortin mRNA levels in the anterior and intermediate lobes of the rat pituitary. *Endocrinology,* 1982, *110,* 1442–1444.

Scharrer, B. General principles of neuroendocrine communication. In F. O. Schmitt (Ed.), *The neurosciences: Second study program.* New York: Rockefeller University Press, 1970.

Scharrer, E. The final common path in neuroendocrine integration. *Arch. Anat. Microsc. Morph. Exp. (Paris),* 1965, *54,* 359–370.

Scharrer, E., & Scharrer, B. Secretory cells within the hypothalamus. In E. Scharrer & B. Scharrer (Eds.), *The hypothalamus and central levels of autonomic function. Research publications: Association for research in nervous and mental diseases* (Vol. 20). New York: Raven Press, 1940.

Scharrer, E., & Scharrer, B. Hormones produced by neurosecretory cells. *Recent Progr. Horm. Res.,* 1954, *10,* 183–240.

Schimmer, B.P. Cyclic nucleotides in hormonal regulation of adrenocortical function. In P. Greengard & G.A. Robison (Eds.), *Advances in cyclic nucleotide research* (Vol. 13). New York: Raven Press, 1980.

Schmitt, F.O., & Worden, F.G. (Eds.), *The neurosciences: Fourth study program.* Cambridge, Mass.: The MIT Press, 1979.

Schmitt, F.O., Dev, P., & Smith, B.H. Electrotonic processing of information by brain cells. *Science,* 1976, *193,* 114–120.

Schmutzler, W., & Freundt, G.P. The effect of glucocorticoids and catecholamines on cyclic AMP and allergic histamine release in guinea pig lung. *Int. Arch. Allergy Appl. Immunol.,* 1975, *49,* 209–212.

Schwartzberg, D.G., & Nakane, P.K. Ontogenesis of adrenocorticotropin-related peptide determinants in the hypothalamus and pituitary gland of the rat. *Endocrinology,* 1982, *110,* 855–864.

Seidman, J.G., Leder, A., Nau, M., Norman, B., & Leder, P. Antibody diversity. *Science,* 1978, *202,* 11–17.

Seif, S.M., & Robinson, A.G. Localization and release of neurophysins. *Ann. Rev. Physiol.,* 1978, *40,* 345–376.

Selye, H. The evolution of the stress concept. *Amer. J. Cardiol.,* 1970, *26,* 298–299.

Selye, H. *Stress without distress.* Philadelphia: J.B. Lippincott Co., 1974.

Sergeeva, V.E. Histotopography of catecholamines in the mammalian thymus. *Bull. Exp. Biol. Med. USSR,* 1974, *77,* 456–458.

Shapiro, H.M., & Strom, T.B. Electrophysiology of T-lymphocyte cholinergic receptors. *Proc. Natl. Acad. Sci. USA,* 1980, *77,* 4317–4321.

Shepherd, G.M. *The synaptic organization of the brain.* New York: Oxford University Press, 1974..

Shute, C.C.D., & Lewis, P.R. Cholinergic and monoaminergic pathways in the hypothalamus. *Brit. Med. Bull.,* 1966, *22,* 221–226.

Siggins, G.R. Neurotransmitters and neuromodulators and their mediation by cyclic nucleotides. In Y.H. Ehrlich, J. Volavka, L.G. Davis, & E.G. Brungraber (Eds.), *Advances in experimental medicine and biology.* New York: Raven Press, 1979.

Silverman, A.J., Knigge, K.M., & Peck, W.A. Transport capacity of the median eminence. I. Amino acid transport. *Neuroendocrinology,* 1972, *9,* 123–132.

Simon, R.H., Lovett, E.J., Tomaszek, D., & Lundy, J. Electrical stimulation of the midbrain mediates metastatic tumor growth. *Science,* 1980, *209,* 1132–1133.

Sklar, L.S., & Anisman, H. Stress and coping factors influence tumor growth. *Science,* 1979, *205,* 513–515.

Sklar, L.S., & Anisman, H. Stress and cancer. *Psychol. Bull.,* 1981, *89,* 369–406.

Sloper, J.J. Gap junctions between dendrites in the primary cortex. *Brain Res.,* 1972, *44,* 641–646.

Smelik, P. G., & Papaikonomou, E. Steroid feedback mechanisms in pituitary-adrenal function. *Progr. Brain Res.,* 1973, *39,* 99–109.

Smith, E. M., & Blalock, J. E. Human lymphocyte production of corticotropin and endorphin-like substances: Association with leukocyte interferon. *Proc. Natl. Acad. Sci. USA,* 1981, *78,* 7530–7534.

Smith, E. M., Meyer, W. J., & Blalock, J. E. Virus-induced corticosterone in hypophysectomized mice: A possible lymphoid-adrenal axis. *Science,* 1982, *218,* 1311–1312.

Snell, G. D. The major histocompatibility complex: Its evaluation and involvement in cell-mediated immunity. *Harvey Lect.,* 1980, *74,* 49–80.

Sofroniew, M. V. Immunoreactive β-endorphin and ACTH in the same regions of the hypothalamic arcuate nucleus in the rat. *Amer. J. Anat.,* 1979, *154,* 283–289.

Solomon, G. F., & Amkraut, A. A. Psychoneuroendocrinological effects on the immune response. *Ann. Rev. Microbiol.,* 1981, *35,* 155–184.

Sotelo, C. Electrical and chemical communication in the central nervous system. In B. R. Brinkley & K. R. Porter (Eds.), *International cell biology.* New York: The Rockefeller University Press, 1977.

Spector, N. H. The central state of the hypothalamus in health and disease: Old and new concepts. In P. J. Morgane & J. Panksepp (Eds.), *Handbook of the hypothalamus. Physiology of the hypothalamus* (Vol. 2). New York: Marcel Dekker, Inc., 1980.

Spector, N. H., & Korneva, E. A. Neurophysiology, immunophysiology and neuroimmunomodulation. In R. Ader (Ed.), *Psychoneuroimmunology.* New York: Academic Press, 1981.

Sperry R. W. Neurology and the mind-brain problem. *Amer. Sci.,* 1952, *40,* 291–312.

Sperry, R. W. A unifying approach to mind and brain: Ten year perspective. In M. A. Corner & D. F. Swaab (Eds.), *Progress in brain research* (Vol. 45) New York: Elsevier Scientific Publishing Co., 1976.

Spiess, J., Rivier, J., Rivier, C., & Vale, W. Primary structure of corticotropin-releasing factor from ovine hypothalamus. *Proc. Natl. Acad. Sci. USA,* 1981, *78,* 6517–6521.

Sprent, J., & Korngold, R. Immunogenetics of graft-versus-host reactions to minor histocompatibility antigens. *Immunol. Today,* 1981, *2,* 189–195.

Stein, M., Keller, S. E., & Schleifer, S. J. The role of the hypothalamus in mediating stress effects on the immune system. In B. A. Stoll (Ed.), *Mind and cancer prognosis.* New York: John Wiley & Sons, 1979.

Stein, M., Keller, S. E., & Schleifer, S. J. The hypothalamus and the immune response. In H. Weiner, M. A. Hofer, & A. J. Stunkard (Eds.), *Brain, behavior and bodily disease.Res. Pub. Assoc. Res. Nerv. Mental Dis.,* (Vol. 59). New York: Raven Press, 1981.

Stein, M., Schleifer, S. J., & Keller, S. E. Hypothalamic influence on immune responses. In R. Ader (Ed.), *Psychoneuroimmunology.* New York: Academic Press, 1981.

Stephens, C. G., & Snyderman, R. Cyclic nucleotides regulate the morphologic alterations required for chemotaxis in monocytes. *J. Immunol.,* 1982, *128,* 1192–1197.

Stepien, H., Kunert-Radek, J., Karasek, E., & Pawlikowski, M. Dopamine increases cyclic AMP concentration in the rat spleen lymphocytes *in vitro. Biochem. Biophys. Res. Commun.,* 1981, *101,* 1057–1063.

Stoll, B. A. (Ed.). *Mind and cancer prognosis.* New York: John Wiley & Sons, 1979.

Strom, T. B., & Carpenter, C. B. Cyclic nucleotides in immunosuppression–neuroendocrine-pharmacologic manipulation and *in vivo* immunoregulation of immunity acting *via* second messenger systems. *Transplant. Proc.,* 1980, *12,* 304–310.

Strom, T. B., George, K., & Lane, M. A. Are immunoregulatory signals governed by temporal changes in neurohormonal receptor expression on T-lymphocytes? *Clin. Res.,* 1979, *27,* 475A. (Abstract)

Strom, T. B., Lane, M. A., & George, K. The parallel, time-dependent, bimodal change in lymphocyte cholinergic binding activity and cholinergic influence upon lymphocyte-mediated cytotoxicity after lymphocyte activation. *J. Immunol.,* 1981, *127,* 705–710.

Strom, T. B., Lundin, A. P., & Carpenter, C. B. The role of cyclic nucleotides in lymphocyte activation and function. *Progr. Clin. Immunol.,* 1977, *3,* 115–153.

Svedersky, L. P., Hui, A., May, L., McKay, P., & Stebbings, N. Induction and augmentation of mitogen-induced immune interferon production in human peripheral blood lymphocytes by N^α-desacetylthymosin α_1. *Eur. J. Immunol.,* 1982, *12,* 244–247.

Szentivanyi, A. The beta-adrenergic theory of the atopic abnormality in bronchial allergy. *J. Allergy,* 1968, *42,* 203–232.

Talal, N. *Autoimmunity: Genetic, immunologic, virologic and clinical aspects.* New York: Academic Press, 1977.

Talal, N. Autoimmunity and the immunologic network. *Arth. Rheum.,* 1978, *21,* 858–861.

Tappaz, M. L., & Brownstein, M. J. Origin of glutamate-decarboxylase (GAD)-containing cells in discrete hypothalamic nuclei. *Brain Res.,* 1977, *132,* 95–106.

Taylor, J. (Ed.), *The collected works of John Hughlings Jackson.* London: Staples Press, 1958.

Thompson, S. A. Localization of immunoreactive prolactin in ependyma and circumventricular organs of rat brain. *Cell Tissue Res.,* 1982, *225,* 79–93.

Tsong, S. D., Phillips, D., Halmi, N., Liotta, A. S., Margioris, A., Bardin, C. W., & Krieger, D. T. ACTH and β-endorphin-related peptides are present in multiple sites in the reproductive tract of the male rat. *Endocrinology,* 1982, *110,* 2204–2206.

Tyrey, L., & Nalbandov, A. V. Influence of anterior hypothalamic lesions on circulating antibody titers in the rat. *Amer. J. Physiol.,* 1972, *222,* 179–185.

Uehara, H., Ewenstein, B. M., Martinko, J. M., Nathenson, S. G., Coligan, J. E., & Kindt, T. L. Primary structure of murine major histocompatibility complex alloantigens: Amino acid sequence of the amino terminal one hundred and seventy-three residues of the H-2K^b glycoprotein. *Biochemistry,* 1980, *2,* 306–325.

Ungerstedt, U. Stereotaxic mapping of the monoamine pathways in the rat brain. *Acta Physiol. Scand.,* 1971, *367 (Suppl.),* 1–48.

Vale, W., Spiess, J., Rivier, C., & Rivier, J. Characterization of a 41-residue ovine hypothalamic peptide that stimulates the secretion of corticotropin and β-endorphin. *Science,* 1981, *213,* 1394–1397.

Van der Gugten, J., Palkovits, M., Wijnen, H. L. J. M., & Versteeg, D. H. G. Regional distribution of adrenaline in rat brain. *Brain Res.,* 1976, *107,* 171–175.

Van der Kar, L. D., & Lorens, W. Differential serotoninergic innervation of individual hypothalamic nuclei and other forebrain regions by the dorsal and median midbrain raphe nuclei. *Brain Res.,* 1979, *162,* 45–54.

Visintainer, M., Volpicelli, J. R., & Seligman, M. E. P. Tumor rejection in rats after inescapable or escapable shock. *Science,* 1982, *216,* 437–439.

Wahl, S. M., Altman, L. C., & Rosenstreich, D. L. Inhibition of *in vitro* lymphokine synthesis by glucocorticoids. *J. Immunol.,* 1975, *115,* 476–480.

Walaas, I., & Fronnum, F. The effect of parenteral glutamate treatment on the localization of neurotransmitters in the mediobasal hypothalamus. *Brain Res.,* 1978, *153,* 549–562.

Waldmann, T.A., & Broder, S. Suppressor cells in the regulation of the immune response. *Progr. Clin. Immunol.,* 1977, *3,* 155–159.

Watson, S.J., & Akil, H. On the multiplicity of active substances in single neurons: β-endorphin and α-MSH as a model system. In D. de Wied & P.A. van Keep (Eds.), *Hormones and the brain.* Lancaster: The MIT Press, 1981.

Watson, S.J., Akil, H., Ghazarossian, V.E., & Goldstein, A. Dynorphin immunocytochemical localization in brain and peripheral nervous system: Preliminary studies. *Proc. Natl. Acad. Sci. USA,* 1981, *78,* 1260–1263.

Watson, S.J., Khachaturian, H., Akil, H., Coy, D.H., & Goldstein, A. Comparison of the distribution of dynorphin systems and enkephalin systems in brain. *Science,* 1982, *218,* 1134–1136.

Wayner, E.A., Flannery, G.R., & Singer, G. The effects of taste aversion conditioning on the primary antibody response to sheep red blood cells and *Brucella abortus* in the albino rat. *Physiol. Behav.,* 1978, *21,* 995–1000.

Weight, F.F. Physiological mechanisms of synaptic modulation. In F.O. Schmitt (Ed.), *The neurosciences: Third study program.* Cambridge, Mass.: The MIT Press, 1973.

Weindl, A., & Joynt, R.J. The median eminence as a circumventricular organ. In K.M. Knigge, D.E. Scott, & A. Weindl (Eds.), *Brain-endocrine interaction: Median eminence: Structure and function.* Basel: S. Karger, 1972.

Weiner, H. Presidential address: Some comments on the transduction of experience by the brain. Implications for our understanding of the relationship of mind and body. *Psychosom. Med.,* 1972, *34,* 355–380.

Weiner, H. *Psychobiology and human disease.* New York: Elsevier North-Holland, Inc., 1977.

Weiner, H., Hofer, M., & Stunkard, A.J. (Eds.), *Brain, behavior and bodily disease.* New York: Raven Press, 1980.

Weiss, S.M., Herd, J.A., & Fox, B.H. (Eds.), *Perspectives on behavioral medicine.* New York: Academic Press, 1981.

de Wied, D., & Jolles, J. Neuropeptides derived from pro-opiocortin: Behavioral, physiological, and neurochemical effects. *Physiol. Rev.,* 1982, *62,* 976–1059.

Wiegant, V.M., & de Wied, D. Behavioral effects of pituitary hormones. In P.D. Hrdina & R.L. Singhal (Eds.), *Neuroendocrine regulation and altered behavior.* New York: Plenum Press, 1981.

Wilkes, M.M., Watkins, W.B., Stewart, R.D., & Yen, S.S.C. Localization and quantification of β-endorphin in human brain and pituitary. *Neuroendocrinology,* 1980, *30,* 113–121.

Wilkinson, C.S., Shiusako, M.F., & Dallman, M.F. Daily rhythms in adrenal responsiveness to adrenocorticotropin are determined primarily by the time of feeding in the rat. *Endocrinology,* 1979, *104,* 350–359.

Williams, J.M., & Felten, D.L. Sympathetic innervation of murine thymus and spleen: A comparative histofluorescence study. *Anat. Rec.,* 1981, *199,* 531–542.

Williams, J.M., Peterson, R.G., Shea, P.A., Schmedtje, J.F., Bauer, D.C., & Felten, D.L. Sympathetic innervation of murine thymus and spleen: Evidence for a functional link between the nervous and immune systems. *Brain Res. Bull.,* 1981, *6,* 83–94.

Witter, A., Gispen, W.H., & de Wied, D. Mechanisms of action of behaviorally active ACTH-like peptides. In J.L. Martinez, R.A. Jensen, R.B. Messing, H. Rigter, & J.L. McGaugh (Eds.), *Endogenous peptides and learning and memory processes.* New York: Academic Press, 1981.

Wurtman, R.J. Neuroendocrine transducer cells in mammals. In F.O. Schmitt (Ed.), *The neurosciences: Second study program.* New York: The Rockefeller University Press, 1970.

Wurtman, R.J. Brain monoamines and endocrine function. *Neurosci. Res. Bull.,* 1971, *9,* 177–297.

Wurtman, R.J., & Anton-Tay, F. The mammalian pineal as a neuroendocrine transducer. *Recent Progr. Horm. Res.,* 1969, *25,* 493–522.

Wybran, J., Appelboom, T., Famaly, J.P., & Govaerts, A. Suggestive evidence for receptors for morphine and methionine-enkephalin on normal human blood T-lymphocytes. *J. Immunol.,* 1979, *123,* 1068–1070.

Xu, G.-J., Hannappel, E., Morgan, J., Hempstead, J., & Horecker, B.L. Synthesis of thymosin β_4 by peritoneal macrophages and adherent spleen cells. *Proc. Natl. Acad. Sci. USA,* 1982, *79,* 4006–4009.

Yates, F.E., & Maran, J.W. Stimulation and inhibition of adrenocorticotropin release. In R.O. Greep and E.B. Astwood (Eds.), *Handbook of physiology: Endocrinology* (Vol. 4, pt. 2). Washington, D.C.: The American Physiological Society, 1974.

Yuwiler, A. Stress, anxiety, and endocrine function. In R.G. Grenell and S. Gray (Eds.), *Biological foundations of psychiatry.* New York: Raven Press, 1976.

Záborszky, L. Afferent connections of the medial basal hypothalamus. In W. Hild, J. Van Limborgh, R. Ortmann, J.E. Pauly, & T.H. Schiebler (Eds.), *Advances in anatomy, embryology and cell biology* (Vol. 69). New York: Springer-Verlag, 1982.

Zimmerman, E.A., & Robinson, A.G. Hypothalamic neurons secreting vasopressin and neurophysin. *Kidney Int.,* 1976, *10,* 12–24.

Hypothalamic, Metabolic and Immune Mechanisms of the Influence of Stress on the Tumor Process

V. M. Dilman and M. N. Ostroumova

Introduction

There is a large body of evidence suggesting that chronic stress and mental depression may influence the induction and progression of tumors. However, the related empirical observations involve a great number of problems concerning the operation and mechanism of stress and mental depression on the one hand, and their effect on tumor processes on the other. First of all, it is necessary to comprehend the way in which the state of chronic stress is maintained in the organism. The production of a stress reaction is known to depend upon the activation of the limbic-hypothalamo-pituitary system. This activation, in its turn, leads to increases in the blood levels of ACTH, cortisol, prolactin, growth hormone, glucose, free fatty acids (FFA), and other factors. According to the negative feedback mechanism these hormone-metabolic shifts should inhibit hypothalamo-pituitary complex activity and thus eliminate the deviation from homeostasis which is required for the production of a stress reaction. However, since the state of stress may be maintained in the organism for rather a long period we can conclude that stress produces changes in hypothalamic regulatory mechanisms which prevent the restoration of homeostasis (Dilman, 1976, 1981). The present paper reports arguments supporting the above conclusion. In particular we point out that it is elevation of the hypothalamo-pituitary-complex threshold of sensitivity to feedback inhibition by glucocorticoids that rules out the restoration of homeostasis in the course of the stress reaction. In the light of this suggestion a resemblance is noted between chronic stress and mental depression, since the latter is also characterized by hypothalamic resistance to glucocorticoid action (Carroll, Curtiss, & Mendels, 1976; Nuller & Ostroumova, 1980).

In addition, our chapter provides data on the resistance of the hypothalamo-pituitary complex to dexamethasone inhibition in cancer patients with tumors in various sites, as well as during normal aging – though there might be some difference in the mechanism of operation of this hypothalamic complex under chronic stress and mental depression on the one hand, and in the course of normal aging on the other. Although a similar metabolic pattern is observed in all of these states, the mere presence of common features in hormone-metabolic patterns of chronic stress, mental depression, normal aging, and tumors of different sites is not sufficient for a conclusion about the influence of metabolic factors on the tumor process. In the present state of scientific knowledge only the construction of tentative models with consideration of the above factors is possible. In this chapter two such models will be discussed – the metabolic immunodepression model characterizing the mechanism of cellular immunity inhibition by metabolic disturbances peculiar to the states we are considering, and the model of cancrophilia, a special term used here to indicate the sum of metabolic disturbances which increase the risk of tumor development.

Finally, we will demonstrate some elements of the mechanism by which the hypothalamic threshold of sensitivity to homeostatic influences is elevated under chronic stress, mental depression and aging. These data might be used for working out the means for elimination of hyperadaptosis – the excessive reaction of the adaptation system observed in chronic stress, mental depression, normal aging, and in many patients with tumors of different sites.

The Syndrome of Hyperadaptosis

To assess the sensitivity of the hypothalamo-pituitary complex to homeostatic inhibition by glucocorticoids, the dexamethasone suppression test was generally used. Instead of the usual dosage of dexamethasone – 1 mg – we administered 0.5 mg of the drug at 11 p.m. For determination of 11-hydroxycorticosteroid (11-OHCS) concentration, blood was sampled at 9 a.m. on the day of dexamethasone administration, and at 9 a.m. on the day following administration. Our former investigations allowed us to suggest resistance to dexamethasone action in patients whose blood level of 11-OHCS after dexamethasone administration remained higher than 10 µg% or was lowered by less than 40% of its initial value.

Table I shows that, according to average figures, patients with tumors in various sites display resistance to the inhibiting effect of dexamethasone. The resistance is observed in 38–67% of the patients, depending on the primary localization of the tumor.

Table I. Effect of Dexamethasone on the Level of 11-Hydroxycorticosteroids in Patients with Cancer, Endogenous Mental Depression, and in Normal Subjects.

Group	No. of cases	Blood 11-hydroxycortico-steroids (μg%)		Inhibition (in %)	Dexamethasone-resistant patients (%)
		basal	after dexamethasone		
Ambulatory Control	85	14.4±0.5	5.0±0.4	65	9
Hospital Control	24	12.3±0.9	8.0±0.9	35	41
Mental Depression	52	20.6±0.8	16.5±0.9	19	69
Endometrial Cancer	57	15.6±1.1	9.9±0.6	37	67
Breast Cancer	13	13.7±1.6	8.6±1.2	37	38
Stomach Cancer	36	15.7±0.7	9.5±0.8	39	61
Colon Cancer	55	15.8±0.6	9.8±0.2	38	60
Lung Cancer	15	15.4±0.8	10.2±1.3	34	44
Prostatic Cancer	70	16.7±1.2	11.3±0.8	32	53

However, the resistance to inhibition by dexamethasone was not specific to cancer patients. The data of the hospital control group – patients without malignant tumors who had been hospitalized in our Institute for clinical examinations – also differed from those of the first control group of subjects who had been studied under ambulatory conditions. The sensitivity to dexamethasone in the hospital control group might have been lowered as a result of emotional stress caused by hospitalization in the oncological clinic. In this respect it may be mentioned that ether stress (Ostroumova, 1978; Zimmerman & Critchlow, 1969) and psychic stress (Blumenfield et al., 1970) increase the resistance of the hypothalamo-pituitary complex to the inhibiting effect of dexamethasone, whereas drugs with a specific anti-alarm effect (benzodiazepines) have the ability to restore sensitivity to glucocorticoids (Nuller & Ostroumova, 1980).

Of course, the tumor itself, by its systemic influence on the organism, may produce an additional reduction of dexamethasone inhibition. According to Saez (1974) breast cancer patients demonstrate a negative correlation between the stage of the disease and sensitivity to the effect of dexamethasone. Our data also show that among patients with stage III–IV stomach cancer dexamethasone has less effect than among those in stages I–II (the blood level of 11-OHCS after dexamethasone was 10.7 ± 0.62 and 6.4 ± 1.40 µg% respectively; $p < 0.01$).

However, the majority of the patients we observed were in good condition, and we do not believe that the resistance to dexamethasone suppression shown in Table I was due to advanced disease. Besides, patients with mental depression showed dexamethasone test responses similar to those of cancer patients (Table I). That finding could serve as evidence for a functional mechanism defining the dexamethasone response (Carroll et al., 1976; Nuller & Ostroumova, 1980).

Of course, additional information is needed in order to analyze the mechanism of resistance to dexamethasone's action. As is known, the regulation of ACTH secretion involves various mechanisms for: (a) basal production of the hormone; (b) the circadian rhythm of its secretion; (c) stress-induced release of ACTH. The basal secretion of ACTH is less sensitive to inhibition by glucocorticoids than the "circadian output" of ACTH, which depends on regulation by extrahypothalamic brain structures (Ceresa et al., 1969). That is why the dosage for administration of dexamethasone at 11 p.m. should be 2–3 times less than that for inhibition of the basal level. We assume that the short-term "night" dexamethasone test involves the extrahypothalamic component of the regulatory system. This component responds to stress and mental depression. The so-called long-term dexamethasone test assesses the basal hypothalamic mechanism of negative feedback. With

Table II. Comparison of the Results of "Long-Term" and "Short-Term" Dexamethasone Test in Healthy Women and in Breast Cancer Patients of Various Ages.

Group	Average Age	No. of cases	"Short-Term" Dexamethasone Test 11-hydroxycorticosteroids (μg%)			"Long-Term" Dexamethasone Test 17-hydroxycorticosteroids (mg/24 hrs)		
			basal	after dexamethasone	% of inhibition	basal	after dexamethasone	% of inhibition
Healthy women:								
young	35.4 ± 0.6	19	13.9 ± 1.2	4.6 ± 1.1	67	4.7 ± 0.4	2.5 ± 0.2	47
middle-aged	50.6 ± 0.6	18	15.0 ± 1.4	5.2 ± 1.3	65	4.9 ± 0.8	3.3 ± 0.2	33
							$p < 0.05$	
Breast cancer patients:								
young	36.5 ± 0.7	13	–	–	–	5.8 ± 0.7	2.1 ± 0.3	63
middle-aged	54.9 ± 0.5	22	–	–	–	5.3 ± 0.4	3.4 ± 0.5	36
							$p < 0.05$	

aging the latter undergoes regular changes (see Dilman, 1981). For evaluation of this aging-associated process dexamethasone is administered at a dosage of 0.125 mg 4 times a day for 2 days, and the excretion of glucocorticoids is measured.

As seen in Table II, in healthy women of two different age groups the administration of 0.5 mg of dexamethasone at 11 p.m. (short-term dexamethasone test) causes the same inhibition of 11-OHCS blood level independently of age, whereas with the long-term test an age-dependent difference in the sensitivity to dexamethasone is observed. The latter test also reveals an increase in the resistance to dexamethasone in breast cancer patients of the older age group. Thus in the course of normal aging an elevation of the hypothalamic threshold of sensitivity to the inhibiting (homeostatic) effect of glucocorticoids appears to occur. The short-term dexamethasone test does not reveal this age-associated phenomenon. However, this test registers the elevation of the sensitivity threshold to inhibition by dexamethasone in many patients with stress, mental depression and cancer.

However, the goal of this paper is not to point out the difference between the tests, but to point out the fact that elevation of the hypothalamic threshold of sensitivity to the inhibiting effect of glucocorticoids

Table III. The Effect of Surgical Intervention on the Level of 11-Hydroxycorticosteroids in Stomach Cancer Patients.

Blood Sampling	Dexamethasone-sensitive patients* aged 51.9±3.8 (n=14)	Dexamethasone-resistant patients* aged 51.5±2.9 (n=8)
Before the operation	14.3±1.3	16.3±1.3
After premedication	14.8±1.9	18.2±2.8
The most traumatic moment of the operation	22.7±1.5	28.1±2.9
Final stage of the operation	28.1±2.6	33.7±1.5
After the operation 1 day	15.5±1.6	18.4±2.3
2 days	16.9±1.6	26.0±4.33
3 days	14.5±1.7	19.1±1.5

* The short-term dexamethasone test was used for the assessment of a patient's sensitivity to dexamethasone inhibition several days before the operation.

(revealed by both long-term and short-term dexamethasone suppression tests) leads to the development of hyperadaptosis, i.e. the excessive and thus undesirable reaction of the adaptive system. Table III shows that in dexamethasone-resistant patients the level of 11-OHCS remains elevated not only during the period of surgical intervention but also for some days following it. This suggests disturbances not only in the "extrahypothalamic component" of the adaptive homeostat but also in the basal feedback mechanism in dexamethasone-resistant patients. Such disturbances lead to excessive 11-OHCS production, i.e. to the development of the syndrome of hyperadaptosis.

A similar phenomenon was observed by Blichert-Toft (1975), who studied the influence of operative stress on 11-OHCS level in two age groups of patients – "young" ones and "older" ones. He found that the same operative stress produced a significantly greater rise in blood cortisol level in older patients than in the young ones. The author explained his results by the slower metabolic removal of cortisol with age. However, he did not take into account the rise in 17-ketogenic steroid excretion with age. This fact means that a real increase in 11-OHCS production occurred in older patients. This phenomenon is consistent with the elevation of the threshold of sensitivity to the inhibiting effect of dexamethasone, which indicates the state of hyperadaptosis.

We can say, then, that hyperadaptosis is created by the elevation of the threshold of sensitivity of the hypothalamo-pituitary complex to homeostatic inhibition in patients with various disturbances – be they chronic stress, mental depression, tumor process, or indeed, in normal aging. Taking into account its age-dependent character, hyperadaptosis is referred to as one of the so-called 10 normal aging-associated diseases, i.e. the diseases resulting from normal aging (Dilman, 1981).

Certainly, in the course of normal aging the absolute blood level of cortisol is not elevated as a rule. Meanwhile, 17-ketosteroid production is known to fall as age advances in both men and women, while the excretion of 17-hydroxysteroids remains unchanged. As a result, the ratio of 17-ketosteroids to 17-hydroxysteroids is lowered. The origin of the age-associated dissociation in hormone production is obscure. However, as both groups of hormones are secreted by the adrenal cortex, this dissociation might be a result of the difference in the sensitivity of various regions of the adrenal cortex to ACTH stimulation. At the same time this dissociation is sure to cause a relative excess of glucocorticoids, which produces a pathogenic effect on the organism. One of the most essential risk factors for breast cancer development is the discriminant function of Bulbrook, which is defined as the ratio of 17-hydroxycorticosteroid levels to those of 17-ketosteroids (Bulbrook & Hayward, 1967). Similar results were obtained when studying patients suffering from endometrial (de Waard et al., 1969) and lung (Rao, 1970) cancers. However, if under basal conditions hyperadaptosis peculiar to normal aging is revealed as a relative hypercorticism, then under the conditions of chronic stress true corticosteroid hyperproduction pertinent to hyperadaptosis is quite obvious.

An analysis of the incidence and severity of postoperative complications in patients with gastrointestinal cancer shows that the mode of hypothalamic regulation assessed by the dexamethasone test has a definite relation to the postoperative course (Ostroumova & Simonov, 1981). In radically operated patients (the degree of surgical intervention being approximately equal in all of them) the majority of severe complications and all the cases of death were observed in dexamethasone-resistant patients (Table IV). Thus hyperadaptosis, leading to the

Table IV. Rates of Postoperative Complications in Patients with Gastro-intestinal Cancer vs the Results of Dexamethasone Test*

Group	Without complications		With complications					
			medium		severe		died	
	A**	B**	A	B	A	B	A	B
Colon cancer								
Dexamethasone-sensitive patients (n = 21)	16	76%	1	5%	4	19%	0	0%
Dexamethasone-resistant patients (n = 31)	11	35% p<0.05	7	23%	5	16%	8	26% p<0.05
Stomach cancer								
Dexamethasone-sensitive patients (n = 16)	14	87%	2	13%	0	0%	0	0%
Dexamethasone-resistant patients (n = 18)	11	61%	2	11%	2	11%	3	16%

* Patients were considered dexamethasone-resistant if after the test the level of 11-hydroxycorticosteroids remained higher than 10μg% or was lowered by less than 40% of its initial value.

** A: number of patients; B: percentage of the total number of patients in the group.

excessive influence of glucocorticoids on the organism, could produce an unfavorable effect on the state of cancer patients.

· Certainly, the direct effect of cortisol is not the only pathogenic factor in hyperadaptosis. Secondary metabolic shifts associated with hyperadaptosis might be of importance, too. For instance, the study of endometrial cancer patients did not show a distinct rise in the basal blood 11-OHCS level (Table I). Meanwhile, the level of 11-OHCS after dexamethasone suppression was significantly higher in endometrial cancer patients than in healthy subjects.

Correspondingly, the results of the dexamethasone test covary with some metabolic parameters (such as body weight, concentration of blood lipids, glucose tolerance) which functionally relate to blood glucocorticoid level (Table V). The 11-OHCS level after dexamethasone load has a statistically significant positive correlation with the basal level of triglycerides and with the concentration of blood sugar 2 hours after glucose load, while the 11-OHCS inhibition rate by dexamethasone correlates negatively with the level of β-lipoproteins. In other words, the elevation of the hypothalamic threshold of sensitivity to the inhibiting effect of glucocorticoids, i.e. the central type of homeostatic failure peculiar to hyperadaptosis (Dilman, 1976, 1981), promotes carbohydrate and lipid metabolic disturbances.

Thus, in the course of normal aging elevation of the hypothalamic threshold of sensitivity to the inhibiting effect of cortisol produces the

Table V. Coefficients of Correlation between Blood 11-Hydroxycorticosteroid Level and Metabolic Parameters in Patients with Endometrial Cancer.

Metabolic parameters	11-Hydroxycorticosteroids		Inhibition (in %)
	basal	after dexamethasone	
Cholesterol	0.28	0.06	−0.03
Triglycerides	0.11	0.52*	−0.31
β-lipoproteins	−0.02	0.39	−0.49*
Glucose (two hours after glucose load)	−0.26	0.49*	−0.13
Excess of body weight (in % from ideal)	−0.05	0.33	0.05

* Correlation is statistically significant.

phenomenon of hyperadaptosis. The clinical features of this syndrome are the same as those pertinent to Itsenko-Cushing's disease, though less pronounced. With advancing age each individual starts to live as if in a state of chronic stress, and that is why he is in many respects helpless when real stress makes its demands on the organism. With aging, and as a result of the development of hyperadaptosis, the stress reaction becomes excessive and thus damaging. In a sense, time is a natural stressor.

Some Hypothalamic Mechanisms of Hyperadaptosis

The similarity of disturbances in regulation of glucocorticoid secretion caused by aging, chronic stress, and depression might indicate a common mechanism in their operation. Physiologically, this mechanism focuses on the elevation of the hypothalamic threshold of sensitivity to homeostatic stimuli. The biochemical basis of this hypothalamic phenomenon is the change in the level and metabolism of neurotransmitters, primarily of biogenic amines. Biogenic amines are among the factors determining the secretion of corticotropin-releasing factor (CRF) in the hypothalamus. Experiments, particularly *in vitro,* show that serotonin stimulates CRF synthesis and secretion rate, while noradrenaline inhibits these processes (Buckingham & Hodges, 1977). Mental depression is associated with a decrease in serotonin and noradrenaline concentrations in the brain (Coppen, 1967; Maas, 1975; Schildkraut, 1965). The stress reaction is released by increases in neuromediator turnover in the central nervous system. As a result, their reserve in the brain might be decreased (Bliss & Zwanzinger, 1966; De Pasquale, Costa, & Scapagnato, 1977). In addition, in the course of normal aging monoamine oxidase activity increases, and biogenic amine concentration correspondingly decreases in the hypothalamic area (Robinson, 1975; Robinson et al., 1972). Thus it is natural to suggest that the elevation of the hypothalamic threshold of sensitivity in inhibition by glucocorticoids occurring in aging, chronic stress and mental depression is caused by the fall in neurotransmitter concentration. In order to assess differentially the influence of the lack of serotonin and noradrenaline on feedback mechanism sensitivity, L-tryptophan and L-DOPA were used in healthy persons and in patients with mental depression, various psychoses, and Parkinson's disease (Nuller & Ostroumova, 1980).

It was found that the above drugs increased the inhibiting effect of dexamethasone (Table VI). The positive influence of L-DOPA on the results of the dexamethasone test might depend on the intensification of noradrenergic processes in the hypothalamus, corresponding to the inhibition of the secretion of CRF (Buckingham & Hodges, 1977) and ACTH (Van Loon et al., 1971) by noradrenaline. L-tryptophan also increased sensitivity to dexamethasone suppression, presumably by means of an increase in the serotonin synthesis rate in the brain.

Table VI. Effect of L-DOPA, L-tryptophan, diazepam and phenazepam on the results of dexamethasone test (Nuller & Ostroumova, 1980).

Preparation		11-Hydroxycortico-steroids (µg%)		Inhibition (in %)
		basal	after dexametha-sone	
L-DOPA, (n = 14)	before treatment	20.6 ± 1.8	11.5 ± 1.4	39 ± 7
	after treatment	19.3 ± 1.9	6.1 ± 0.9*	52 ± 10
L-tryptophan, (n = 20)	before treatment	20.1 ± 1.5	12.0 ± 1.5	40 ± 7
	after treatment	20.0 ± 1.9	8.2 ± 1.4*	59 ± 4*
Diazepam, (n = 6)	before treatment	23.4 ± 2.1	20.1 ± 2.3	12 ± 12
	after treatment	16.4 ± 1.8*	6.2 ± 1.1*	63 ± 4*
Phenazepam, (n = 27)	before treatment	20.8 ± 1.4	14.4 ± 1.1	24 ± 8
	after treatment	14.9 ± 1.3*	6.7 ± 0.9*	55 ± 5*

* Difference is statistically significant.

It should be noted that biogenic amines do not produce the same effect on the secretion of hypothalamic hormones and on the sensitivity of the hypothalamus to homeostatic stimuli.

Many data provide convincing evidence for both a stimulating and an inhibiting effect of serotonin on the system responsible for glucocorticoid secretion (Imura et al., 1973; Krieger & Rizzo, 1969; Vermes, Telegdy, & Lissák, 1972; Vernikos-Danellis, Berger, & Barchas, 1973). It is probable that in the brain there are several populations of serotoninergic neurons which differ in their final effect on hypothalamic CRF secretion. Serotonin seems to stimulate CRF secretion in the hypothalamus, while in other structures of the brain, particularly in the hippocampus, which also contains a number of receptors to glucocorticoids, serotoninergic processes increase the inhibiting effect of dexamethasone.

Thus, our data show that the dexamethasone test might also serve as one of the criteria for determining biogenic amine concentrations (or their efficiency) in the hypothalamus. In other words, the dexamethasone test might prove a "window" through which one could peep into an area inaccessible to direct inspection.

It turns out that the administration of tranquilizers might also contribute to the study of the mechanism of hyperadaptosis. Anti-alarm therapy by benzodiazepines – diazepam and phenazepam – in patients with an alarm-depressive syndrome had not only a beneficial effect, but also normalized sensitivity of the hypothalamo-pituitary complex to inhibition by dexamethasone (Table VI). This property of benzodiazepines might be associated with their ability to lower monoamine turnover in the brain and prevent monoamine depletion (Dominic, Sinha, & Barchas, 1975).

The increase in catecholamine and serotonin concentrations under the influence of anti-alarm drugs may also be explained in this way. Elimination of stress leads to elimination of the inhibiting influence of catecholamines on insulin secretion. This is supported by some data obtained in our laboratrory. According to studies by Kovaleva, phenazepam increases blood insulin-like activity (measured by the diaphragmatic method) from 566 ± 91 to $797 \pm 107 \mu U/ml$. The concentration of triglycerides, which is a marker for the biological effect of insulin, also rises from 159 ± 12.1 to $203 \pm 22 mg\%$ ($p < 0.01$). Meanwhile, insulin increases the uptake of amino acids, thus improving the supply of the brain with catecholamine and serotonin precursors (Fernstrom & Wurtman, 1971).

Summing up the data reported here, we may suggest that the age-associated decline in biogenic amine levels in the hypothalamus (which causes elevation of the hypothalamic threshold of sensitivity to the inhibiting effect of cortisol) leads to the development of the phenomenon of hyperadaptosis.

The process of aging is also accompanied by concealed mental depression expressed, first of all, by changes in one's mood. To some extent, aging-dependent low spirits are close to the phenomenon of hyperadaptosis, i.e., they represent a regular process caused by the age-associated decrease in biogenic amine levels in the brain. Hyperadaptosis and latent mental depression are two manifestations of the same phenomenon. Unlike the changes caused by chronic stress, however, they develop (more or less rapidly) in everyone according to the program of the organism's development – the manifestation of the law of deviation of homeostasis (Dilman, 1981). In their turn, stressor factors may promote the process of aging and the development of mental depression by causing an additional fall in biogenic amine concentrations. As a result, adaptative processes are impaired. In the following, the model for the influence of hyperadaptosis on the tumor process is discussed.

The Syndrome of Metabolic Immunodepression and Cancrophilia

There are at least three general conditions contributing to cancer development: an increase in the proliferative pool of somatic cells, a decrease in the activity of cellular immunity and macrophage function, and finally, damage to the DNA repair system. These conditions may occur independently of each other, and not infrequently only one of them is sufficient for an increase in cancer incidence. The most typical examples of the first condition are the development of endometrial cancer caused by an excess of estrogens, and of thyroid cancer caused by an excess of thyroid-stimulating hormone. The increase in tumor incidence resulting from persistent administration of immunodepressants (Penn, 1975, 1978) may serve as an illustration of the second condition. The third of these conditions is illustrated by the increase in the incidence of skin cancer in individuals with genetic deficiencies in DNA repair (Setlow, 1978).

A number of arguments allow us to suggest that the increase in the influence of each of these cancer-promoting factors may be caused by the same metabolic disorder, i. e., to suggest the concept of cancrophilia (Dilman, 1977, 1978, 1981). The main feature of this hormone-metabolic disturbance is the shift towards the predominant utilization of free fatty acids (FFA) instead of glucose as an energy substrate.

Here we shall consider this concept briefly in light of the mechanism of the development of metabolic immunodepression (Dilman, 1978, 1981).

It was found that an improvement of immune function in middle-aged subjects could be achieved by normalization of carbohydrate and lipid metabolism. The administration of the anti-diabetic biguanide, phenformin, and the hypolipidemic drug, clofibrate, in patients with atherosclerosis essentially normalized the level of lipidemia. It also increased the blast transformation of lymphocytes and the phagocytic and lysosomal activity of macrophages (Dilman et al., 1977; Nemirovski et al., 1978). The improvement of metabolic parameters in patients with diabetes mellitus was also accompanied by an increase in cellular immune activity (Nemirovski, Ostroumova, & Dilman, 1980).

Other evidence for the existence of the phenomenon of metabolic immunodepression is our finding of a negative correlation between the state of cellular immunity on the one hand and carbohydrate and lipid metabolism on the other (Poroshina et al., 1980). Concentrations of blood cholesterol, triglycerides, β-lipoproteins and FFA were chosen for the evaluation of metabolic parameters. The absolute number of T-lymphocytes, phytohemagglutinin (PHA)-induced blast transformation, and phagocytic and lysosomal macrophage activity were the immune parameters investigated. Negative correlations were found between the total indices of metabolic and immune patterns (Table VII). We take this as another indication of an immune impairment caused by some kind of metabolic shift, and call this phenomenon metabolic immunodepression (Dilman, 1977, 1978). In primary breast cancer patients the correlation is absent (see Table VII), due, we believe, to an inhibitory effect on the immune system produced by the tumor itself.

It is of interest to mention here some data obtained in experiments on obese hyperlipidemic insulin-resistant mice (ab & db) with lowered glucose tolerance. These animals demonstrated a decrease in skin graft rejection and in lymphocyte killer function (Chandra & Au, 1980; Fernandes et al., 1978a; Mandel & Mahmud, 1978; Meade, Sheena, & Mertin, 1979). Similar decreases in immune activity were not found in studies of lymphocytes in cell culture. Hence, the authors just cited concluded that the impairment of immunity had been caused by the metabolic environment of immunocompetent cells *in vivo*.

It should be noted, however, that it is rather difficult to interpret data from studies involving the whole organism, because any disturbance in lipid and carbohydrate metabolism is accompanied by a change in hormonal background which, in its turn, may result in the development of immunodepression. Thus for convenience we shall discuss the *in vitro* literature on the immunodepressive properties of the metabolic factors mentioned above.

Various classes of lipoproteins are known to inhibit mitogen-induced blast transformation of lymphocytes *in vitro* (Chisari, 1977; Curtiss & Edgington, 1976; Morse, Witte, & Goodman, 1977). The inhibition of lymphocyte proliferation by human serum sampled from patients with hypertriglyceridemia has been shown to depend on the increased blood concentration of very low density lipoproteins (Waddell, Taunton, & Twomey, 1976). Lipoproteins obtained from the serum of mice receiving a high calorie diet are known to inhibit lymphocyte blast transformation (Kollmogen et al., 1979). The lymphocyte blast transformation rate can be restored when lipoproteins are eliminated from the cell culture (Waddell et al., 1976; Hui, Berebitsky, & Harmony, 1979).

A number of functions of immunocompetent cells, such as sensitivity to activation stimuli (Rivnay, Globerson, & Shinitzky, 1978), proliferation activity (Chen, 1979), cytotoxity (Heininger, Brunner, & Cerottini, 1978), chemotaxis, and phagocytosis (Pike & Snyderman, 1980) depend

Table VII. Comparison of Immune and Metabolic Parameters Assessed as Scores in Healthy Women and Breast Cancer Patients.

Group	No. of cases	Age	Total index of immunity	Total index of metabolism	Coefficient of correlation	p
Controls:						
young women	20	22 ± 0.9	23.7 ± 1.0	18.8 ± 1.1	−0.57	<0.01
middle-aged women	19	55 ± 2.4	19.3 ± 1.0	25.0 ± 1.1	−0.56	<0.02
Primary breast cancer patients	37	53 ± 1.5	16.8 ± 0.7*	26.9 ± 0.8	−0.23	>0.05
Breast cancer patients in clinical remission	30	58 ± 1.3	14.8 ± 1.2*	26.8 ± 1.1	−0.42	<0.02

* Difference from the corresponding age control is statistically significant.

on intracellular cholesterol metabolism. The saturation of lymphocyte membranes with cholesterol by means of cholesterol-lecithin liposomes impairs the blastogenic reaction of lymphocytes (Alderson & Green, 1975; Rivnay et al., 1978). Despite the rather effective self-regulatory system of cholesterol metabolism, the concentration of cholesterol in lymphocytes is known to rise as age advances and in patients with ischemic heart disease (Kovaleva & Dilman, 1981). A probable cause for this process might be changes of hormone-metabolic background in such patients. In particular, the stimulation of very low density lipoprotein transport into cells under the influence of insulin is accompanied not by a fall, but by an increase in the activation of endogenous cholesterol synthesis in cultured human lymphocytes (Nakayama et al., 1979). Thus, hormones are responsible for regulatory changes that could lead to enrichment of lymphocyte membranes with lipid components.

Increased blood levels of saturated and unsaturated fatty acids also inhibit lymphocyte blast transformation (Meade & Mertin, 1978). Unsaturated fatty acids, being the precursors of prostaglandins, influence the immune system by increasing the prostaglandin synthesis rate (Meade & Mertin, 1978). It should be noted that immunodepression which arises through the system "unsaturated fatty acids-prostaglandins" differs from metabolic immunodepression, which is assumed to be connected with the ensuring of energy and dynamic needs in the course of the organism's development (Dilman, 1981). Finally, increased blood insulin level, which diminishes the number of insulin receptors on the plasma membranes of lymphocytes and monocytes (Archer, Gorden, & Roth, 1975), may also contribute to metabolic immunodepression.

We also attach importance to the fact that metabolic immunodepression involves changes in T-immunity and macrophage activity, but seems to increase the activity of the system of humoral immunity. Elimination of metabolic immunodepression is believed to decrease the enhanced activity of the humoral immune system. This might have some relation to the decrease in the incidence of the aggressive autoimmune disorders which is found in mice fed calorie-restricted diets (Fernandes et al., 1978b). The findings discussed above suggest that such common disorders as hyperlipoproteinemia, hypercholesterolemia, hyperinsulinemia, and elevated blood concentrations of FFA can lead to metabolic immunodepression. However, it should be noted that none of these factors alone is capable of inducing the syndrome of metabolic immunodepression. The syndrome seems rather to be caused by the total effect of these hormonal and metabolic factors. We have already mentioned that hyperlipoproteinemia is often accompanied by a rise in blood cortisol level, and hence the role in the inhibition of cellular immunity of metabolic factors on the one hand, and of the rise in cortisol level on the other, is still obscure. However, it seems unlikely to be mere chance that metabolic disturbances contributing to the genesis of metabolic immunodepression are intensified by hypercorticism (see Table V). Generally, hyperadaptosis causing either a relative or an absolute excess in cortisol production leads to a decrease in glucose utilization and, correspondingly, to an increase in the utilization of FFA as the energy substrate. This in turn not only activates the operation of the system of gluconeogenesis, but also induces metabolic immunodepression. Moreover, there is evidence that the lymphocytolysis caused by glucocorticoids involves a toxic effect of FFA on lymphocytes (Turnell, Clarke, & Burton, 1973).

Cancer patients frequently manifest metabolic disturbances pertinent to metabolic immunodepression. In our laboratory we studied blood lipid levels of primary oncological patients. A rise in triglyceride concentration and a fall in high density lipoprotein level turned out to be the most pronounced metabolic disorders in patients with endometrial, breast, lung, and colon cancer (Table VIII) (Dilman, Berstein et al., 1981). Barclay and Skipski (1975) observed a fall in a certain fraction of high density lipoproteins not only in cancer patients but also in families with high risk of cancer.

It should be emphasized that the hormone-metabolic pattern peculiar to metabolic immunodepression is likely to provide favorable conditions for cell proliferation, i.e., for another parameter of the cancrophilia syndrome. The data on this subject seem sufficiently convincing, though they are indirect (Dilman, 1981).

Activation of cell division requires insulin (and other serum growth factors). It also requires enhanced cholesterol synthesis in the cell (Kandutsch & Chen, 1978) or its enhanced uptake by the cell from blood, since cholesterol is required for daughter cells as a component of plasma membranes. Low density lipoproteins are chiefly responsible for cholesterol transport. Naturally, certain amounts of FFA are also necessary for cell proliferation. Thus, hyperlipidemic serum stimulates cell proliferation (Chen et al., 1977). It is interesting in this connection to take into consideration the data obtained in our laboratory from patients with phenotypical hyperlipoproteinemia of the IIb type, which is characterized by increased levels of both cholesterol and triglycerides (markers of hyperinsulinemia). Blood somatomedin activity in such patients was 2–2.5 times higher than normal (Vasiljeva et al., 1980).

We also found an association between elevated cholesterol concentrations in serum and lymphocytes on the one hand, and decreased activity of the DNA repair system on the other (Dilman & Revskoy, 1981). Should this interrelation be confirmed, and should the rate of

Table VIII. The Level of Lipidemia in Oncological Patients (Dilman et al., 1981).

Group	No. of cases	Age	Total Cholesterol (mg%)	Triglycerides (mg%)	Total β-lipoproteins (U/ext.)	Cholesterol HDL (mg%)
Controls:						
women	45	51±1	246±8	109±4	459±20	59±2
men	35	48±1	241±5	139±9	538±24	53±3
Breast cancer	48	53±1	251±7	156±10*	586±15	51±1*
Lung cancer:						
(men)	113	58±0.7	214±4*	163±6*	552±12	45±2*
Colon cancer:						
women	24	56±2	243±6	149±11*	580±21*	56±3
men	18	55±2	253±8	152±12	566±29	48±3
Stomach cancer:						
women	20	52±2	255±15	152±15*	581±29*	51±3*
men	22	52±2	227±9	138±8	542±28	49±3*

* Difference from the corresponding age control is statistically significant (p<0.05).

DNA repair be improved by normalization of metabolic disturbances, then we will have convincing evidence for the idea that all three factors of cancrophilia are induced by the same hormone-metabolic shift. Hence, according to this conceptualization, cancrophilia is a syndrome in which certain hormone-metabolic shifts (the lowering of glucose tolerance, hyperinsulinemia, enhanced FFA utilization, and hypercholesterolemia) induce an increase in the pool of proliferating cells, metabolic immunodepression, and a decrease in the activity of the DNA repair system, thus increasing the risk of cancer development.

Some epidemiologic studies indirectly support the role of cancrophilia as a background for cancer development. These studies show that a high calorie diet is associated with an increase in the incidence of breast and colon cancer (Gori, 1979; Wynder, 1980). Correspondingly pharmacologic interventions (such as the anti-diabetic drug, phenformin, and the hypolipidemic drug, clofibrate) aimed at normalization of lipid and carbohydrate metabolism, have been shown to decrease the rate of tumor induction by carcinogens (Dilman et al., 1974). Phenformin was also shown to increase the lifespan of experimental animals (rats and mice) by 20–25%, while the incidence of malignant tumors in these animals was lowered (Dilman & Anisimov, 1980). These data support the concept of the syndrome of cancrophilia and its role in cancer induction.

It should be noted that cancrophilia involves certain conditions promoting the development of cancer, but not the mechanism of malignant transformation of the cell.

Stress, Mental Depression and Cancer

To a great extent the premorbid characteristics of an individual determine his response to strong psychic overloads. Longitudinal observations on the emotional status of women suffering from cancer show that the risk of tumor development is increased under the influence of strong emotional stress, and especially in persons with less stable nervous systems (Hagnell, 1966). Nevertheless, the suppression of strong emotions also contributes to cancer promotion (Editorial, 1979). Certain features of temperament are known to influence the formation of various neurotic states caused by severe psychosocial traumas. It is remarkable that a great number of oncological patients seem to have suffered from severe chronic stress or prolonged alarm states and mental depression approximately 5–10 years before the detection of a tumor.

For example, 250 breast cancer patients were questioned as to whether they had taken tranquilizers in the period 10 years before the diagnosis of a tumor. Those who did receive the drugs displayed a greater amount of metastasis to lymphatic nodes and had more relapses 12 months following their radical surgery than did those who had not suffered formerly from stress and mental depression (Stoll, 1976). This study indicated an increased risk of cancer in subjects prone to alarm and depressive states.[1]

It is also believed by a great number of oncologists that cancer prognosis and treatment response are much better in optimistic, well-balanced patients, than in those who are passive, depressed, or have unstable psychic reactions. These interrelations can be considered in light of the concepts of hyperadaptosis and cancrophilia.

As for the stress reaction, its occurrence requires an increased energy supply, which is attained in the following way. The complex of lipolytic and contra-insulin hormones prevailing in blood during stress (epinephrine, growth hormone, ACTH, prolactin, and cortisol) diminishes glucose utilization, and hence FFA becomes the predominant energy substrate. The effect of lipolytic hormones in combination with the rise in FFA blood concentration causes an impairment of glucose tolerance. Tumor cells readily use FFA as an energy substrate (Lankin, 1973). The increase in the rate of cholesterol synthesis is another pathogenic factor contributing to cell proliferation subsequent to enhanced FFA utilization. FFA transport into the liver provides for the synthesis of triglycerides and very low density lipoproteins, which are transformed in the blood to low density lipoproteins. The latter transfer cholesterol into cells. In addition, the synthesis of cholesterol within cells from acetyl-coenzyme-A (which is a product of FFA metabolism) may contribute to the total increase in cholesterol synthesis rate. Thus, enhanced lipolysis leads to an increase in cholesterol concentration in the cell, providing the ground for intensified division of both normal and malignant cells.

Patients with mental depression often demonstrate lowered sensitivity to the action of insulin and decreased glucose tolerance accompanied by reactive hyperinsulinemia (Mueller & Heininger, 1969). Insufficient glucose utilization leading to the predominant use of FFA as an

---

[1] Some experiments have not found a protective effect of tranquilizers or an accelerating influence of stress on the tumor process. It was shown that stress delays the development of DMBA-induced breast cancer (Newberry & Sengbusch 1979; Bhattacharyya & Pradhan, 1979). In addition the administration of diazepam promoted tumor growth (Horrobin et al., 1979). Such unexpected results might be caused by the inhibiting influence of stress on the secretion of insulin and gonadotropins, and correspondingly, estrogens. Insulin particularly activates cell division in mammary glands. Hence, a decrease in its level might diminish the output of DMBA-induced tumors (Shafie, Cho-chung, & Gullino, 1979), whereas an increase in its concentration under the influence of diazepam might lead to tumor progression.

energy substrate, in combination with hyperinsulinemia, as a rule causes a rise in blood cholesterol and triglyceride concentrations. It is believed that in patients suffering from mental depression immunity is impaired, which might occur in many cases through the mechanism of metabolic immunodepression as we discussed it above.

At the same time, in light of the data concerning the role played by the hypothalamus in the immune response (Besedovsky & Sorkin, 1977; Korneva, Klimenko, & Shkhinek, 1978), it would be interesting to put forward another hypothesis. According to this the elevation of the hypothalamic threshold of sensitivity caused by aging, chronic stress, or mental depression may influence the activity of the anti-tumor immune reaction. It has recently been shown that the process of immunization is accompanied by an increase in the activity of neurons in the hypothalamic ventromedial nuclei (Korneva et al., 1978). Meanwhile, for some time during immunoactivity the blood concentration of adrenal corticoids is raised, and the levels of thyroid hormones are lowered (Besedovsky, Del Rey, & Sorkin, 1979; Besedovsky & Sorkin, 1977). Thus a hormonal background is formed which diminishes the immune response to the consequent administration of another antigen. This phenomenon is thought to be involved in the mechanism of antigenic competition (Besedovsky et al., 1979; Besedovsky & Sorkin, 1977). Concentrations of cholesterol and triglycerides have also been shown to rise during immunization (Di Perri, 1975; Mathews & Feery, 1978). Hence, the direct influence of the hypothalamus on the system of immunity may be associated with changes in the hormone-metabolic pattern. In this regard, it is natural to ask whether the hypothalamic threshold of sensitivity to tumor-associated antigens is changed by normal aging, stress, and mental depression. Changes of this kind might introduce an important modulating element into the formation of the organism's antitumor response.

Conclusions

The generation of a stress reaction requires the disturbance of homeostasis. However, because of the mechanisms of self regulation which are characteristic of the neuroendocrine system, a stable deviation from homeostasis can be achieved only by an elevation of the threshold of sensitivity of the central regulatory structures – primarily the hypothalamo-pituitary complex – to homeostatic stimuli. In other words the activation of this complex causes its set-point of sensitivity to homeostatic stimuli to change. As a result, a constant deviation of homeostasis occurs. Any such persistent deviation of homeostasis can be considered pathologic.

The two peculiarities of "stress disease" should be pointed out. Firstly, the elevation of the hypothalamic threshold is caused by decreases in biogenic amine concentrations in the hypothalamus, which might lead to the development of mental depression under conditions of chronic stress. In its turn, the excess cortisol secretion caused by these factors acts to lower hypothalamic biogenic amine levels (Curzon, 1969; Lapin & Oxenkrug, 1969). Thus a vicious circle is formed which maintains the individual in the states of chronic stress and mental depression. Secondly, the homeostatic disturbance required for the manifestation of the stress response leads to metabolic immunodepression and, finally, to cancrophilia.

The causes of this interrelation lie deep in the physiological processes controlling the development and growth of an organism. They are discussed in detail elsewhere (Dilman, 1981). Generally speaking, just as anti-stressor reactions cannot be achieved without homeostatic disturbances, so also the organism's growth and development (in both the embryonic and post-embryonic periods) are impossible without constant departure from homeostasis. In essence, stability rules out development. In the embryonic period the departure from homeostasis is produced by virtue of hormone synthesis by the fetal-placental system, the production of these hormones (for instance, chorionic somatomammotropin) increasing with a rise in the weight of the placenta. As a result of these normal influences, the departure from homeostasis required by pregnancy occurs in the maternal organism. An essential component of this disturbance is an increase in FFA utilization which, in combination with the excess of insulin and lowered glucose tolerance, induces hyperlipidemia in the maternal organism. The latter is responsible for the excess of cholesterol which is used by the fetal-placental system for cell proliferation and steroid hormone synthesis. At the same time, there arises metabolic immunodepression which prevents the fetus from being rejected as an antigenically foreign entity.

In the postnatal period the departure from homeostasis required for the organism's growth and development is carried out by another pathway whose key element is a hypothalamic mechanism, namely the change of the set-point of the hypothalamic threshold of sensitivity to regulatory homeostatic stimuli (Dilman, 1979, 1981). During the organism's development the elevation of the hypothalamic sensitivity threshold provides a higher level of regulation by increasing the capacity of the main homeostatic systems (i.e., the reproductive, adaptation, and energy systems). However, when development is completed these hypothalamic disturbances keep progressing, thus creating a ground for age-associated pathology. The program of organismic development is immediately transformed into the mechanism of natural (or normal) diseases. Hyperadaptosis can itself be considered one of those diseases. The key factor in its development is the age-associated elevation of the hypothalamic threshold of sensitivity to the inhibitory effect of cortisol (as revealed by the dexamethasone suppression test).

There is a certain difficulty in distinguishing hyperadaptosis from the complex of other age-associated diseases, since hyperadaptosis is an indispensable mechanism of the other diseases. Hyperadaptosis might be observed in patients with obesity, diabetes mellitus, arterial hypertension, atherosclerosis, cancer, and especially mental depression. However, hyperadaptosis is not a mere component of the main age-associated diseases. It is an independent disease of regulation in the adaptive homeostat. In the course of normal aging it exists as a disease *sui generis*, but for reasons mentioned above, chronic stress may contribute to its formation by the exhaustion of adrenergic and serotoninergic brain mechanisms. This linkage of hyperadaptosis to internal phenomena involved in growth and development on the one hand, and to external environmental factors on the other, precludes making a completely clear distinction between hyperadaptosis as a component of other adaptational diseases, and hyperadaptosis as a disease *sui generis* (Dilman, 1981).

Thus, chronic stress, mental depression, and the conditions conducive to cancer induction and progression may be characterized by a number of common signs. These signs are: a decrease in biogenic amine concentrations in the hypothalamus, a deficiency in homeostatic regulation, and a metabolic shift to enhanced utilization of FFA as fuel. As a result, cellular immunity and macrophage function are lowered. Meanwhile, a metabolic pattern peculiar to these states is likely to promote the division of malignant as well as normal cells. It might also inhibit the activity of the DNA repair system. The confluence of these three conditions – immunodepression, stimulation of cell division, and deficiency in DNA repair – forms the syndrome of cancrophilia. From this point of view it is clear why stress and mental depression should be associated with an enhancement of tumor induction and progression.

The concepts we have outlined may have implications for oncological practice. There may be uses for depressants and other drugs which increase biogenic amine concentrations in the hypothalamus (e. g. tryptophan, or mazindol – an anorexic that increases the reuptake of noradrenaline) or normalize hypothalamic control mechanisms. In addition anti-diabetic biguanides and hypolipidemic preparations which could normalize the metabolic pattern associated with aging may improve the immune response and eliminate some cancrophilic factors. In sum, there is now a good rationale for pharmacological intervention to correct alarm and depressive-like states (and, first of all, hyperadaptosis), and to normalize metabolic disturbances in cancer patients.

References

Alderson, J. C. E. & Green, C. Enrichment of lymphocytes with cholesterol and its effect on lymphocyte activation. *FEBS Lett.,* 1975, *52,* 208–211.

Archer, J. A., Gorden, P., & Roth, J. Defect in insulin binding to receptors in obese man: Amelioration with calorie restriction. *J. Clin. Invest.,* 1975, *55,* 166–174.

Barclay, M. & Skipski, V. P. Lipoprotein in relation to cancer. In K. K. Carrol (Ed.), *Progress in biochemical pharmacology. Lipids and tumours.* Basel: S. Karger, 1975.

Besedovsky, H. O., Del Rey, A., & Sorkin, E. Antigenic competiton between horse and sheep red blood cells as a hormone-dependent phenomenon. *Clin. Exp. Immunol.,* 1979, *37,* 106–113.

Besedovsky, H. O. & Sorkin, E. Network of immune-neuroendocrine interactions. *Clin. Exp. Immunol.,* 1977, *27,* 1–12

Bhattacharyya, A. K. & Pradhan, S. E. Effect of stress on DMBA-induced tumor growth, plasma corticosterone and brain biogenic amine in rats. *Res. Commun. Chem. Pathol. Pharmacol.,* 1979, *23,* 107–116.

Blichert-Toft, M. Secretion of corticotrophin and somatotrophin and by the senescent adenohypophysis in man. *Acta Endocrinol. Kbh.,* 1975, *78,* Suppl. 195, 1–157.

Bliss, E. L. & Zwanziger, J. Brain amines and emotional stress. *J. Psychiat. Res.,* 1966, *4,* 189–198.

Blumenfield, M., Rose, I., Richmond, H., & Beering, S. C. Dexamethasone suppression in basic trainees under stress. *Arch. Gen. Psychiat.,* 1970, *23,* 299–304.

Buckingham, J. C. & Hodges, J. R. Production of corticotrophin releasing hormone by the isolated hypothalamus of the rat. *J. Physiol.* (Lond.), 1977, *272,* 469–479.

Bulbrook, R. D. & Hayward, J. L. Abnormal urinary steroid excretion and subsequent breast cancer. *Lancet,* 1967, *1,* 519–522.

Carroll, B. J., Curtis, G. C., & Mendels, J. Neuroendocrine regulation in depression. *Arch. Gen. Psychiat.,* 1976, *33,* 1039–1044.

Ceresa, F., Angeli, A., Boccuzzi, G., & Molino, G. Once-a-day neurally stimulated and basal ACTH secretion phases in man and their response to corticoid inhibition. *J. Clin. Endocrinol. Metab.,* 1969, *29,* 1074–1082.

Chandra, R. K. & Au, B. Spleen hemolytic plaque-forming cell response and generation of cytotoxic cells in genetically obese (C 57 Bl/6J *ob/ob*) mice. *Internat. Arch. Allergy Appl. Immunol.,* 1980, *62,* 94–98.

Chen, R. M., Getz, G. S., Fisher-Dzoga, K., & Wissler, R. W. The role of hyperlipidemic serum in the proliferation and necrosis of aortic medial cells *in vitro. Exp. Mol. Pathol.,* 1977, *26,* 359–374.

Chen, S.-H. Enhanced sterol synthesis in concanavalin A-stimulated lymphocytes: Correlation with phospholipid synthesis and DNA synthesis. *J. Cell. Physiol.,* 1979, *100,* 147–157.

Chisari, F. V. Immunoregulatory properties of human plasma in very low density lipoproteins. *J. Immunol.,* 1977, *119,* 2129–2136.

Coppen, A. The biochemistry of affective disorders. *Brit. J. Psychiat.,* 1967, *113,* 1237–1264.

Curtiss, L. K. & Edgington, T. S. Regulatory serum lipoproteins: Regulation of lymphocyte stimulation by a species of low density lipoprotein. *J. Immunol.,* 1976, *116,* 1452–1458.

Curzon, G. Tryptophan pyrrolase: A biochemical factor in depressive illness. *Brit. J. Psychiat.*, 1969, *115*, 1367–1379.

Dilman, V. M. The hypothalamic control of aging and age associated pathology: The elevation mechanism of aging. In: A. V. Everitt and J. A. Burgess (Eds.), *Hypothalamus, pituitary and aging*. Springfield: Thomas, 1976.

Dilman, V. M. Metabolic immunodepression which increases the risk of cancer. *Lancet*, 1977, *2*, 1207–1209.

Dilman, V. M. Ageing, metabolic immunodepression and carcinogenesis. *Mech. Ageing Dev.*, 1978, *8*, 153–173.

Dilman, V. M. Hypothalamic mechanisms of ageing and of specific age pathology. V. A model for the mechanism of human specific age pathology and natural death. *Exp. Gerontol.*, 1979, *14*, 287–300.

Dilman, V. M. *The Law of Deviation of Homeostasis and diseases of aging*. PSG Publishing Co., 1981.

Dilman, V. M. & Anisimov, V. N. Effect of treatment with phenformin, diphenylhydantoin or L-DOPA on life span and tumour incidence in C3H/Sn mice. *Gerontology*, 1980, *26*, 241–246.

Dilman, V. M., Berstein, L. M., Ostroumova, M. N., Tsyrlina, Y. V., & Golubev, A. G. On the peculiarities of hyperlipidemia in tumour patients. *Brit. J. Cancer*, 1981, *43*, 637–643.

Dilman, V. M., Berstein, L. M., Zabezhinski, M. A., & Alexandrov, V. A. Effect of phenformin on DMBA-induced breast cancer in the rat. *Probl. Oncol.*, 1974, *9*, 94–98 (in Russian).

Dilman, V. M., Ostroumova, M. N., Blagosklonnaya, Y. V., Nemirovski, V. S., Uskova, A. L., Lvovitch, E. G., Berstein, L. M., Tsyrlina, E. V., & Bobrov, Y. F. Metabolic immunodepression. Normalizing influence of phenformin. *Human Physiology*, 1977, *3*, 579–586 (in Russian).

Dilman, V. M. & Revskoy, S. Y. The rise of cholesterol level in blood and in lymphocytes as a factor of age-associated impairment of DNA repair. *Human Physiol.*, 1981, *1*, 125–129 (in Russian).

Dominic, J. A., Sinha, A. K., & Barchas, J. D. Effect of benzodiazepine compounds on brain amine metabolism *Eur. J. Pharmacol.*, 1975, *32*, 124–127.

Editorial: Mind and Cancer. *Lancet*, 1979, *1*, 706–707.

Fernandes, G., Handwerger, B. S., Yunis, E. J., & Brown, D. M. Immune response in the mutant diabetic C57BL/Ks-db+ mouse. *J. Clin. Invest.*, 1978a, *61*, 243–250.

Fernandes, G., Yunis, E. J., Miranda, M., Smith, J., & Good, R. A. Nutritional inhibition of genetically determined renal disease and autoimmunity with prolongation of life in *kdkd* mice. *Proc. Nat. Acad. Sci. USA*, 1978b, *75*. 2888–2892.

Fernstrom J. D. & Wurtman, R. J. Brain serotonin content: Increase following ingestion of a carbohydrate diet. *Science*, 1971, *174*, 1023–1025.

Gori, G. B. Dietary and nutritional implications in the multifactorial etiology of certain prevalent human cancers. *Cancer*, 1979, *43*, Suppl., 2151–2161.

Hagnell, O. The premorbid personality of persons who develop cancer in a total population investigated in 1947 and 1957. *Ann. N. Y. Acad. Sci.*, 1966, *125*, 846–855.

Heininger, H. J., Brunner, K. T., & Cerottini, J.-C. Cholesterol is a critical cellular component for T-lymphocyte cytotoxicity. *Proc. Nat. Acad. Sci. USA*, 1978, *75*, 5683–5687.

Horrobin, D. F., Ghayur, T., & Karmali, R. A. Mind and cancer. *Lancet*, 1979, *1*, 978.

Hui, D. Y., Berebitsky, G. L., & Harmony, J. A. K. Mitogen-stimulated calcium ion accumulation by lymphocytes: Influence of plasma lipoproteins. *J. Biol. Chem.* 1979, *254*, 4666–4673.

Imura, H., Nakai, Y., & Yoshimi, T. Effect of 5-Hydroxytryptophan (5-HTP) on growth hormone and ACTH release in man. *J. Clin. Endocrinol. Metab.*, 1973, *36*, 204–206.

Kandutsch, A. A., Chen, H. W., & Heiniger, H.-J. Biological activity of some oxygenated sterols. *Science*, 1978, *201*, 498–501.

Kollmogen, G. M., Sansing, W. A., Lehman, A. A., Fischer, G., Longley, R. E., Alexander, S. S., Jr., King, M. M., & McCay, P. B. Inhibition of lymphocyte function in rats fed high-fat diets. *Cancer Res.*, 1979, *39*, 3458–3462.

Korneva, E. A., Klimenko, V. M., & Shkhinek, E. K. *Neurohumoral supply of immune homeostat.* Leningrad: "Nauka" Publ., 1978. (in Russian)

Kovaleva, I. G. & Dilman, V. M. Age-associated increase of cholesterol level in lymphocytes of peripheral blood: Relation to specific age pathology. *Human Physiol.*, 1981, *1*, 120–124. (in Russian)

Krieger, D. T. & Rizzo, F. Serotonin mediation of circadian periodicity of plasma 17-hydroxycorticosteroids. *Am. J. Physiol.*, 1969, *217*, 1703–1707.

Lankin, V. Z. High fatty acids and tumor energy turnover. *Actual Probl. Modern Oncol.*, 1973, *3*, 112–120. (in Russian)

Lapin, I. P. & Oxenkrug, G. F. Intensification of the central serotoninergic processes as a possible determinant of the thymoleptic effect. *Lancet*, 1969, *1*, 132–136.

Maas, J. W. Biogenic amines and depression. *Arch. Gen. Psychiat.*, 1975, *32*, 1357–1361.

Mandel, M-A. & Mahmoud, A. A. F. Impairment of cell-mediated immunity in mutation diabetic mice (db/db). *J. Immunol.*, 1978, *120*, 1375–1377.

Mathews, J. D. & Feery, B. J. Cholesterol and immune response to influenza antigens. *Lancet*, 1978, *2*, 1212–1213.

Meade, C. J. & Mertin, J. Fatty acids and immunity. *Adv. Lipid Res.*, 1978, *16*, 127–165.

Meade, C. J., Sheena, J., & Mertin, J. Effects of the obese (ob/ob) genotype in spleen cell immune function. *Int. Arch. Allergy Appl. Immunol.*, 1979, *58*, 121–127.

Morse, J. H., Witte, L. D., & Goodman, D. S. Inhibition of lymphocyte proliferation stimulated by lectins and allogeneic cells by normal plasma lipoproteins. *J. Exp. Med.*, 1977, *146*, 1791–1803.

Mueller, P. S. & Heininger, G. R. Insulin tolerance test in depression. *Arch. Gen. Psychiatry*, 1969, *21*, 587–594.

Nakayama, H., Kiematu, M., Kurihara, Y., Manda, N., Sasaki, T., & Nakagawa, S. The effect of insulin on cultured human lymphocytes: Examination of the activity of 3-hydroxy-3-methylglutaryl coA reductase (HMGR) and low density lipoprotein (LDL) receptor activity. *J. Lipid Res.*, 1979, *20*, 1047–1048. (Abstract)

Nemirovski, V. S., Ostroumova, M. N., Blagosklonnaya, Y. V., Uskova, A. L., Freindlin, I.-S., Lvovitch, E. G., Tsyrlina, E. V., & Dilman, V. M. The improvement of functional morphological parameters of mononuclear cells caused by miscleron. *Probl. Oncol.*, 1978, *4*, 65–68. (in Russian)

Nemirovski, V. S., Ostroumova, M. N., & Dilman, V. M. The interrelation of blood lymphocyte and monocyte function and the level of some lipids and 11-hydroxycorticosteroids in diabetic patients. *Probl. Endocrinol.*, 1980, *2*, 8–12. (in Russian)

Newberry, B. H. & Sengbush, L. Inhibitory effect of stress on experimental mammary tumors. *Cancer Detect. Prev.*, 1979, *2*, 225–233.

Nuller, J. L. & Ostroumova, M. N. Resistance to the inhibiting effect of dexamethasone in patients with endogenous depression. *Acta Psychiat. Scand.,* 1980, *61,* 169–177.

Ostroumova, M. N. Age-associated decrease in hypothalamo-pituitary complex sensitivity to the inhibiting effect of dexamethasone: The influence of stress, polypeptide pineal extract and phenformin. *Probl. Endocrinol.,* 1978, *6,* 59–64. (in Russian)

Ostroumova, M. N. & Simonov, N. N. The resistance to the inhibiting effect of dexamethasone and risk of postoperative complications in patients with colon cancer. *Probl. Oncol.,* 1981, *4,* 48–52. (in Russian)

De Pasquale, A., Costa, G., & Scapagnato, C. Noradrenaline e serotonina cerebrali dopo stressa antigeno nel ratto: Influenza della resina di "Cannabis". *Riv. Farmacol. Ter.* 1977, *1,* 71–78.

Penn, I. Incidence of malignancies in transplant recipients. *Transplant. Proc.,* 1975, *7,* 323–326.

Penn, I. Malignancies associated with immunosuppressive or cytotoxic therapy. *Surgery,* 1978, *85,* 492–501.

Di Perri, T. Iperlipoproteinemie ed immunità. *Minerva Med.* 1975, *66,* 3397–3405.

Pike, M. C. & Snyderman, R. Lipid requirements for leukocyte chemotaxis and phagocytosis: Effects of inhibitors of phospholipid and cholesterol synthesis. *J. Immunol.,* 1980, *124,* 1963–1969.

Poroshina, T. E., Fedorov, S. N., Ostroumova, M. N., & Dilman, V. M. The comparison of metabolic and immune parameters in breast cancer patients. *Probl. Oncol.* 1980, *8,* 24–27. (in Russian)

Rao, L. G. S. Discriminant function based on steroid abnormalities in patients with lung cancer. *Lancet,* 1970, *2,* 441–445.

Rivnay, B., Globerson, A. & Shinitzky, M. Perturbation of lymphocyte response to concanavalin A by exogenous cholesterol and lecithin. *Eur. J. Immunol.,* 1978, *8,* 185–189.

Robinson, D. S. Changes in monoamine oxidase and monoamines with human development and aging. *Fed. Proc.,* 1975, *34,* 103–107.

Robinson, D. S., Nies, A., Davis, J. N. Bunney, W. E., Davis, J. M., Colburn, R. W., Bourne, H. R., Shaw, D. M., & Coppen, A. J. Ageing, monoamines and monoamine-oxidase levels. *Lancet,* 1972, *1,* 290–291.

Saez, S. Corticotropin secretion on relation to breast cancer. In B. A. Stoll (Ed.), *Mammary cancer and neuroendocrine therapy.* Butterworth & Co., 1974.

Schildkraut, J. J. The catecholamine hypothesis of affective disorders: A review of supporting evidence. *Am. J. Psychiatry,* 1965, *122,* 509–522.

Setlow, R. B. Repair deficient human disorders and cancer. *Nature,* 1978, *271,* 713–717.

Shafie, S. M., Cho-Chung, Y. S., & Gullino, P. M. Cyclic adenosine 3′5′-monophosphate and protein kinase activity in insulin-dependent and -independent mammary tumors. *Cancer Res.,* 1979, *39,* 2501–2504.

Stoll, B. A. Psychosomatic factors and tumour growth. In B. A. Stoll (Ed.), *Risk factors in breast cancer.* Chicago: William Heinemann Med. Books, 1976.

Turnell, R. W., Clarke, L. H., & Burton, A. F. Studies on the mechanisms of corticosteroid-induced lymphocytolysis. *Cancer Res.,* 1973, *33,* 203–212.

Van Loon, G. R., Scapagnini, U., Moberg, G. P., & Ganong, W. F. Evidence for central adrenergic neutral inhibition of ACTH secretion in the rat. *Endocrinology,* 1971, *89,* 1464–1469.

Vasiljeva, I. A., Berstein, L. M., Ostroumova, M. M., & Dilman, V. M. Effect of phenformin and clofibrate on the blood somatomedin activity level in breast cancer patients. *Probl. Oncol.* 1980, *9,* 34–36. (in Russian)

Vermes, I., Telegdy, G., & Lissák, K. Inhibitory action of serotonin on hypothalamus-induced ACTH release. *Acta Physiol. Acad. Sci. Hung.,* 1972, *41,* 95–98.

Vernikos-Danellis, J., Berger, P., & Barchas, J. D. Brain serotonin and pituitary-adrenal function. *Progr. Brain Res.,* 1973, *39,* 308–309.

de Waard, F., Thyssen, J. H. H., Veeman, W., & Sander, P. C. Steroid hormone excretion pattern in women with endometrial carcinoma. *Cancer,* 1969, *22,* 988–993.

Waddell, C. C., Taunton, O. D., & Twomey, J. J. Inhibition of lymphoproliferation by hyperlipoproteinemic plasma. *J. Clin. Invest.,* 1976, *58,* 950–954.

Wynder, E. L. Dietary factors related to breast cancer. *Cancer,* 1980, *46,* 899–904.

Zimmerman, E. & Critchlow V. Negative feedback and pituitary-adrenal function in female rats. *Am. J. Physiol.,* 1969, *216,* 148–155.

Variables in Behavioral Oncology: Overview and Assessment of Current Issues

Benjamin H. Newberry, Annabel G. Liebelt and David A. Boyle [1]

Introduction

We refer to the area defined by interest in the relationships between psychosocial variables and neoplastic diseases as behavioral oncology – the behavioral medicine (Miller, 1981) of cancer. Thus construed, behavioral oncology is the interdisciplinary field concerned with the integration of biomedical and behavioral knowledge relevant to cancer.

The field can be subdivided, imperfectly, by taking cancers and their sequelae as either dependent or independent variables. First, when cancer is the independent variable, the field deals with its direct and indirect psychosocial consequences, direct consequences being due to the disease itself rather than to its diagnosis or therapy. The second subdivision deals with cancers as dependent variables which may be affected by psychosocial factors. There are two partially independent means by which such effects on cancer can occur. In *external loop* ((EL) situations, behavior exposes the organism to exogenous agents (ExA) with the capacity to alter neoplastic outcomes. The second type of psychosocial effect on cancer is the *internal loop* (IL) effect. In IL cases, psychosocial factors affect endogenous aspects of host resistance.

Behavioral oncology deals with extremely complex interacting systems. Neoplasms express series of complex and varied processes often over long periods of time. These processes occur in even more complex

[1] Data presented in this paper were collected during research supported in part by the American Cancer Society, Ohio Division; National Institutes of Health Biomedical Research Grant program; and the Research Council of Kent State University. The authors thank Anita Lash, Diane Dinardo, and Patricia John for their invaluable assistance in preparing the manuscript. We thank the Upjohn Co. for DMBA emulsion.

hosts. Hosts, particularly humans, interact with complex environments. A priori, it is unlikely that simple generalizations in this field will apply broadly enough to contribute prominently to cancer control, particularly where IL effects are concerned.

This chapter will present a general framework and will assess specific issues which we see as relevant to some current preoccupations of the field. The discussion will be limited in several ways. The focus will be on possible IL effects, though EL effects and cancer as independent variables will not be wholly ignored. We cannot review or integrate the many behavioral and biomedical literatures that contribute to behavioral oncology. A review would require far too much space. Integration is presently impossible; the quantitative, interdisciplinary knowledge required is not available. Space will not permit detailing the results and implications of even the fraction of the literature we will be able to cite. Instead of review and integration we will use the devices of discussing general classes of variables and of illustrating by example the range of specific factors requiring attention. Given present knowledge such discussion is necessarily speculative at points. To a considerable extent, therefore, we deal with possibilities – with seemingly relevant effects whose magnitudes and generality are unclear.

An Extended Stimulus-Organism-Response (S-O-R) Framework for Behavioral Oncology Variables

Adapting an interactional S-O-R framework to behavioral oncology by including disease processes allows some organization of relevant variables and illustrates some general sequences of events by which psychosocial factors may be related to cancer. Figure 1 depicts such a framework. It presents ten very general classes of variables organized under the even more general headings of environment, organism, and response. It depicts 25 potentially relevant relationships between pairs of variable classes and implies very large numbers of extended sequences. (The numbers at the heads of arrows will be used in the text to identify relationships.)

"Others" (Oth) refers to individuals or groups whose neoplastic disease is not under consideration but who may affect the person whose disease is at issue. Exogenous agents (ExA) are environmental factors which may affect the organism or its pathology and whose effects in this regard are non-psychological, i.e., are exerted by relatively direct action on tissues. Psychosocial stimulation (PsyS) represents environ-

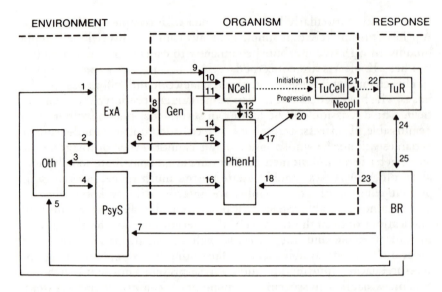

Fig. 1: Schematic of relationships among general variable classes potentially relevant to behavioral oncology. Abbreviations are as follows: Oth = other persons or groups; ExA = exogenous agents; PsyS = psychosocial stimulation; Gen = genome; NCell = normal target cell; PhenH = Phenotypic host; TuCell = tumor cell; TuR = tumor response; Neopl = neoplastic processes; BR = overt behavioral response. Numbers at the heads of arrows are used in the text to refer to particular relationships.

mental factors whose effects are primarily psychological, i.e., mediated via sense receptors. Obviously, some stimuli may serve as both ExA and PsyS (e.g., tobacco smoke). The genome (Gen) is separated from the rest of the organism primarily to emphasize that the origin of differences relevant to cancer need not be in the environment. Gen is taken, somewhat arbitrarily, to be fixed. Thus somatic mutations or alterations in gene expression will not be considered genomic. The phenotypic host (PhenH) is the cancer host or potential host as it is developing under the influences of Gen and environment. For our purposes, all aspects of organism structure and function are considered under PhenH except overt behavior, Gen, and those elements most directly involved in the disease process. Neoplastic processes (Neopl) are represented in a compromise fashion in Figure 1. Normal target cells (NCell) are cells whose neoplastic transformation is at issue. They are normal at least in the sense that with present methods those that do transform appear similar in morphology and function to those that do not. Some distinctions among Neopl are indicated by differentiating among

NCell, TuCell (tumor cell or transformed cell), and TuR (the response or "behavior" of the neoplasm), and by including some relationships among them (19, 21, 22). At the same time, however, influences on Neopl are represented generally (9, 20, 24) because we cannot describe here even what is known about tumor development[2] and because the locus of effects often cannot be described with precision. We will use the term *tumor system* to refer to the complex of host-plus-neoplasm since tumors are often restricted to particular hosts and cannot be studied separately. Behavioral response (BR) in Figure 1 refers to overt behavior; covert behavior is taken for convenience as part of PhenH.

Figure 1 illustrates some of the things which make behavioral oncology complex. Since each variable class contains large numbers of specific variables which interact with each other and with variables in other classes, and since each variable class serves in both independent and dependent variable capacities, it is likely that a large number of relationships are relevant to behavioral oncology. These relationships are dynamic in terms of both the number of (possibly opposing) effects any specific variable may have and the number of temporal sequences which may occur. Such a depiction of relationships illustrates the number and types of factors which must be controlled to demonstrate that an association between a psychosocial factor and a neoplastic outcome is causal. As will be apparent below, the shortage of adequately controlled studies is a major problem in IL behavioral oncology.

Figure 1 is in no meaningful sense a theory. Like other "models" which appear in behavioral literatures, it points to variables which need attention without being precise about their relationships. Thus it both oversimplifies and makes rather arbitrary distinctions.

In the following sections we will briefly describe some of the relationships involving each variable class and its specific variables. Under each variable class we will consider relationships in which it acts as dependent variable. This is arbitrary, of course; each class also serves as independent variable. Some of the relationships are obvious, of questionable importance, or relatively tangential to our main concern of IL effects; these will be treated very briefly. Those more central to our main topic will be dealt with more extensively, but even there we will present examples rather than a survey of the relevant research.

---

[2] We will use the term tumor development to refer to any of a variety of outcome variables which reflect neoplastic processes. The term should not be taken to imply reference to any particular stage of the neoplastic process.

Environment

Others (Oth)

Of particular relevance when Oth is taken as dependent variable are reactions to the host's disease and its sequelae (e.g., Cohen, Cullen, & Martin, 1982). The impacts on Oth are important as outcomes in themselves and as sources of comfort or distress to the host. The behavior of the host is one obvious source of effects on Oth (5: BR→Oth). Another source of influence is host appearance (3) either deriving from the disease (e.g., weight loss, visible neoplasms, visible effects of surgery) or independent of Neopl (e.g., host age, sex, beauty).

Exogenous Agents (ExA)

With cancer, the most obvious ExA are chemical carcinogens, procarcinogens, promoters, radiation, oncogenic viruses, and chemotherapeutic agents. However, a wide variety of other things are probably directly or indirectly relevant as well (e.g., nutritional factors, drugs, cosmetics, nononcogenic infectious agents, and physical objects such as those produce trauma).

In Figure 1, ExA is affected by Oth (2), by BR (1), and by other aspects of PhenH (6). Oth alter exposure to ExA just as they alter other aspects of the environment. BR often brings about ExA exposure; drug intake, smoking, working in hazardous areas, and contacting persons who transmit infections are examples. PhenH characteristics may affect at least the effective level of exposure. Skin pigmentation, gastrointestinal characteristics, and respiratory tract characteristics are examples.

Something which might be considered a PhenH → ExA sequence is host effect on ExA after they have been incorporated. The most obvious example of this would be the metabolism of carcinogens and procarcinogens ("Mechanisms," below).

Psychosocial Stimulation (PsyS)

In Figure 1, PsyS is considered to be influenced by BR (7) and Oth (4). Behavior brings the individual into contact with parts of the environment and alters that environment. Other individuals provide stimulation both in themselves and by their manipulations of the physical environment.

In behavioral oncology, there has been an emphasis on "stressful" stimulation. However, "stressor" and "stress" have only connotative meaning. Components of the "stress" response often fail to covary or respond to "stressors" as would be expected (e. g., Brady, 1975; Mason, 1971, 1975; Sandman et al., 1973). Studies of "stress" and cancer have often failed to assess putative "stress" mediation adequately, and there is no reason to assume that nonspecific responses to demands (Selye, 1976) are more important than specific ones in neoplastic disease. To reflect these problems we will speak of presumably stressful stimulation (PSS) rather than "stressor" (Newberry, 1981a) and apologize to the reader for yet another abbreviation.

Organism

Genome (Gen)

The only influence on Gen in Figure 1 is that of ExA (8). Given our consideration of the genome as fixed, this effect refers to gametes or very early embryos.

Phenotypic Host (PhenH)

In IL behavioral oncology the core relationships are those among PsyS and/or host psychological characteristics, the host physiologic milieu in which Neopl take place, and the Neopl themselves. Thus in general, sequences of the form (20) or (16–20) are central.

We can do no more than hint at the number of PhenH factors which are relevant to oncogenesis and host-tumor interaction. The nervous, endocrine, and immune systems are those most often considered (e. g., Lloyd, this volume). Unfortunately, each of these systems is being revealed as much more complex than was known a few years ago, and their interactions are being revealed as so intimate and numerous that it is difficult even to consider them separately. Many discussions (e. g., Ader, 1981a; Anisman & Sklar, in press; Krieger & Hughes, 1980; Lloyd, this volume; Meltzer & Fang, 1976; Snyder, 1980) and specific findings illustrate the vast range of influences which occur among these systems.

Nor should consideration stop with the nervous, endocrine and immune systems. We have already noted the relevance of carcinogen-activating and -deactivating enzymes and body surface characteristics. General metabolic factors and the cardiovascular system are probably relevant at various points in the networks of events leading to neoplastic outcomes.

NCell → PhenH (13). For completeness, we have included in Figure 1 the effect of NCell on the host. Since the effect of one or a few normal cells is usually small, we will say no more about it.

Gen → PhenH (14). Genetically determined host characteristics are relevant to behavioral oncology beyond differences in the transforming genes themselves. We have mentioned general appearance (e.g., 3). More directly involved are the large numbers of physiologic parameters under genetic influence. Among these are differences in pituitary-mammary and -gonadal axes (e.g., Bardin, Liebelt, & Liebelt, 1966; Huggins, Oka, & Fareed, 1972), catecholamine biosynthesis (Weinshilboum, 1983), responses to PSS (e.g., McCarty, Chiueh, & Kopin, 1978), basal levels and inducibility of relevant enzymes (e.g., Bürki, Liebelt, & Bresnick, 1975), and DNA repair capacity (e.g., Bamborschke et al., 1983). In some cases highly specific genetic determinants of host resistance to tumor are known, as in Marek's disease (Briles et al., 1983).

ExA → PhenH (15). In addition to their direct effects (9, 10), ExA may act relevantly through their effects upon the host and the subsequent effects of host factors on tumor development (12, 20) or other classes of variables (e.g., 15–23–1–9). The exact means by which ExA act is often not known.

Oncogenic agents have effects other than their direct ones. They may affect endocrine organs (e.g., Huggins & Morii, 1961; Liebelt, Liebelt, & Lane, 1964), the immune system (see Hewitt, 1978) and perhaps the nervous system (Balitsky & Vinnitsky, 1981). Nononcogenic infectious agents probably act in several ways, through alterations in endocrine activity, blood flow, body temperature, and host cell division.

Drugs have importance beyond their direct effects on Neopl. Antibiotics affect infectious agents and gut flora. Exogenous hormones will have effects similar to those of their endogenous counterparts. Psychoactive agents are potentially relevant in several ways, since they may alter peripheral physiology, cognitive processes, and behavior. Many psychoactive drugs affect the CNS transmission systems which control hypothalamic and pituitary hormone outputs (e.g., Wurtman & Fernstrom, 1976). Among drugs of seeming relevance are phenothiazines (e.g., Byck, 1975), benzodiazepines (e.g., Lahti & Barsuhn, 1974), caffeine (e.g., Henry & Stephens, 1980), and the broad groups of sympathomimetics, catecholamine antagonists, anesthetics, and analgesics (see Gilman, Goodman, & Gilman, 1980).

PsyS → PhenH (16). External stimuli affect almost all aspects of the organism's physiology via the CNS, endocrine, immune, and cardiovascular systems. The immune system will be considered below ("PSS, Immunodepression, and Tumor Enhancement"). Here we give a few examples of relationships involving other host systems, concentrating on the effects of PSS.

Regarding the endocrine system, PSS seems able to increase pituitary-adrenocortical and sympathomedullary activity, prolactin, thyroid-stimulating hormone, growth hormone, glucagon (e.g., Curtis, 1979), antidiuretic hormone (Corson & Corson, 1976), melanocyte-stimulating hormone (Sandman et al., 1973), progesterone (Plas-Roser & Aron, 1981), and β-endorphin (Guillemin et al., 1978). Insulin (Curtis, 1979) and testosterone (e.g., Mason, 1975) may be reduced in response to PSS, the latter effect probably reflecting gonadotropin decreases.

There are subtleties to the effects of PSS. Interaction among neural and endocrine responses to PSS is illustrated by the involvement of opioids, not only as elements of the response but as modulators of other elements, both neural (Watkins & Mayer, 1982) and humoral (e.g., Van Vugt, Bruni, & Meites, 1978). Opioid systems' responses are in turn influenced by hormonal factors (e.g., MacLennan et al., 1982). Hormonal effects on psychological processes are well known (e.g., De Wied et al., 1976). Interactions between the cardiovascular system and others are illustrated by the finding that the baroreceptor response may reduce the emotional/motivational response to PSS (Dworkin et al., 1979). The conditionability of hormonal responses such as corticosteroid increases (Ader, 1976) and decreases (Coover, Sutton, & Heybach, 1977), of stress-induced analgesia (Watkins & Mayer, 1982) and of immune responses (Ader, 1981b) is further testimony to the complexity and plasticity of responses to PSS.

Several aspects of response to PSS are not understood well enough to be used in predicting total effects upon the organism. Temporal factors are one example relevant to cancer. Truly long-term effects have not received enough study even in animals, yet present knowledge suggests that there is much to be learned. Adaptation seems to vary with the particular type of PSS (e.g., Anisman, 1978; Henry, Ely et al., 1975) and to be capable of taking nonmonotonic forms (e.g., Brady, 1975; Henry, Ely et al., 1975). In a particular PSS episode, not enough is known about the time course of physiologic responses. Particularly when rebounds occur (e.g., Davidson, Smith, & Levine, 1978), the initial response misleads as to the total effect. If some other event, such as a critical period in tumor development, occupies a brief period, then its precise time of occurrence in relation to the time course of the PSS response can determine the magnitude or direction of any effect.

Another important aspect of PSS is the organism's ability to control or cope with it. We will discuss coping in relation to immune function and tumor development below ("PSS, Immunodepression, and Tumor

Enhancement," and "Stimulus-Based Hypotheses"). We need to note here that the availability of coping responses is thought critical to many aspects of PSS response. In some instances, coping opportunity has essentially eliminated some aspect of response to PSS (e. g., Jackson, Maier, & Coon, 1979; MacLennan & Maier, 1983).

While coping can dampen response to PSS, the boundary conditions for such effects are not yet clear. The expected effects do not always occur (e. g., Murison, Isaksen, & Ursin, 1981; Rosellini & Seligman, 1978), and effects attributed to controllability may be due at least in part to other factors (e. g., Burger & Arkin, 1980; Lubow, Rosenblatt, & Weiner, 1981). Operationalization of coping/controllability can present problems. In infrahuman studies, intermediate degrees of controllability have not often been deliberately studied, and it may be difficult to characterize degree of controllability. In forced swimming, for example, an animal cannot prevent the onset or bring about the offset of its confinement to the water but can effectively prevent its drowning. An animal in a shock escape situation cannot prevent shock onset or escape the test chamber. The degree of control in these cases is unclear.

Neopl → PhenH (17). The effects of neoplastic disease on the host must be considered a major issue in behavioral oncology. These effects are important whether the concern is with quality of life as an endpoint or with desease course itself and psychosocial influences upon it.

Cancers have great effects upon their hosts. Some of these are obvious, such as alterations in appearance, obstruction of lumina, and anorexia. Less obvious changes include those in electrolytes (Cameron & Hunter, 1983), endocrine function, lipid regulation, protein synthesis, glucose metabolism and availability, blood volume (Dilman & Ostroumova, this volume; Liebelt & Liebelt, 1967b; Shapot, 1979), and the hemostatic system (Donati et al., 1977). Compounds produced by tumors which participate in these effects include ectopic hormones (e. g., Lippman, 1982), growth factors capable of inducing growth in normal cells (Sherwin et al., 1983), growth inhibiting factors (De Wys, 1972), and factors which increase vascular permeability (Senger et al., 1983).

Neopl affect the immune system in several ways. Leukocytosis and alterations in leukocyte ratios can accompany non-lymphoreticular neoplasms (e. g., Delmonte, Liebelt, & Liebelt, 1966). Antigenic tumors and oncogenic viruses can stimulate the immune system. The hormonal and nutritional changes brought about by tumor development will also have effects. Immunodepression frequently accompanies neoplastic disease in humans (e. g., Jassem & Serkies, 1980; Nimberg et al., 1975) and infrahumans (see Stutman, 1975).

CNS and psychological function are likely to be affected by Neopl in several ways – by the hormonal changes to which we have alluded, by interoceptive stimulation resulting from peripheral changes (and, in humans at least, by the interpretations the person makes of these), and by small metastases to the brain as noted by Fox (1978). Balitsky and Vinnitsky (1981) suggested that Neopl interfere with the hypothalamic activation required for optimal immune function. If correct, this idea suggests that relationships between the immune and nervous systems (e.g., Besedovsky & Sorkin, 1981; Stein et al., 1981) may be of significance in cancer.

BR → PhenH (18). The effects of overt behavior on the organism may be relevant in at least two ways. Exercise has well known effects, as in cardiopulmonary conditioning and its concomitants. It affects body temperature and immune function (Cannon & Kluger, 1983) and can reduce the adrenocortical response to PSS (Starzec et al., 1979). Psychologically, a person's interpretation of his/her behavior is relevant. Attitudes, motivation, self-perception, and psychophysiologic responses are influenced by behavior so as to make them consistent with behavior (e.g., Zimbardo, 1969). Thus to the extent that physiologic responses are influenced by interpretations of events, BR forms a class of events whose interpretation may affect Neopl.

Neoplastic Processes (Neopl)

The development of malignancy begins by definition with non-transformed cells. Transformation or initiation is a function of the characteristics of NCell, the actions of ExA on the cell, and the milieu provided by the host. A transforming characteristic is produced or expressed under these influences.

Transformation often if not always involves a modification of nucleic acid function due to mutation, alterations in gene expression or addition of viral material (e.g., Bishop, 1982; Oppenheimer, 1982). Cellular oncogenes are apparently conserved and may function in normal processes (Goyette et al., 1983). Allelic differences occur at oncogene loci, with some alleles capable of producing transformation and other not (Muschel et al., 1983).

Chemical and radiation carcinogenesis may operate through alterations in either the genetic material or oncogene expression (e.g., Farber, 1981; Oppenheimer, 1982). Hormonal stimulation can produce transformation in susceptible cells (e.g., Furth, 1975) and enhance the effects of initiating agents (e.g., Liebelt & Liebelt, 1967a), at least at high levels. Inert substances can induce transformation (e.g., Brand, 1976) or direct transformation by systemically distributed carcinogens (Konstantinidis, Smulow, & Sonnenschein, 1982). It is worth noting that there is now a fair and growing amount of evidence for virus involvement in some human cancers (e.g., Popovic et al., 1983).

Oncogenic agents can interact. This is best known in the initiation-promotion sequence (e.g., Diamond, O'Brien, & Baird, 1980) but occurs among initiating agents as well. For example, methylcholanthrene inhibits carcinogenesis by 2-acetylaminofluorine but not by its metabolite N-hydroxy-2-acetylaminofluorine (Miller, Miller, & Hartman, 1961) and increases mammary cancer incidence in mice carrying mammary tumor virus, probably by activating or hastening viral transformation (e.g., Moore, 1975).

Space does not permit describing the subsequent events in tumor development which result in frank and/or disseminated disease. We can only give examples which suggest possibilities for psychosocial influences on the outcome. The behaviorally-oriented reader can consult many sources for entrances into the relevant literature (e.g., Becker, 1975; Farber, 1981; Fidler & Hart, 1982; Sklar & Anisman, 1981a).

ExA → Neopl (9). In addition to the well-known oncogens and antitumor therapeutic agents, ExA which are less often considered relevant can apparently affect Neopl – either directly (9) or via their effects on PhenH (15–20) – and thus participate in EL effects. We have already alluded to some of the indirect effects of ExA, as in discussing their influences on the host. It should be noted that it is not always known whether an effect is direct or indirect; *in vivo* studies may not distinguish between the two, and with some ExA both types of effects may occur. We will consider exogenous hormones in the next section since they may reflect possibilities for IL influences. Here we mention some other types of ExA.

Among drugs capable of affecting Neopl at least under some circumstances are phenothiazines (e.g., Pearson et al., 1969), benzodiazepines (Horrobin & Trosko, 1981 – though this idea is controversial, Jackson & Harris, 1981), thiopental (Lundy et al., 1978), isobutyl nitrate, a component of some incense (Hersh et al., 1983), ethanol (see Committee on Diet, Nutrition and Cancer, 1982), and caffeine (Nomura, 1983).

Ordinary nutritional factors represent another group of ExA which may modulate Neopl, though human data are not conclusive (Enstrom, 1982). Tumor development at certain sites may be increased by high fat, protein, and/or caloric intake (see Committee on Diet, Nutrition, and Cancer, 1982). In a recent animal study, type of fat was found to be important (Chan, Ferguson, & Dao, 1983). Vitamin C, vitamin E, selenium (Committee on Diet, Nutrition, and Cancer, 1982), and vitamin A compounds (Committee on Diet Nutrition, and Cancer, 1982; Seifter, 1976) appear capable of protective effects.

Nononcogenic infectious agents may have several types of influence.

Viral infection can alter TuCell antigens (Zbar et al., 1983). Lactate de-hydrogenase-elevating (LDH) virus has been shown to affect murine tumors, perhaps via interferon (Riley, 1966) or corticosterone (Riley et al., 1981). More general effects of infection might also influence Neopl. Increased body temperature may be anti-oncogenic (Bull, 1982). Farber (1981) has noted that cell division may reduce the likelihood that car-cinogenic alterations in DNA will be successfully repaired.

  PhenH → Neopl (20). The basic idea of IL effects on cancer implies variations in host resistance, and thus host effects on Neopl either di-rectly or through modifications of ExA activity. We will consider im-munologic influences below ("PSS, Immunodepression, and Tumor En-hancement") and will briefly mention some other possibilities here.

  Regarding CNS function, Sklar and Anisman (e.g., 1981a; Anisman & Sklar, in press) have argued that brain neurotransmitter levels and activities are related to host resistance, with norepinephrine and dopa-mine depletion particularly associated with tumor enhancement. They have reviewed considerable amounts of data seemingly consistent with this hypothesis. Balitsky and Vinnitsky (1981) have suggested that hy-pothalamic activation inhibits tumor development via immunoenhance-ment. Turkevich (1958) discussed the Pavlovian nervous system typolo-gy, associating "strong unequilibrated" and "weak" nervous systems with tumor enhancement.

  We know of few studies which directly examine CNS factors in tu-mor hosts. Cotzias and Tang (1977) found that levels of brain adenyl-ate cyclase induced in mice by dopamine strongly predicted strain inci-dence of mammary tumors. Bhattacharyya and Pradhan (1979) found slight but significant decreases in diencephalon-midbrain norepineph-rine associated with inhibition of rat mammary tumors by PSS.

  The relationship of hormones to Neopl is an area of great interest. We have noted that hormones can sometimes act as initiating agents, but post-initiation effects are probably more relevant to IL phenomena. Hormonal influences are best known in neoplasms derived from highly hormonally-responsive tissue (e.g., Iacobelli et al., 1980). However, en-docrine effects are complex and extend beyond the most obvious tu-mor/hormone combinations. We can present only a few examples of endocrine effects here. The reader is referred to Furth (1975), Iacobelli et al. (1980), Lippman (1982) and an issue of *Cancer Research* (1978, *38,* 11, Part 2) for more information.

  DMBA rat mammary tumors are responsive to prolactin and gonadal hormones (e.g., Dao, 1972), but the direction of effect depends on hor-mone levels (Heise & Gorlich, 1966; Huggins, Briziarelli, & Sutton, 1959). There are great differences among individual tumors in response to gonadal steroids (Garcia & Rochefort, 1978). Prolactin enhances rat mammary tumor development after induction but protects against induction (see Smithline, Sherman, & Kolodny, 1975), indicating the importance of periods of tumor development. Antidiuretic hormone stimulates growth of WRK-1 rat mammary tumor cells *in vitro* (Monaco et al., 1980). Rat mammary tumors are apparently also responsive to insulin (Heuson & Legros, 1972).

Mouse mammary tumors *in vivo* are often independent of the pituitary-gonadal axis once they appear. However, tumors of strain RIII are responsive to pregnancy and lactation hormones (Foulds, 1969; Liebelt et al., 1968). *In vitro* growth of S115 mouse mammary tumor cells is enhanced by androgens, but culture without androgens renders them less responsive (Yates, Couchman, & King, 1980). Like those of rats, mouse mammary tumors may be insulin-responsive (Puckett & Shingleton, 1972).

The pituitary-gonadal axis influences leukemias. Mouse leukemias are inhibited by gonadal hormones. The effect is greater in males than females (Kirschbaum & Liebelt, 1955; Kirschbaum, Liebelt, & Falls, 1955; Liebelt & Liebelt, 1962). Corticosteroids are associated with inhibition of lymphoid neoplasms, though there are wide differences in sensitivity (see Claman, 1972).

Adrenal corticoids affect non-lymphoid neoplasms as well. Rat mammary tumors can be enhanced by adrenalectomy (Daniel & Prichard, 1967) and inhibited by exogenous glucocorticoid (see "Tumor System Specificity" below). Corticoids bind to progesterone receptors in rat mammary tumors (Goral & Wittliff, 1976), enhance replication of mouse mammary tumor virus (Parks, Scolnick, & Kozikowski, 1974), and slow tumor growth by inhibiting angiogenesis and tumor collagenase (Gross et al., 1981). Deoxycorticosterone can protect against the tumor-enhancing effects of PSS in some tumor systems (see Seifter, 1976). Work on hormonal requirements for serum-free tumor cell cultures (Sato, 1980) may shed interesting light on cancers' endocrine sensitivities.

Endogenous factors other than hypophyseal and steroid hormones can affect Neopl. Gluthathione reacts with some carcinogens and can thereby alter their activity. Reduced glutathione produces regression of rat liver tumors (Novi, 1981). Epinephrine, 5-hydroxytryptamine, and histamine reduce growth of P815 mastocytoma cells *in vitro*, the effects being markedly increased by theophylline (Keller & Keist, 1973). Prostaglandins affect a variety of tumors, sometimes enhancing and sometimes inhibiting growth (Bennett, 1980). The hemostatic system may be relevant to metastasis. There are apparently several types of possible effects, including aggregation of blood-borne neoplastic cells, platelet effects on vascular permeability, and activity of fibrin to inhibit release of cells from tumors but facilitate arrest and growth of metastatic cells (Donati et al., 1977).

BR → Neopl (24). It is possible that behavior can act rather directly on tumors. Contact with physical objects or forces exerted by muscular contraction might dislodge cells and so contribute to metastasis (Bammer, 1981). Tumors on or near the body surface might be affected by palpation or scratching.

TuR → TuCell (21). This sequence represents the effects of tumor cells or tumors upon themselves or each other. Equilibria in heterogeneous TuCell populations (Fidler & Hart, 1982) are an example. Sugarbaker, Thornthwaite, and Ketcham (1977) have reviewed data showing that tumors often inhibit each others' growth. They favored tumor-produced mitosis inhibitors as mediators of the effect. Tumors may also secrete factors which promote their own growth (Sherwin et al., 1983).

Response

Overt behavioral responses (BR) and the behavior of tumors (TR) in terms of growth, invasion, metastasis, and substance production are major classes of outcome variable in behavioral oncology. BR as an endpoint relates to quality of life issues and TR to disease outcome.

Behavioral Response (BR)

Overt behavior in Figure 1 is affected by PhenH (23) and by Neopl (25). The effect of PhenH is the O-R sequence of the behavioral S-O-R model and needs no explication at this point. The effect of Neopl on BR is included for completeness – to depict the possibility of direct alterations of motor response by tumor masses.

Tumor Response (TuR)

To differentiate TuR from the neoplasm itself is somewhat artificial but is helpful in depicting the self-feedback and mutual influences in Neopl (21) and in representing a group of dependent variables. TuR is represented in Figure 1 as affected by TuCell (22) and as included within the complex of Neopl to be affected by other variable classes (9, 20, 24). The dependence of Tur on these variables has been discussed above.

Although we tend to speak of tumor development in general terms, the particular dependent variable chosen for study can influence the interpretation of findings. Spontaneous regression of rat mammary tumors was found to be increased by neonatal thymectomy, but other measures of tumor development were unaffected (Gunn, Carr, & Currie, cited in Scott, Christian, & Currie, 1967). Dechambre (1981) found that PsyS which increased ascites volume in mice also lengthened survival time, presumably because toxic lysate was released when tumor cells were destroyed. Sugarbaker, Cohen, and Ketcham (1970) found that cortisol failed to affect growth of Walker 256 or its pulmonary metastases, but did increase visceral metastases.

Conclusions

The enumeration of relevant variable classes and their relationships illustrates the variety of influences acting on cancers. These influences interact and the number of specific variables is great. Thus there are very large numbers of ways in which psychosocial factors *might* influence cancers. It remains to be seen whether they actually do so and do so to a practically significant degree. Most of the possibilities have received little attention, either empirically or in published discussions.

An Assessment of Internal Loop Psychosocial Effects on Cancer

Having looked at the general classes of variables which seem to require consideration, we will attempt to evaluate some aspects of the field. We will concentrate on IL effects and on the particular role of PSS. The framework presented in the preceding section serves as background. After presenting the extant literature and its methodologic problems in very general terms, we will address more specific issues. These latter reflect what we believe to be the most important issues in the field at present as represented (sometimes by their near absence) in recent reviews and discussions. In places we will be somewhat critical. Authors have often been cautious about their suggestions, but there has been a tendency for certain possibilities to be stressed repeatedly and for others to be omitted or mentioned only in passing. This may be producing a premature consolidation of belief about what questions and phenomena are most important.

Research on Internal Loop Behavioral Oncology

There have been a number of reviews and discussions pertinent to IL effects (e.g., Anisman & Sklar, in press; Bieliauskas & Garron, 1982; Borysenko, 1982a, 1982b; Fox, 1978, 1981, 1983; LaBarba, 1970; Levy, 1983; Morrison & Paffenbarger, 1981; Newberry, 1981a; Peters & Mason, 1979; Riley, 1979b, 1981; Sklar & Anisman, 1981a, 1981b). The reader is referred to these for citations of the numerous studies which have appeared.

Animal Research

The basic characteristics of animal IL research are clearly apparent. Nearly all studies considered to be a part of this literature have been conceptualized by their authors or by commentators in terms of "stress" or PSS. PSS frequently has significant and strong effects on Neopl. Both tumor enhancement and tumor inhibition by PSS have been reported with impressive frequency. Among tumors reported as having been enhanced by PSS, and among those reported as having been inhibited, are found a wide variety of tumor systems. Tumor enhancement by PSS seems to have been reported most often in rapidly developing mouse tumors which are transplanted or virally induced. Inhibition by PSS has been reported most frequently with slowly developing chemically induced tumors in rats. However, there are exceptions to this generalization, and more importantly there have been lamentably few direct comparisons of tumor systems.

A wide varietey of PSS types have been reported as effective, including electric shock, restraint, infection, temperature extremes, social disruption, demanding learning tasks, and exposure to predators. These types of stimulation have been presented at many intensities, for many durations, and with different timing relative to stages of Neopl. However, there has been rather little systematic study of PSS parameters.

Despite its large number of studies and variables, the animal PSS-cancer literature lacks clear conclusions of useful generality. This has been noted in nearly every commentary on the area. We know that important effects occur when animal tumor systems are subjected to PSS but are unable to offer confirmed, systematic accounts of these effects at any level of analysis. As Peters and Mason (1979, p. 113) put it, "It is apparent from the literature reviewed that experimental support can be found for essentially any view concerning the effect of stress on neoplasia."

Because decisive human research in this area is quite difficult to do, some burden falls on animal research to clarify possibilities. It is therefore appropriate to mention some methodologic issues which bear upon the disarray of the animal research and upon its role in IL behavioral oncology.

There are unavoidable limitations to the applicability of infrahuman findings to human IL effects. One problem is differences between animal and human tumors. A difficulty in attempting to list the differences is our meager knowledge of early events in human oncogenesis. Autochthonous experimental tumors are usually induced by large doses of chemical carcinogens or laboratory viruses in especially susceptible species/strains; transplanted tumors' characteristics may alter with repeated passage (e.g., Hewitt, 1978).

Discussion of differences between human and experimental tumors has often focused on tumor antigenicity. Induced laboratory tumors are often more antigenic than "spontaneous" ones (Hewitt, 1978). Inoculation of oncogenic viruses may provoke immune responses to viral antigens, creating the possibility of immunologic priming against both the virus particles and tumor cells which express viral antigens. Prehn (1976) has noted that transplantation of tumor cells may produce greater immune reactions than would occur if the same cells grew autochthonously. Allogeneic tumors, of course, are of limited relevance.

Differing effects of PSS may also reduce the comparability of animal studies to human situations. Experimental tumors usually develop more rapidly than human cancers. This may change the possibilities for PSS effects because humans may go through more physiologic changes during tumor development than is possible with experimental tumors. Also, in many animal studies some groups are subjected to quite unusual and severe treatments (Peters & Mason, 1979; Riley, 1979b). These extremes are helpful in basic research on PSS response but may relate poorly to the everyday life of humans. Finally, cognitive differences between humans and lower animals may limit comparability in IL effects. Human responses to PSS can be attenuated or increased by interpretations of situations or psychological defenses (e.g., Cohen & Lazarus, 1979), and it is not clear that comparable phenomena occur in animals.

Fox (e.g., 1981) has pointed out limitations in the inferences which may be drawn for humans from infrahuman studies but has indicated as well that many of the basic processes in human oncogenesis are paralleled in animal models. The efficiency of animal studies and the basis of much tumor biology in animal models compel their use in behavioral oncology. At the same time, we must avoid simple generalizations from animal to human.

The interpretation of animal IL studies has been hampered by avoidable difficulties as well as inherent ones. One avoidable problem is investigators' tendency to use idiosyncratic combinations of tumor system and PSS. When investigators using both different tumor systems and different PSS obtain different effects on tumor, the reasons for the divergent findings are unknown. Greater comparability of studies is much needed.

Insufficient attention has been given to physiologic mediation of IL effects. Many PSS-tumor studies have not obtained data on mediation. Others have used crude or inconclusive methods such as adrenal weight or thymicolymphatic involution, presumably because better ones were not available (e.g., Newberry, 1978; Newberry et al., 1972, 1976, submitted). Even if such measures happen to reflect the actual mediators, they may be too insensitive to detect important differences. Even when optimal measures of putative mediators are taken, they are only correlational. Covariation between tumor outcome and suspected mediators in response to PSS need not mean that the suspected mediators are in the causal sequence leading to tumor effects. Additional methods such as pharmacologic or surgical techniques to mimic or block the hypothesized mediational sequences are needed. Even these must be interpreted with care, however, because many will have effects different from those the investigator would ideally like to produce. In studying adrenal corticoid mediation, for example, adrenalectomy, exogenous hormone administration, and blocking biosynthesis as with metyrapone all have effects which differ from those of PSS-induced corticoid increases.

An overlooked point about mediation is that reliance on mediational data from animals (or humans) not subject to the Neopl under consideration is highly questionable. The many effects of Neopl and oncogenic agents on hosts ("Neopl → PhenH," above) suggest that hosts' responses to PSS need not be the same as in organisms not so insulted. Yet generalizations from uninsulted organisms to hosts are frequently made.

In this area as in any other, some published studies have weaknesses in design or analysis. It has often been forgotten that studies of crowding, or other conditions in which animals in a treatment condition are housed together, are hierarchical and must be so analyzed. Other problems have been absent control groups (particularly where sampling over time is involved, the initial time sampling often being the only control value obtained), absent or inadequate statistical analyses, and questionable dependent variables (see, e.g., Newberry, 1981b). Two relatively recent reports which have been overinterpreted subsequent to their publication deal with rodent mammary tumors and are therefore conspicuous to us. Nieburgs et al. (1979) reported in two experiments that chronic handling, tail shock, or cold swim for 5 minutes every 96 hours enhanced rat mammary tumor development. However, no statistical tests were reported, and the differences appear small enough to be due to chance (Newberry, 1981b). Riley (1975) is frequently cited as demonstrating that protective housing delays the onset of mouse mammary tumors. However, the animals in the presumably stressful conventional housing were housed with males, unlike those in the protected housing. Riley reported data for parous and non-parous animals separately, but even among non-parous females, tumor development could have been affected by the males in a variety of ways. Indeed, Riley and colleagues (Riley et al., 1981) have themselves reported that housing with, or even in proximity to, males produces a large and very prolonged corticosterone elevation in female mice. The hormonal effects of blocked pregnancy or pseudopregnancy could also have contributed to the observed effect on tumor.

Human Research

The inherent difficulties of human research relevant to IL effects have resulted in a literature more instructive in its methodologic reviews (e.g., Bieliauskas & Garron, 1982; Cox & Mackay, 1982; Fox, 1978; Greer & Morris, 1978; Morrison & Paffenbarger, 1981; Perrin & Pierce, 1959) than in meaningful findings.

Human research has suffered from avoidable methodologic flaws similar to those of animal studies. However, unlike animal PSS-cancer research which utilizes experimental manipulation, human studies are largely restricted to correlational data. As Figure 1 and its discussion indicate, large numbers of variables must be controlled to demonstrate that associations between psychosocial factors and Neopl represent causal IL sequences. Two groups of alternative explanations to be ruled out are (a) effects of Neopl and their sequelae on psychosocial predictor variables, and (b) effects of ExA on Neopl and/or psychosocial predictors.

Clearly, the longer the interval between the taking of predictor measures and diagnosis, the safer the conclusion that Neopl-related factors are not affecting the supposed predictors. Unfortunately, long-term prospective studies will miss effects which occur later in tumor development. When life events are studied, it is useful to remember not only time intervals but also that events which are more independent of subjects' personalities and behavior are less likely to be confounded with direct or indirect Neopl effects. Although human IL cancer studies have seldom investigated physiologic mediation, the risk of generalizing from studies of mediators in tumor-free subjects exists as it does in animal research.

Confounds with ExA exposure are as troublesome as Neopl confounds. ExA with well-known effects, such as tobacco, are less of a problem than the larger numbers whose effects are less obvious or less studied. It is not unreasonable to suspect that some combinations of drugs, diet, and nononcogenic infectious agents can tip the balance toward host or Neopl. Thus large numbers of ExA need to be assessed in human studies. This requires large sample sizes, particularly since interactions should be included as predictors.

The earliest human studies to appear were retrospective. Tarlau and Smalheiser (1951) and Bacon, Renneker and Cutler (1952), for example, drew rather psychodynamic conclusions about the personalities of breast and cervix patients. These reports contributed to a presumption of psychosocial causation, as their authors resisted the interpretation that the psychological characteristics they observed were a result of illness. Interestingly, Bacon et al. recommended prophylactic psychotherapy for persons whose personality organizations indicated risk. Greene and colleagues (e. g., Greene, 1966) concluded from unstructured interviews that loss and the resulting sense of hopelessness and helplessness may be among the conditions determining the development of leukemia and lymphoma.

Such retrospective studies, though important in drawing attention to the possibility of IL effects, suffer from possible contamination by Neopl effects, ExA effects, researcher bias, and non-replicable predictor variables (cf. Brown, 1974; Fox, 1978). Lacking control groups, they do not even demonstrate associations between cancer and psychosocial variables.

Well conducted semi-prospective case-control studies can remove confounding with certainty of diagnosis and researcher bias (Greer & Morris, 1978), though other confounds remain. Muslin, Gyarfas, and Pieper (1966) did a well controlled semi-prospective study of psychological loss in patients admitted for breast biopsy. No significant differences were found in loss experience between subjects with malignant and benign biopsies. The care taken by Muslin et al. in subject selection and matching, objective definition and standardized measurement of loss, and blind assessment contrasts greatly with many other studies. Schmale and Iker (1966) applied a semi-prospective approach in an investigation of hopeless affect in women with suspicious cervical smears. For subjects who were judged by one of the investigators as expressing hopelessness, a malignant biopsy was predicted. The hit rate was better than chance. As with Muslin et al. (1966), this study is adequate in subject selection and blind assessment. However, the use of a nonstandard interview renders the results difficult to interpret (Bieliauskas & Garron, 1982).

There is an interesting case in which two independent research programs using semi-prospective designs produced apparently converging findings. Kissen and colleagues (e.g., Kissen, Brown, & Kissen, 1969) found that lung cancer patients had lower Maudsley or Eysenck Personality Inventory (EPI) neuroticism than did other chest patients. They interpreted this as suggesting a diminished outlet for emotional discharge as an element in the etiology of lung cancer. Greer and Morris (1975) arrived at similar conclusions from their study of breast patients admitted for biopsy. Prior to surgery, Greer and Morris gave a number of measures, including the EPI and structured interviews with each patient and a close relative. The interviews indicated abnormal suppression or extreme expression of anger and other feelings in patients with malignant biopsies.

The convergence of the Kissen et al. and Greer and Morris conclusions might be interpreted as evidence for an etiologic influence of emotional inhibition on Neopl. However, Fox (1978) pointed out that Kissen's interpretation of his findings is questionable. Fox cited Eysenck (1965) to the effect that low neuroticism is more likely to mean low emotionality than poor emotional discharge. Moreover, Greer and Morris (1975) found that their patients with malignant biopsies did not differ significantly on neuroticism from those with benign lesions. In other words, two groups of investigators have interpreted conflicting results as meaning the same thing. While it seems clear that both groups found something, there is little to suggest that the findings are consistent.

A few prospective investigations have appeared. While prospective data remain correlational, such studies seem necessary for assigning IL etiologic significance to psychosocial factors. Perhaps the best-known prospective research in this area has been by Thomas and colleagues (e.g., Thomas, Duszynski, & Shaffer, 1979). They followed 1337 medical students for up to 30 years. Questionnaire data were gathered with the object of assessing psychological precursors of suicide, mental illness, hypertension, coronary disease, and cancer. Subjects who later developed malignancies had felt significantly less close to their parents than had healthy subjects. A later study (Duszynski, Shaffer, & Thomas, 1981) investigated actual traumatic events and subsequent tumor incidence, and found no significant association. This suggests that the reported associations with closeness to parents involve attitudes rather than actual events. The conclusions of Thomas et al. are problematic because of uncertain questionnaire validity and inappropriate statistical analyses (Fox, 1978).

Hagnell (1966) collected personality data from inhabitants of a small Scandinavian town using reportedly well validated measures (Cox & Mackay, 1982). Ten years later, women who had been assessed as having exaggerated emotional reactions had a greater cancer incidence (cf.

Greer & Morris, 1975; Kissen et al., 1969). Possible shortcomings in the Hagnell study are the 10-year prospective period, which may be too short, and uneven data analysis (Fox, 1978).

Shekelle et al. (1981) used a prospective approach with archival data to investigate MMPI depression and cancer mortality. Data were obtained on 2020 employees from a longitudinal study of coronary disease. Depression, as measured by the MMPI, was associated with a twofold increase in odds of cancer death – an association that persisted over the 17-year follow-up period and after adjustment for some major cancer risk factors. Although combining of cancer sites and the unavailability of more ExA data might be criticized, the major problem of interpretation is that this study stands alone. No other work of such quality has been reported.

The available data provide some, but very far from compelling, evidence for IL effects on human cancer. Positive results in studies with relatively few methodologic problems are too limited to indicate which psychosocial factors might be important. Given the quality of the evidence, it is understandable that some authors have concluded that no IL effect exists or have strongly emphasized cautiousness (e.g., Bieliauskas & Garron, 1982; Fox, 1978, 1983; Morrison & Paffenbarger, 1981). Other authors have been more tolerant. They have tended to minimize or ignore methodologic problems in some studies (animal and human), exclude studies with negative findings, and/or fail to adequately evaluate the strength of conclusions. The result can be an impression (possibly unintended) that IL effects on human cancer are close to firmly demonstrated (see, e.g., Baltrusch, 1978; Borysenko, 1982a; Cox & Mackay, 1982; Simonton & Simonton, 1975).

We feel compelled to mention the issue of psychotherapy for cancer patients. It is accepted practice to offer psychotherapy with the object of improving overall quality of life (Wellisch, 1981) or reducing adverse effects of medical therapies (Burish & Carey, this volume). However, any exaggeration of the case for human IL effects might encourage psychotherapy for intervention in the disease process.

Some (e.g., Achterberg et al., 1977; Simonton & Simonton, 1975) have advocated psychotherapy for the disease itself, and they have appeared willing to emphasize any data which support their position and downplay any which do not. Fiore (1979) described in the *New England Journal of Medicine* his own experience with neoplastic disease. This author is apparently a psychotherapist and made a number of sound recommendations in that regard. However, he referred to associations between helplessness/depression and cancer and to improving immunologic control of malignancy via imagery as though these ideas were well supported by data. Others have been more cautious. Borysenko (1982a) mentioned IL disease course interventions as well as the life-quality and adverse-reaction uses of psychotherapy. She cited studies relating prognosis to behavioral variables. Survival time has been suggested to be positively correlated with rated amount of adjustment needed to cope with the disease (Rogentine et al., 1979), a fighting spirit (Achterberg et al., 1977), or strong denial (Greer, Morris, & Pettingale, 1979). Some studies have gone to considerable length to control for ostensible severity of disease (e.g., Rogentine et al., 1979). However, even if psychological variables were demonstrated to influence prognosis, clinical trials would be required to show that therapeutic alteration of such variables changes disease course.

There are serious ethical issues in doing psychotherapy without adequate evidence for efficacy (Strupp, 1978). These issues may be particularly serious when the object is to alter serious medical disorders. Holland and Rowland (1981) noted, for example, that psychotherapy of the Simonton sort may intensify patients' guilt feelings if the therapy fails. There is sufficient justification for clinical trials, and they have been called for (e.g., Borysenko, 1982a; Cunningham, 1982), but using psychotherapy to improve cancer outcome without proper trials puts therapists in a position uncomfortably similar to that of laetrile advocates prior to confirmation of experimental findings and adequate trials with that supposed therapy.

There is a side advantage to studying post-diagnosis psychological interventions' impacts on disease course. Such studies could, and should, be truly experimental. Thus to the extent that preclinical tumor development shares characteristics with post-diagnosis development, positive results from good psychotherapy trials would add greatly to the general case for IL effects on human cancer.

PSS, Immunodepression, and Tumor Enhancement

An hypothesis of wide interest and impact links PSS and such related things as extremes in emotional state to an enhancement of tumor development via immunodepression. This general viewpoint has frequently been mentioned favorably (e.g., Baltrusch, 1978; Bammer, 1981; Borysenko, 1982a; Fiore, 1979; Lewis & Phillips, 1979; Locke, 1982; Riley, 1979b, 1981; Riley, Fitzmaurice, & Spackman, 1981, 1982; Rosch, 1979; Visintainer, Volpicelli, & Seligman, 1982). These authors differ in the centrality of the PSS-immunodepression-tumor-enhancement hypothesis to their presentations and in the consideration they give to other possibilities. However, it is easy to come away from the group of such papers with the impression that (a) tumor enhancement is the most likely effect of PSS on tumor development, and (b) immunodepression is the most likely mediator of that enhancement.

There is evidence consistent with these ideas, though it is not as conclusive or unmixed as the frequency of its discussion might suggest. Three lines of evidence are frequently cited: impairment of immune function by PSS, immunologic control of cancer, and PSS effects on cancer. We have already noted that PSS effects on cancer are quite varied.

Immune Impairment by PSS

It is clear that PSS can affect the immune system, often in ways which suggest impairment of its capability. Several human studies have been cited to this effect. These studies also suggest, however, that immunodepression by PSS may not be a straightforward phenomenon. Bartrop et al. (1977) found that lymphocyte response to mitogens was inhibited by bereavement but delayed hypersensitivity was not. Palmblad (1981) reported increased interferon production by a 72-hour sleep deprivation which inhibited neutrophil phagocytosis. Locke and Kraus (1982) reported low natural killer (NK) cell activity in subjects with high life readjustment plus high scores on a symptom checklist (taken as indicating low coping), but the highest NK activity in subjects reporting high readjustment and high coping (low symptoms), suggesting that moderately demanding conditions might actually enhance NK function. They also reported that only one-year readjustment participated in this relationship; one-month and two-week scores were not related to NK activity. In a study of preparation for a critical examination (Dorian et al., 1981) and the 72-hour sleep deprivation study of Palmblad and colleagues (Palmblad, 1981), there was some evidence for a rebound of immune function above baseline after the PSS episode.

Numerous infrahuman studies have dealt with effects of PSS on the immune system. A number of reviews discuss this work (e.g., Ahlqvist, 1981; Borysenko & Borysenko, 1982; Claman, 1972; Dannenberg, 1979; Herberman, 1982; Monjan, 1981; Solomon, Amkraut, & Rubin, 1979). Rather than repeating their citations of a large number of studies, we will note some conclusions and particular findings which seem germane to IL effects on neoplasia.

More clearly than in humans, PSS and PSS-responsive hormones have been shown capable of reducing immune function in animals. Antibody levels, susceptibility to anaphylaxis, lymphocyte proliferation, graft-versus-host response, phagocytosis, and NK activity are among the dependent variables which can be so affected. However, as most of the authors cited above have noted at least in passing, PSS and PSS-responsive factors do not inevitably inhibit immune function. The effect varies with the specific mediating factor considered, organism characteristics, time, characteristics of the PSS, and the aspects of immune function studied.

Two frequently mentioned mechanisms for down-regulation of immune function by PSS are glucocorticoids and catecholamines, but their functions are not particularly simple. Regarding the traditional glucocorticoid effects (e.g., Dougherty & White, 1943), indices of cell number such as circulating lymphocytes, or weights of thymus, spleen, or nodes are probably poor indices of immune function. Their deficiencies may relate in part to differences in corticoid resistance at different stages of lymphocyte maturation. Claman (1972) has noted, for example, that immature cortical thymocytes are sensitive while mature T cells, activated or inactivated, are resistant.

Lymphocytes of different species vary greatly in sensitivity to glucocorticoids (Claman, 1972). Moreover, cortisol, the primary corticoid of resistant species, is more potent as a glucocorticoid than corticosterone, the primary corticoid of the sensitive rat and mouse. These species differences argue for cautious, quantitative interpretations of glucocorticoid effects, particularly effects of cortisol or synthetic glucocorticoids on sensitive species.

Sex and strain differences are also relevant. Females may have greater antibody response than males, greater ability to reject weakly antigenic allografts (Ahlqvist, 1981), and less inhibition of antibody response by glucocorticoids (Branceni & Arnason, 1966). Lymphocytes from female C57BL/6 mice show reduced response to concanavalin A (conA) at lower cortisol concentrations than males (Monjan, 1981). Monjan and colleagues found that the enhancement of lymphocyte stimulation which occurred with low cortisol levels in BALB/c mice did not occur in C57BL/6 and that cells from immunized BALB/c had greater numbers of β-adrenergic receptors.

Glucocorticoids can potentiate aspects of immune function at certain concentrations. Adolph and Swetly (1979) found that corticoids can increase interferon production in lymphoid cells at concentrations which reduce DNA synthesis. Monjan and colleagues (Monjan, 1981) found that below approximately 100 ng/ml cortisol increased thymidine incorporation in BALB/c lymphocytes stimulated with conA or lipopolysaccharide (LPS). At 100 ng/ml lymphocyte reactivity approximated control values, while above 100 ng/ml it was reduced. Similar effects occurred in a mixed lymphocyte reaction.

If corticoid effects on immunologic variables such as those studied by Monjan et al. parallel the traditional glycogen deposition or antiinflammatory indices of glucocorticoid potency, cortisol might have effects equivalent to corticosterone concentrations roughly three times as high, and corticosterone is the natural glucocorticoid of mice. Further, corticosterone is relatively more potent as a mineralocorticoid (Haynes & Murad, 1980). Mineralocorticoids may possibly have immunoenhancing ("prophlogistic") effects (see Selye & Heuser, 1956); thus it is conceivable that results with corticosterone would differ more from those with cortisol than even their disparity in glucocorticoid potency would suggest.

There are also possible complications with catecholamines. Though β-adrenergic stimulation often impairs immune function, α-adrenergic stimulation may have an opposite effect, possibly by reducing cyclic adenosine-3′, 5′-monophosphate (cAMP) (Ahlqvist, 1981; Locke & Kraus, 1982). Substances which increase cAMP may have positive effects on thymocyte maturation (Ahlqvist, 1981). Immunization may allow an increase in lymphocyte DNA synthesis to be produced by β-adrenergic stimulation (Sandberg et al., 1978).

Some hormones thought to increase under PSS are seemingly immunoenhancing. These include growth hormone, thyroid hormones, and prolactin (Ahlqvist, 1981; Berczi et al., 1981; Monjan, 1981). Insulin may be immunoenhancing (Ahlqvist, 1981), but its secretion is thought to be reduced by PSS (Curtis, 1979).

Temporal factors are another influence on immune system response to PSS and related substances. The changes in reactivity of lymphocytes with their maturation are an illustration. The apparent decline in immune function with age (see, e.g., Monjan, 1981; Riley et al., 1982) is another. The duration or onset time of PSS is important in determining its effect on the immune system; we have noted such effects in human studies, and they occur in animals also.

Perhaps the best-known animal work indicating the importance of time is that of Monjan and colleagues (Monjan, 1981; Monjan & Collector, 1977). They showed that lymphocytes from mice exposed to intense sound for 35 days had an enhanced response to conA and LPS. A similar pattern occurred for lymphocyte toxicity to P815 mastocytoma cells. Sound PSS for fewer days reduced these responses below control levels. Interestingly, extension of sound PSS beyond 35 days produced a reversion of mitogen activation toward baseline levels in these studies, suggesting a triphasic effect.

Other characteristics of PSS might influence its effect on the immune system. Exercise, which might be considered "stressful," produces pyrogenic activity capable of increasing cytotoxicity and neutrophil recruitment (Cannon & Kluger, 1983). The evidence for immunoenhancement by low levels of cortisol suggests that overall PSS severity might be important (cf. Keller et al., 1981). Similarly, controllability might be expected to reduce the effects of PSS on immune function.[3]

Compound PSS – the occurrence of an additional source of PSS when the organism is being or has been subjected to others – is relevant, though there has been little systematic work on it. Among the best known arguments on compound PSS are those of Riley and colleagues (e. g., Riley, 1975, 1979 a). Their data indicate that routine aspects of animal housing have large effects on corticosterone in mice, and they suggested that these conditions will affect immune function. They emphasized the problems that these background factors might pose for interpreting experimental results. Functional relationships between PSS parameters and outcomes cannot be fully understood if very mild conditions cannot be obtained, particularly when the relationship between a PSS parameter and a dependent variable is nonmonotonic. On the other hand, low stimulation conditions are artificial and could pose problems of interpretation.

Monjan (1981) illustrated the subtleties of compound PSS. Retroorbital bleeding shortly before harvesting splenic lymphocytes dramatically increased their thymidine incorporation. This is opposite to the effect of acute (3–5 days) sound PSS (Monjan & Collector, 1977). In addition, retroorbital bleeding reversed the inhibitory effect of sound PSS applied for 1–8 days. Monjan's findings indicate that acute PSS can have an immunoenhancing effect and that the effect depends upon the particular characteristics of the stimulation.

It seems that no simple generalizations can describe the immune system's response to PSS. The effect seems to depend on the immunologic parameter studied, on several sets of temporal factors and on the quantitative characteristics of the stimulation. Stein (1983) has recently suggested that at present the complexity of relationships between psychological/neural factors and the immune system argue against simple generalizations or attempts at application. When considering disease outcomes in this context, it is necessary to remember that human lives involve multiple demands and multiple types of stimulation whose onsets and offsets follow each other in complex patterns over long periods of time. Immunodepression with PSS seems to have appeared in the literature more often than immunoenhancement, but we do not know what reported effects best reflect actual occurrences in everyday life.

---

[3] As this chapter was being typeset, a report appeared indicating that inescapable electric shock inhibits lymphocyte thymidine uptake in response to mitogens. That inhibition did not occur with escapable shock or restraint, as compared to no-treatment controls. (M. L. Laudenslager, S. M. Ryan, R. C. Drugan, R. L. Hyson, S. F. Maier. *Science,* 1983, *221,* 568–570.)

Immune System Effects on Cancer

A PSS-immunodepression-tumor-enhancement hypothesis presupposes that the immune system exerts significant and general inhibitory effects on tumor development. However, as in most other areas involving behavioral oncology, tumor-immune interactions appear capable of subtlety and of permitting conflicting outcomes for the host.

Acquired Immunity. For the antigen-dependent arms of the immune system to modulate tumor proliferation and spread, tumor cells must be antigenic. Many tumor cells are antigenic (e.g., Baldwin & Price, 1975; Kennett, Jonak, & Byrd, 1982; Levine, 1982; Reif, 1982). These determinants may be of several origins: viral antigens, reappearing embryonic antigens, new antigens resulting from transforming genes, increases in normal proteins, and complexes of foreign and normal protein.

However, tumor antigens may often be weak or undetectable (e.g., Fidler & Kripke, 1980; Kobayashi, 1979; Old, 1982; Prehn, 1976). Related to this is the phenomenon of "sneaking through" (Prehn, 1976). Small inocula of experimental tumor cells may grow more rapidly than larger inocula due to partial immunologic tolerance. Prehn argued that if a small dose of relatively antigenic tumor cells fails to provoke an immune response, the few weakly antigenic cells of autochthonous tumors are unlikely to do so.

There is also evidence that immune responses can enhance tumor development. Prehn (1976) cited several such findings, indicating, for example, that immune spleen cells enhance growth of transplanted tumors, that thymus grafting restores susceptibility to chemical carcinogenesis in the skin of nude athymic mice, and that the injection of normal spleen cells into experimentally immunodepressed animals can accelerate chemical carcinogenesis. Prehn suggested that such reactions would characterize weak immune responses to tumor. The mechanisms by which the immune system can enhance neoplastic processes and the generality of such phenomena seem far from clear. Black (1980) discussed blocking antibody on tumor cells, occupation of antibody by circulating antigen, and increases in suppressor cell activity. Lewis et al. (1977) noted in addition that anti-antibodies can develop in cancer hosts. These kinds of effects may indicate a strong immune response and therefore be separate from the enhancement by weak immune reactions postulated by Prehn (1976).

Another body of evidence concerns tumor development in naturally, medically, or experimentally immunodepressed individuals. If immunologic control of cancer is a strong, general phenomenon, such individuals should be highly susceptible to a wide variety of malignancies. This area has been discussed extensively (e.g., Keast, 1981; Melief &

Schwartz, 1975; Stutman, 1975). The evidence is not uniform, but it fails at present to confirm the idea of a strong, general immunologic inhibition of cancer. Among the points made by the authors just cited are the following: There are cases in which tumor development is well controlled by specific immunity, particularly with tumors induced by certain animal viruses. However, the negative evidence is considerable. Immunodeficient nude and pituitary dwarf mice show strong resistance to many tumors. Thymectomy often produces little or no increase in tumor development and in some tumor systems can have the opposite effect, actually increasing host resistance. Immunodepressed humans do not show the increases in cancer incidence which would be expected. Many of the human reports suffer from methodologic inadequacies such as difficulties in population definitions, sampling deficiencies, and possible inadequate diagnoses. Lymphoreticular malignancies seem to account for most if not all of the well substantiated increases in cancer among immunodepressed humans, and these may reflect the assault imposed on the immune system rather than deficient immunologic control of malignancy in general.

The types of findings which we have summarized have led to questions about the generality of immune surveillance and control of cancer by antibody-mediated immune mechanisms (see Keast, 1981; Melief & Schwartz, 1975; Prehn, 1976; Stutman, 1975; Wunderlich, 1982). It is likely that these mechanisms do sometimes serve as significant curbs to neoplastic disease, but they need not do so in general and may have the opposite effect, reducing rather than increasing host resistance.

Non-Specific Immunity. With discouragement about specific immunity has come increasing attention to non-specific or natural immunity against tumor. Discussion has concentrated on macrophages and NK cells. These cells can participate in antibody-dependent cytotoxicity, but they also display anti-tumor activity that does not require specific immunity.

Macrophages/monocytes are activated to kill tumor cells by a variety of agents, including interferon, other lymphokines, and LPS. This effect is rather specific to tumor cells, and a variety of tumor types are affected (Alexander, 1977; Chirigos et al., 1981). NK cells are reactive against tumor cells and a number of other types. They respond to and produce interferon; they proliferate in response to T cell growth factor (Herberman, 1982). Herberman and Ortaldo (1981) have presented a very useful comparison of NK cells with other immune effector cells. It may be that natural controls are most important for incipient primary tumors while metastasis is more under the control of specific immunity (Alexander, 1977).

The activity of activated macrophages and NK cells can be inhibited by PSS or PSS-responsive humoral factors. Pavlidis and Chirigos (1980) demonstrated that both immobilization and corticosteroids inhibited the action of activated mouse macrophages against tumor cells. Herberman (1982) cited a considerable amount of evidence on PSS-related inhibition of NK activity. Animal shipment, glucocorticoids, and catecholamines can all depress NK activity. A complex association between NK activity and human life readjustment has been suggested (Locke & Kraus, 1982).

However, even including the important functions of natural immunity, it remains unclear whether immunologic control is great in a large proportion of cancers. Several things seem important to us from the perspective of a PSS-immunodepression-tumor-enhancement hypothesis. One is the generality and strength of natural effector-cells' antitumor activity. Herberman and Ortaldo (1981) indicated that NK cells are far from equally reactive against all tumors and that the evidence for NK activity against autochthonous tumors is spotty. LoBuglio et al. (1981) found great differences among tumor cell types in susceptibility to human monocyte toxicity. Also, it does not seem at all clear how adding natural effector cells to our consideration of the PSS-immunodepression hypothesis reduces the force of evidence that specific immune function can *enhance* tumor development.

Summary and Conclusions

The idea that PSS will enhance tumor development by inhibiting anti-tumor immune function seems to be very popular. Behavioral oncology discussions which include this idea sometimes seem to imply by their cursory treatment of other possibilities that this particular effect has been demonstrated to be so general and strong a phenomenon that other outcomes and mechanisms may be regarded as relatively unimportant. Validation of any hypothesis about mediation of PSS effects necessitates elimination of alternative explanations. We are aware of no evidence clearly requiring the attribution of an *in vivo* PSS influence on tumor to immunologic mediation.

Any outcome is at least conceivable. PSS might enhance tumor development by either immunodepression or immunoenhancement; PSS might inhibit tumor development by either immunodepression or immunoenhancement. To know whether one of those outcomes is predominantly likely requires a statistically representative sample from the possible combinations of tumor system, PSS, and temporal relations. It is likely to be some time before such a sample accrues. Indeed, even the identification of immune effector cells as mediators need not mean that immunologic effects are involved, since those cells have other functions as well (Fidler, 1980).

The major attraction of the PSS-immunodepression-tumor-enhancement idea is its generality. If neoplasms are uniformly and effectively antigenic, if PSS uniformly impairs anti-tumor immune functions, and if no other mechanisms operate effectively, the biologic diversity of cancers can be ignored and general conclusions drawn. Very general conclusions seem unlikely, but the possibility of even moderately broad generalizations demands that PSS-immune-cancer relationships be pursued vigorously. Our only concern is that other possibilities not be ignored in this pursuit.

Stimulus-Based Hypotheses: PSS Severity and Related Variables

It has been suggested that specific characteristics of PSS are critical to the *direction* of its effect on Neopl. Physical severity (Turkevich, 1958), unpredictability (Henry, Stephens, & Watson, 1975b; Sklar & Anisman, 1981a), uncontrollability (Anisman & Sklar, 1982; Sklar & Anisman, 1981a, 1981b), and acuteness – or lack of opportunity for adaptation – (Ray & Pradhan, 1974; Sklar & Anisman, 1981a, 1981b) have been mentioned. In each case, it was suggested that PSS which is relatively severe (physically severe, unpredictable, uncontrollable, acute) would be more likely to enhance tumor development relative to controls, whereas relatively mild PSS would be more likely to inhibit.

Sklar and Anisman have a particularly well-developed view (Anisman & Sklar, 1982; in press; Sklar & Anisman, 1979, 1980, 1981a, 1981b; Sklar, Bruto, & Anisman, 1981). They have emphasized controllability and chronicity (and have also considered social conditions and mentioned predictability and intensity). They hypothesize that acute, uncontrollable PSS will generally enhance tumor development and that chronic uncontrollable PSS is more likely to inhibit, though they acknowledge that other factors may also have effects. Controllability will prevent tumor enhancement by acute PSS and may inhibit tumor development. They emphasize CNS neurochemical effects as mediators. Anisman and Sklar (in press) refer to the possibility that "moderate" PSS may mobilize resources (presumably in terms of increased synthesis and/or decreased utilization of CNS amines) and be protective (cf. Turkevich, 1958). Regarding chronicity, Anisman & Sklar (in press) have noted that its effects cannot be due merely to simple adaptation. Simple adaptation should merely equate tumor development under chronic PSS to that of controls. They suggest increased brain amine synthesis, decreased utilization after PSS episodes, and receptor subsensitivity as active processes differentiating chronic PSS organisms from those not subjected to PSS.

Hypotheses such as those of Sklar and Anisman, Turkevich (1958), Henry, Stephens et al. (1975) and Ray and Pradhan (1974) are interesting partly because of a similarity among them. If one risks abstracting from them, they seem to suggest that the general aversiveness or degree of physiologic disruption produced by PSS determines the direction of tumor response vis-à-vis controls. If we use a term like "functional intensity" for this general aversiveness/disruptiveness, the hypothesis is that tumor development is a J-shaped function of PSS functional intensity (see Figure 2). This is an oversimplification on our part. It is very clear that different types of PSS can produce different patterns of peripheral effects. Thus, any suggestion of nonspecificity in responses to PSS is risky. Nevertheless, the similarity of the suggestions regarding physical severity, unpredictability, uncontrollability, and acuteness is in-

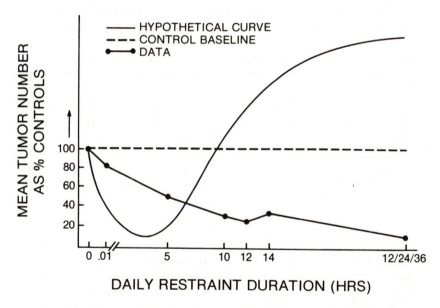

Fig. 2: Cross-experiment relationship between restraint duration and development of the DMBA-induced rat mammary tumor. The duration of .01 refers to running animals through restraining tubes. The 12/24/36 designation refers to a combination of durations selected as the maximum tolerable restraint severity (Boyle, 1982). The smooth curve represents a J-function of the type emerging from published hypotheses regarding PSS functional intensity and tumor development, and is shown for comparison.

triguing, and the more so since these hypotheses represent almost the only attempts to account systematically for the fact that PSS can both enhance and inhibit tumor development.

Physical Severity

Simple parameters of physical severity such as the intensity of PSS or the duration of single episodes have not had extensive study. No consistent pattern has emerged from what has been done.

Over a number of studies, Newberry and colleagues have used a variety of restraint durations with the DMBA rat mammary tumor (Boyle, 1982; Newberry et al., 1976). These conditions have ranged from merely running animals through restraining tubes (unpublished data) to a combination of 12, 24, and 36-hour restraint periods which was at the limit of animals' tolerance (and which also reduced predictability) (Boyle, 1982). Figure 2 plots the effects of varying durations as proportions of control tumor counts. It also portrays a hypothetical J-curve of the type which seems to emerge from the various hypotheses we mentioned above. As Figure 2 indicates, the more severe the conditions, the greater the tumor inhibition. Obviously, cross-experiment comparisons with a single type of PSS are inconclusive, but we have not been able to shift the PSS effect from inhibition to enhancement with these manipulations.

Newberry et al. (1972) found inhibition of the DMBA rat mammary tumor by intense (5–7 mA) electric shock which, like Boyle's (1982) extended restraint durations, seemed close to animals' limits of tolerance. On the other hand, Sklar and Anisman (1979) found that neither the duration of shock sessions nor the intensity of the shock affected P815 mouse mastocytoma; all shock conditions produced equal enhancement.

Unpredictability

Unpredictability increases PSS aversiveness (e. g., Seligman, Maier, & Solomon, 1971), but few experiments have studied the effects of simple predictability manipulations on tumor. Henry, Stephens et al. (1975) employed colony social disruption induced by force breeding in the study which led to their hypothesis that PSS predictability determines the direction of tumor response. In their situation, however, predictability could not be separated from other PSS parameters or from the hormonal consequences of force breeding on mouse mammary tumors (Liebelt & Liebelt, 1967a). Soviet writers (Kavetsky, Turkevich, & Balitsky, 1966; Turkevich, 1958) have cited studies to the effect that signaled PSS can enhance tumor development in comparison with both no-PSS and UCS-only controls.

In an attempt to extend the Henry, Stephens et al. (1975) finding, Newberry et al. (submitted) compared predictable restraint (PR) (Newberry et al., 1976) and a varied, unpredictable regimen (VU) using the DMBA rat mammary tumor and the spontaneous (viral) C3H/HeJ mouse mammary tumor. In the VU condition, restraint, exposure to unfamiliar conspecifics, and a Noble-Collip type drum were used, each with three possible durations. One-third of the VU animals received each stimulation type on each day. Within the constraint that all treatments be completed within a 16-hour laboratory day, treatment onset time was independently randomized for each treatment type on each day. The conditions of the studies prevented experimenter activities from serving as reliable cues to the stimulation animals would receive. Daily PR and VU were given from 38 to 125 days of age in the rat study and from 59 to 445 days of age in the mouse study.

Figure 3 presents tumor incidence data for both systems and mean final tumor counts for the rat system. (Tumor counts are not meaningful in the mouse system; only one mouse developed more than one tumor.) In the rat system both types of PSS inhibited tumor development. Both significantly reduced tumor count. Tumor incidence was also reduced. The incidence effect did not reach the .05 level but has been significant in other experiments (Newberry et al., 1976). In the mouse system, PR had no effect, and VU significantly enhanced tumor development, i.e., increased incidence. These results need to be confirmed with other manipulations, since the PR and VU conditions differed in several ways. However, it may be that predictability is important for mouse mammary tumors and not for rat mammary tumors.

Controllability

There are two studies clearly implicating controllability. Sklar and Anisman (1979) found that inescapable footshock enhanced P815 mouse mastocytoma, whereas escapable shock had no effect. Visintainer, Volpicelli, and Seligman (1982) found a very similar effect with the rat Walker 256. Sklar and Anisman (1980) attributed an effect of fighting to controllability. Mice changed from isolation to grouped housing developed smaller P815 tumors if they fought regularly. Fighting among female mice was associated with inhibition of murine sarcoma virus tumors (Amkraut & Solomon, 1972). On the other side of the controllability ledger, Marsh, Miller, and Lamson (1959) found that ac-

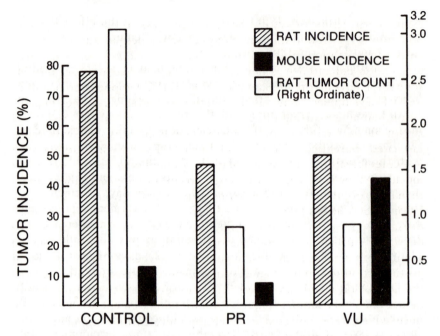

Fig. 3: Comparison of rat and mouse mammary tumor response to two varieties of PSS. PR refers to predictable restraint; VU refers to a varied, unpredictable regimen of stimulation, under which neither the type, the duration, nor the onset time of daily treatment was predictable (see text). Tumor count data are not presented for the mouse tumor system, since only one mouse developed multiple tumors.

tive avoidance conditioning inhibited Ehrlich carcinoma in mice. They found the same effect with restraint, which is seemingly less controllable.

When PSS affects Neopl, controllability should often modify its effects. However, we know too little about both controllability and cancer for confident conclusions.

Chronicity

A few more studies have manipulated PSS chronicity or related timing variables than is the case for other PSS parameters. Sklar and Anisman (1979) found that one and five days of shock after P815 inoculation enhanced tumor development, but ten days had a slight inhibitory effect. Sklar, Bruto, and Anisman (1981) found adaptation to the enhancing effects of shock on P815, but tumor inhibition with larger numbers of shock days did not occur in these studies. Amkraut and Solomon (1972) found that three days of shock before murine sarcoma virus administration inhibited tumor, but the same regimen after virus inoculation enhanced it. Riley et al. (1982) reported that dexamethasone seven days before implantation of 6C3HED lymphosarcoma inhibited its development whereas dexamethasone seven days after implantation had an enhancing effect.

Not all data relevant to chronicity have been consistent with those just cited. Burchfield, Woods, and Elich (1978) exposed rats daily to −20°C temperatures before inoculation of lymphoma or polyoma, after inoculation, or both. All cold-exposed groups developed smaller tumors than controls, the effect being strongest in animals given only preinoculation PSS. Matthes (1963) exposed mice to hungry ferrets daily for 10 days. Groups began exposure three days before, on the day of, or five days after Ehrlich ascites implantation. All three PSS groups developed significantly smaller tumors than controls. Newberry (1978) found that postinduction restraint was necessary to and sufficient for inhibition of the DMBA rat mammary tumor. In the experiments comparing rat and mouse mammary tumors (Figure 3) tumor enhancement occurred in the mice, which were subjected to much the more chronic stimulation.

The effects of repeated PSS should depend upon the relations between temporal patterns of physiologic changes and periods of tumor development. If mediating responses return to baseline with repeated PSS, either asymptotically or on their way to a rebound, there will be a period during which PSS will exert no effect on tumor. If the mediators rebound, there will be a period in which effect on tumor is in the direction opposite to that produced by acute PSS. If tumor response to mediators changes abruptly as mediator activities change (as in thresholds for tumor effects) then the time periods for different tumor responses to the PSS will be different than when the response of the tumor to the mediator is more graded. Added to such considerations are changes in physiologic responses over individual PSS episodes and in tumor and tumor cell characteristics over time (Fidler & Hart, 1982; Griswold & Green, 1970; Kiang et al., 1982). It should be clear that without good knowledge of the tumor system and mediators involved, no relationship between tumor response and PSS chronicity can be surprising.

Conclusions

The tumor effects which have occurred with variations in physical severity, predictability, controllability, and chronicity of PSS are not consistent. The data as a whole do not support any general hypothesis for any of these variables. The inconsistencies must be due in part to differences in basic types of PSS and to parametric differences in the "functional intensity" variables themselves. Therefore it is premature to conclude that no important generalizations occur with these variables, although there would seem to be rather restrictive boundary conditions on any such generalizations.

It is well to remember that these variables are related to each other in practical ways. The observed effect of any one as an independent variable will depend partly on the constant levels chosen for the other functional intensity variables, including laboratory background variables. In some cases, particularly if a complex function relates functional intensity to tumor development, the values of the constant variables could force the manipulated variable to produce almost any effect. The possible complications from variables usually held constant are illustrated by the finding of Sklar and Anisman (1980) that footshock enhances P815 mastocytoma in group housed mice but not in mice housed singly.

Tumor System Differences

Neither of the most mentioned views on PSS-tumor relationships has solid support. The data certainly suggest that some variables have been left out or underemphasized. Interestingly, neither the PSS-immunodepression-tumor-enhancement nor the PSS-characteristics view deals systematically with differences among cancers, except for the idea that a PSS-immunodepression-tumor-enhancement mechanism cannot operate with neoplasms which are free from immune system control (Riley, 1981). Other tumor system factors, such as hormone responsiveness, type of inducing agent, and rate of development (e. g., Newberry, 1981a; Riley, 1979b; Sklar & Anisman, 1981a), have been noticed, but the notice has had little impact. It is almost as though the diseases themselves have been eliminated from attempts to understand IL effects upon them.

Considering Neopl from the perspective of Figure 1, we should expect tumor systems to differ in their relationships to host psychological characteristics and PsyS. A great number of biologic factors are related to psychosocial variables; a great number are also related to Neopl. Cancers differ in their histiogenesis and gross behavior; they have great and varied effects upon hosts.

Evidence that tumor systems differ in responses to endogenous and exogenous factors likely to be related to psychosocial variables is plentiful, though we know of no thorough compilation of this evidence. We have already noted that different types of leukemias are differentially sensitive to corticoids (see Claman, 1972) and that tumors differ in susceptibility to immunologic control ("Immune System Effects on Cancer"). We give here a few additional examples.

Heterogeneity among the cells of individual neoplasms develops with progression (Fidler & Hart, 1982). The cells differ in many ways, including hormone receptors, antigenicity, and tendency to invade and metastasize. Disparate cells influence each other, sometimes to produce an equilibrium in the population. Disruption of the equilibrium, as by selective killing of some subpopulations, may release certain cell types to proliferate. Possibly related to the heterogeneity and equilibria discussed by Fidler and Hart (1982) are cyclic changes in tumor characteristics. Kiang et al. (1982) found that over 22 serial transplantations the frequency of polyploidy, number of progesterone receptors, and amount of thymidine kinase activity in hormonally induced mammary tumors alternately increased and decreased, while hormone responsiveness steadily declined. Decreases in hormone sensitivity with tumor age are not uncommon (e. g., Griswold & Green, 1970) and may reflect cell surface changes which also contribute to metastasis (Poste, 1977).

In terms of endogenous factors, it has been found that interferon (and α-difluoromethyl ornithine, an inhibitor of polyamine synthesis) inhibits B-16 melanoma but not Lewis lung tumor or L1210 leukemia (Sunkara et al., 1983). Botazzi et al. (1983) found that macrophage chemotaxic activity varied greatly over human and mouse tumor cell lines. Leukemia induced by methylcholanthrene is inhibited by cortisone and enhanced by gonadectomy, but skin tumors induced by the same compound show the opposite responses (Liebelt & Liebelt, 1962). Like autochthonous tumors, different types of experimental tumor cells establish metastases at preferred sites (e. g., Liebelt et al., 1968), even when injected into the same organ (Sugarbaker, 1952).

Riley and colleagues (e. g., Riley 1981, Riley et al., 1982) found enhancing effects of glucocorticoids on tumors, including enhancement of 6C3HED lymphosarcoma by dexamethasone and of Moloney virus sarcomas by corticosterone. In an attempt to generalize those findings, Newberry et al. (submitted) studied the effect of dexamethasone on the DMBA rat mammary tumor. In two experiments using different daily doses, dexamethasone significantly inhibited tumor development (Figure 4), a finding opposite to those of Riley et al. with mouse sarcomas.

The effects of ExA other than hormones, including oncogenic agents, also illustrate tumor system differences. The effect of interferon on virus-transformed 3T3 cells depends on the virus (Bakhanashvili, Wreschner, & Salzburg, 1983). With 18 skin paintings, thymic tissue was more susceptible than extra-thymic cells to the leukemogenic ac-

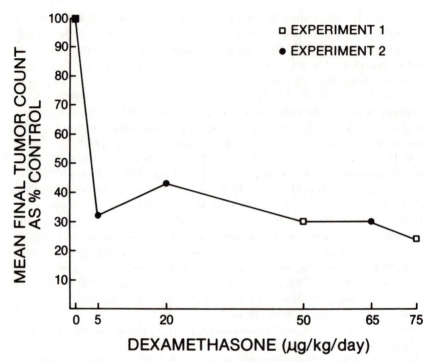

Fig. 4: Effect of dexamethasone on the DMBA-induced rat mammary tumor. Two experiments using different daily doses of dexamethasone are represented. Animals received DMBA by caudal IV at 50, 53 , and 56 days of age for a total of 6 mg. Dexamethasone, in a 1% carboxymethylcellulose suspension, was administered by gastric instillation from 60 to 120 days of age. Vehicle control (0) was run in both studies.

tion of methylcholanthrene; with 36 paintings that difference did not occur (Kirschbaum & Liebelt, 1955).

Major tranquilizers enhance development of DMBA rat mammary tumors (Pearson et al., 1969) but have little or no effect on transplanted mouse mammary tumors (Cranston, 1958). Riley and colleagues have used the nononcogenic LDH virus as a means of inducing "stress" (Riley et al., 1982). Their studies strongly suggest tumor system differences. LDH virus-enhanced development of 6C3HED lymphosarcoma, Moloney virus sarcoma, and a partially histoincompatible B-16 melanoma. It had no effect on a histocompatible B-16 (Riley et al., 1982). The virus inhibited development of spontaneous (viral) mouse mammary tumors (Riley, 1966).

Potentially relevant tumor system differences have been seen in the effects of even biologically similar neoplasms on their hosts. Transplantable CE 1460 mammary tumors in CE mice produced marked leukocytosis with a great increase in the ratio of myeloid to lymphoid cells and with extramedullary hematopoiesis in several organs. On the other hand, transplantable BALB/c 2301 mammary tumor in BALB/c animals produced large fluctuations in platelet levels with no change in erythroid-myeloid ratio and no foci of extramedullary hematopoiesis. The factors elaborated by these two tumors represent differences in genetic origin of tumor rather than tissue of origin since each tumor had its specific effects in CE × BALB/c F_1hybrids (Delmonte, Liebelt, & Liebelt, 1966). Senger et al. (1983) found differences between guinea pig hepatocarcinoma lines in their vascular permeability effects. Tumor lines 1 and 10 both produced high human serum albumin extravasation when injected subcutaneously, but only line 10 did so when given intraperitoneally. The effects of Lewis lung carcinoma on platelets and fibrinogen are greater with intramuscular than with intravenous injection (Donati et al., 1977). B-16 melanoma sublines differ considerably in their degradation of host membranes and connective tissue (Nakajima et al., 1983). The differences are related to differences in metastatic potential and apparently result from differences among sublines in the production of degrading enzymes.

Though host and tumor components of tumor systems often cannot be separated, some evidence suggests host involvement. Rat strains differ in inducibility of mammary tumors by estrogens (Stone et al., 1979) and DMBA (Huggins, Oka, & Fareed, 1972). The effect of methylcholanthrene on mouse mammary tumor incidence varies considerably both within and between groups of high and low MTV strains and between groups with varying hormonal backgrounds (Liebelt & Liebelt, 1967a). The high-leukemia AKR mouse strain shows lower adrenocortical activity than the low-leukemia C3H strain (Metcalf, 1960). Strain differences in brain adenylate cyclase response to L-DOPA relate strongly to mouse mammary tumor incidence (Cotzias & Tang, 1977).

The diversity of findings in the literature certainly suggests animal tumor system differences in responses to PsyS, but few close comparisons of systems have been made. What has been done indicates the importance of tumor system. We have noted the differences found by Riley et al. in tumor systems' responses to the "stress" of LDH virus infection. Molomut, Lazare, and Smith (1963) reported that auditory PSS delayed methylcholanthrene tumors in DBA/1 mice but not in A/Jax. The Newberry et al. (submitted) comparison of rat and mouse mammary tumors' responses to restraint and varied stimulation (Figure 3) also indicates tumor system differences. It goes beyond that to suggest a system-by-PSS *interaction:* What enhances one tumor inhibits another. Even seemingly minor differences in tumor system can be critical. Anisman and Sklar (in press) report that the effect of PSS on P815 mastocytoma depends upon the load of tumor cells given. With high numbers of cells, shock enhances tumor development, but with low numbers it has no effect.

It is clear that tumor systems differ sufficiently in responses to endogenous host factors, to relevant ExA, and to PsyS for their characteristics to be given careful attention in both empirical work and systematization attempts. Fox (1978) made a similar point in warning against combining sites in human studies. Even authors who have themselves found relevant tumor system effects have tended in their discussions to deemphasize them and propose generalizations which largely ignore them.

When we consider possible mechanisms below, additional reasons for including tumor system differences will be apparent. We note here that one probable reason for authors in behavioral oncology deemphasizing tumor systems is the absence of clear evidence on mechanisms. Not knowing how psychosocial variables exercise their effects makes it almost impossible to deal systematically with differences in tumor systems' responses.

Mechanisms

Although demonstration of IL effects and their boundary conditions is necessary, the usefulness of IL behavioral oncology will depend considerably on understanding mechanisms. It might be possible to conceptualize and study IL effects on cancer at a purely psychological level of analysis. However, with such clearly biologic endpoints, genuinely psychobiologic models are almost necessary.

Nevertheless, although we will not emphasize it here, the psychological side of good explanations will have to be solid for practical purposes of prediction in human cancer if for no other reason. This requires the careful selection and manipulation of variables known to be important psychologically (and ethologically) in addition to manipulations chosen for biologic significance, parametric completeness, or convenience.

In considering biologic mediators of IL effects, it is necessary to know that the effects are IL ones. As we have noted, this is a major problem in human research. It is something of a problem in animal studies as well. It has been noted (e.g., Borysenko, 1982a; Newberry, 1981b; Riley, 1979b) that PSS effects on animal tumors could be a consequence of altered food intake. Severe food restriction can inhibit development of a variety of experimental tumors (e.g., Tannenbaum,

1940). Thus a possible food confound seems more likely when PSS inhibits tumor and when the PSS manipulation obviously prevents eating (e.g., Newberry, 1978; Newberry et al. 1976).

Newberry, Mactutus, and Gerstenberger (unpublished observations) found that food and water deprivation produced the same inhibition of DMBA rat mammary tumors as did restraint, but that restrained animals actually consumed more food than controls. These findings and other considerations suggest either that small changes in feeding pattern have significant EL effects or that the psychological effects of food restriction (cf. Welker, Garber, & Brooks, 1977) are important. In the latter case the effect would be IL. In any case, the role of food intake in animal PSS-cancer relationships needs more attention.

Assuming, as is likely, that many PSS effects are IL, it must be remembered that, even if it is linear, the mediation is a multistage process. It runs from exteroceptors to events in the immediate milieu of tumor cells, target cells, carcinogens, or viruses. Thus even when a mediator is identified, the question remains of where in the network of influences it operates. CNS factors, for example, will usually be rather far removed from the final effects.

The question of peripheral mediating factors has received much discussion, but the range of things discussed has been rather limited. For example, Borysenko (1982b, pp. 46–47) listed four specific possibilities: hormonal transformation, reduced immune surveillance against new tumors, increased growth of established or arrested tumors by endocrine changes or immunodepression. Borysenko indicated that other, unspecified, factors might also participate in enhancing established or arrested tumors. As we have noted ("PSS, Immunodepression, and Tumor Enhancement"), it has sometimes appeared to be assumed that only immunologic mechanisms require serious attention as proximal mediators.

Given the amount we do not know, it is useful to be speculative about possible mechanisms. We will organize our speculations by rough stages of tumor development, drawing largely on studies cited previously. The reader should note that we are confining ourselves to IL cases and that even within that restriction, we do not claim exhaustiveness.

Preinitiation

Prior to initiation, endogenous host factors might act to alter levels of initiating agents. PSS can increase levels of glutathione, which affects carcinogen metabolism (Boyd, Sasame, & Boyd, 1981). Polycyclic aromatic hydrocarbon activation is affected by PSS-responsive hormones (Bengtsson & Rydström, 1983). Hormones may regulate the replication of oncogenic viruses (Parks et al., 1974). When PsyS alters immune function, oncogenic viruses may be more or less likely to be eliminated.

Initiation and Promotion

Early in oncogenesis, the actions of initiating agents on target cells may be modifiable by IL processes. Target cell mitotic rates may alter the effects of carcinogens, as when cell division preserves DNA changes (Farber, 1981). The immune system may alter target cell mitosis by modulating nononcogenic infections. Hormones may alter mitotic rates; this may be how preinduction prolactin protects against chemically induced mammary tumors (see Smithline, Sherman, & Kolodny, 1975). Changes in energy substrates may also affect mitosis.

Glucocorticoids can inhibit the incorporation of viral genes into cellular genomes (Gupta & Rapp, 1977). Since the general mechanism of steroid action involves regulation of gene expression by steroid-receptor complexes, it is possible that steroids affect cellular oncogene expression. Perhaps this occurs in hormone-induced transformation. Compounds operating via cyclic nucleotide mechanisms could be involved in activating or deactivating transforming proteins. It is also possible that psychosocial factors influence the DNA repair system. Dilman and Ostroumova (this volume) speculate that this might follow from metabolic changes produced by PSS. Promoters may be subject to metabolic activation or deactivation in ways similar to initiating carcinogens.

Later Premetastatic Growth and Progression

PsyS-responsive hormones affect proliferation of some tumor cells directly (Furth, 1975; Iacobelli et al., 1980; Lippman, 1982). Other factors which affect intracellular regulators such as cyclic nucleotides may also act directly (Cho-Chung et al., 1981; Keller & Keist, 1973). Steroids can retard tumor growth by inhibiting angiogenesis and collagenolysis (Gross et al., 1981).

Tumor cell nutrition may be affected not only by vascularization, but also by regional differences in blood supply. Auerbach and Auerbach (1982) have documented striking regional differences in neoplastic growth. In a variety of tumor types and host strains, tumorigenesis is greater in anterior than posterior body regions. The effect occurs with intradermal, subcutaneous, and intraperitoneal tumors. Auerbach and

Auerbach note that several mechanisms may contribute to these effects. Their discussion of vascular mediation suggests that the blood redistribution produced by PSS might affect tumor development.

As we have seen, immune response to tumor cells is probably an important mediator of IL effects. Immunologic effects need not be direct, however. If PsyS-induced immunomodulation allows viral infection of tumor cells, their antigenicity and subsequent susceptibility to immunologic control may be increased (Zbar et al., 1983). If immunodepression increases the severity of infections, the resulting rise in body temperature may be antitumorigenic (Bull, 1982). Immunologic (or other) attacks on a subpopulation of tumor cells may release others from inter-subpopulation controls (Fidler & Hart, 1982), resulting in tumor enhancement in the long run.

Metastasis

We are unaware that extensive attention has been given to mechanisms of IL effects on metastasis, except as they are similar to premetastatic mechanisms. However, there may well be mechanisms which are peculiar to metastatic spread. The hemostatic system, blood turbulence, and vascular endothelial condition affect metastasis (Donati et al., 1977). Cortisol increases metastases of Walker 256, but has no effect on the primary (Sugarbaker et al., 1970). Intense sound and avoidance conditioning reduce spleen weights in viral leukemia, possibly indicating reduced splenic infiltration. Adrenalectomy prevents that effect (Jensen, 1968).

Discussion

As even a cursory look at the literature reveals, there are many candidates for IL mediating mechanisms. However, these are merely candidates. We reiterate that no mechanism for IL effects is so well supported by data as to compel acceptance, although evidence for immunologic mediation in at least some cases is now rather strong (e. g., Greenberg, Dyck, & Sandler, this volume).

Given the many possibilities, the question is which mediators do in fact act significantly. One part of this question is quantitative. *How much* do psychosocial factors affect mediators, and *how much* effect do those physiologically attainable changes have on Neopl? Relatively little effort has been directed at these issues. An elaboration of the quantitative question concerns the summation of various effects. If there are many mediating sequences, what is the resultant? Corticosteroids, for example, might act to depress or enhance immune function, to increase some oncogenic virus titers, to reduce incorporation of some viral genes, to alter levels of other hormones, and to act directly on some tumor cells. How do these effects add to each other and to the effects of other mediators?

There is probably a complex balance of psychosocially responsive host factors acting upon Neopl, and the outcome probably depends on the balance. This is illustrated by findings of Peters and Kelly (1977) in which both dexamethasone and ACTH enhanced tumor development, but adrenalectomy failed to eliminate the effect of surgical trauma. This kind of interaction highlights the need for quantitative study of mediation.

A further issue deals with host factors whose relations to psychosocial variables are little studied. PsyS might affect blood turbulence, hemostatic factors, or vascular endothelium, either directly or via its effects on other processes such as atherosclerosis and blood pressure. Intracellular regulators might be influenced by psychosocial variables. Polyamines, for example, may protect against carcinogen-induced transformation (Tofilon et al., 1982) but enhance proliferation of neoplastic cells (Luk et al., 1982). Do polyamine concentrations vary with psychosocial factors? Cyclic nucleotides also modulate Neopl (Cho-Chung et al., 1981) and in at least in some types of cells are affected by circulating PsyS-responsive factors such as catecholamines. What effects of psychosocial factors on cyclic nucleotides occur in tumor cells? There are many such questions. Tentative answers for some of them undoubtedly exist in the huge literatures relevant to behavioral oncology. A systematic comparison of (a) factors affected by psychosocial variables, and (b) factors influencing Neopl would surely produce valuable ideas.

The issue of tumor-system differences runs through all consideration of possible IL mediating mechanisms. In some cases, the importance of tumor system is obvious. Hormonal and immunologic control of oncogenic virions is irrelevant if neither virions nor viral antigens are involved. Possibilities for IL effects on nonantigenic and antigenic tumors must be different. Preinitiation and initiation/promotion effects cannot occur in transplanted tumors, except where transplantation from an autochthonous host is employed and that host is subjected to psychosocial manipulations. Allogeneic, and probably multiply passaged syngeneic, transplanted tumors are importantly different from others. Certain questions are irrelevant to tumors that do not metastasize, others to neoplasms that do not grow as solid tumors. However, it is the more subtle tumor differences which are more important, precisely because they are more likely to be overlooked. Differences in tumor-released substances, small differences in antigenicity or nutrient requirements, unexpected differences in hormone responsiveness, and liability to nononcogenic infections are examples.

The host component of tumor systems cannot be overlooked. Basal and/or responsivity differences in almost any biologic function are potentially important. Strain and species differences are obviously critical. Individual differences are less well known to be important but can scarcely fail to be.

Rate of tumor development (and/or latent period) is a tumor system variable which, like the frequent inseparability of host and tumor, constrains what can be known. Post-induction or post-transplantation effects of chronic conditions cannot be studied in rapidly developing tumors. Slowly developing tumors may not show effects of acute conditions unless there is a brief critical period. When the relevant Neopl are gradual, acute events may not occupy a sufficient proportion of tumor development time for their effects to be easily detected. Often it is not possible to do comparable studies of tumor systems with different tumor development rates. One or more of such variables as host age, duration of exposure to experimental treatment, proportion of tumor development time occupied by experimental treatment, or time between treatment and tumor appearance cannot be held constant (Newberry, 1981b).

General Discussion

It should not escape the reader that our intent in this chapter is to contribute to a broadening of the scope of discussion in behavioral oncology. Too much research has been inadequately controlled, reported, or interpreted. Some discussions, even relatively recent ones, give altogether insufficient attention to inconsistent or negative findings, methodologic questions, or the plethora of mediational possibilities. Within a framework emphasizing the probable complexity of phenomena in this field, we have attempted to present both sides of some critical questions. We have attempted, if we erred, to err on the relatively neglected sides of issues.

The following propositions are offered by way of summary and general discussion.

1. At the level of general variable classes, it is apparent that a large number of interacting sequences might relate psychosocial variables to neoplastic processes. Environmental, host psychobiologic, and behavioral factors, in interaction with each other and with neoplastic processes themselves, provide very large numbers of possibilities for relationships between psychosocial variables and neoplastic outcomes (Figure 1).

2. It is useful to distinguish between (a) situations in which behavior affects exposure to relevant exogenous agents (external loop effects), and (b) situations in which psychosocial variables affect neoplastic processes via alterations of endogenous factors (internal loop effects). Demonstration of either type of effect requires controlling for the other.

3. Evidence for internal loop psychosocial effects on human cancer is presently inadequate. This is due to both the difficulty of obtaining truly adequate data on these very complex processes by correlational means and to avoidable methodologic flaws. Prospective studies suffer from difficulties in controlling for the effects of the disease on the supposed predictor variables, and the effects of exposure to large numbers of potentially relevant exogenous agents. Retrospective studies have, in addition, problems of contamination by knowledge of diagnosis, effects of therapy, and response of others to patients' cancers.

4. It is virtually certain that internal loop psychosocial effects occur in experimental cancers. Presumably "stressful" stimulation and manipulations of "stress" hormones have frequently been shown to affect animal neoplasms.

5. Presumably "stressful" stimulation can both enhance and inhibit tumor develoment. Both effects have been reported with considerable frequency in animal studies. It is not known whether one effect is more important than the other, despite implications in published discussions that enhancement is the more important.

6. The stimulation boundary conditions for tumor enhancement and inhibition are not known. Even in animal research, parametric studies, studies comparing qualitatively different experimental conditions, and studies designed to relate to psychological theory have been uncommon or insufficiently programmatic. This is changing, however. There is reason to believe, for example, that controllability of aversive stimulation is important in some cases.

7. The biologic mechanisms mediating internal loop psychosocial effects on neoplastic processes are unknown. There has been an emphasis on the idea that immunodepression induced by "stress" will generally enhance tumor development, but this seems an oversimplification. It is seemingly possible for immunodepression to inhibit tumor development and for "stress" to enhance immune function. There are many other possible mechanisms which have received much less attention and are much further from confirmation. The literature discussed in this chapter suggests that mediation may involve numerous processes and a balance of interacting influences.

8. Tumor system differences are probably critical to internal loop psychosocial influences on cancer. Tumors differ greatly in their responses to the types of host factors which might mediate internal loop effects.

Host differences and differences in stage of tumor development are also relevant. There have been few close comparisons of different tumors' responses to psychosocial conditions, but they have provided evidence for differences, including interactions between tumor system and psychosocial variables. We propose a principle of tumor system specificity: In the absence of evidence to the contrary, it should be assumed that different tumor systems respond to psychosocial factors in different ways and/or through different mechanisms.

9. *It is reasonable to adopt a very tentative working hypothesis that internal loop psychosocial factors affect neoplastic processes in humans.* The variety of conditions under which animal tumors are responsive to psychosocial variables, the number of potential mediators, and the suggestive evidence of human studies combine to suggest such an hypothesis. It has not been confirmed, and it cannot now be predicted how strong such effects might be. However, it is not implausible that internal loop psychosocial effects critically influence the incidence of clinically significant cancers and their course.

References

Achterberg, J., Matthews-Simonton, S., & Simonton, O. C. Psychology of the exceptional cancer patient: A description of patients who outlive predicted life expectancies. *Psychother. Theory Res. Pract.,* 1977, *14,* 416–422.

Ader, R. Conditioned adrenocortical steroid elevations in the rat. *J. Comp. Physiol. Psychol.,* 1976, *60,* 1156–1163.

Ader, R. (Ed.). *Psychoneuroimmunology.* New York: Academic Press, 1981(a).

Ader, R. Conditioned immunopharmacologic responses. In R. Ader (Ed.), *Psychoneuroimmunology.* New York: Academic Press, 1981(b).

Adolph, G. R., & Swetly, P. Glucocorticoid hormones inhibit DNA synthesis and enhance interferon production in a human lymphoid cell line. *Nature,* 1979, *282,* 736–738.

Ahlqvist, J. Hormonal influences on immunologic and related phenomena. In R. Ader (Ed.), *Psychoneuroimmunology.* New York: Academic Press, 1981.

Alexander, P. Innate host resistance to malignant cells not involving specific immunity. In S. B. Day, W. P. L. Myers, P. Stansly, S. Garattini, & M. G. Lewis (Eds.), *Cancer invasion and metastasis: Biologic mechanisms and therapy.* New York: Raven Press, 1977.

Amkraut, A. A., & Solomon, G. F. Stress and murine sarcoma virus (Moloney)-induced tumors. *Cancer Res.,* 1972, *32,* 1428–1433.

Anisman, H. Neurochemical changes elicited by stress: Behavioral correlates. In H. Anisman & G. Bignami (Eds.), *Psychopharmacology of aversively motivated behavior.* New York: Plenum, 1978.

Anisman, H., & Sklar, L. S. Stress provoked neurochemical changes in relation to neoplasia. In S. M. Levy (Ed.), *Biological mediators of behavior and disease: Neoplasia.* New York: Elsevier Biomedical, 1982.

Anisman, H., & Sklar, L. S. Stress as a moderator variable in neoplasia. In G. E. Schwartz, B. Tursky, & L. White (Eds.), *Placebo: Clinical phenomena and new insights.* New York: Guilford Press, in press.

Auerbach, R., & Auerbach, W. Regional differences in the growth of normal and neoplastic cells. *Science,* 1982, *215,* 127–134.

Bacon, C. L., Renneker, R., & Cutler, M. A psychosomatic survey of cancer of the breast. *Psychosom. Med.,* 1952, *14,* 453–460.

Bakhanashvili, M., Wreschner, D. H., & Salzberg, S. Specific antigrowth effect of interferon on mouse cells transformed by murine sarcoma virus. *Cancer Res.,* 1983, *43,* 1289–1294.

Baldwin, R. W., & Price, M. R. Neoantigen expression in chemical carcinogenesis. In F. F. Becker (Ed.), *Cancer: A comprehensive treatise* (Vol. 1). New York: Plenum, 1975.

Balitsky, K. P., & Vinnitsky, V. B. The central nervous system and cancer. In K. Bammer & B. H. Newberry (Eds.), *Stress and cancer.* Toronto: C. J. Hogrefe, 1981

Baltrusch, H. J. F. Psychosomatic cancer research: Present status and future perspectives. In *Psychologie et cancer: Comptes rendu des 2me Journées Medicales sur les Problemes Psychologique en Rapport avec le Cancer.* Paris: Masson, 1978.

Bamborschke, S., O'Connor, P. J., Margison, G. P., Kleihues, P., & Maru, G. B. DNA methylation by dimethylnitrosamine in the Mongolian gerbil *(Meriones unguiculatus):* Indications of a deficient, noninducible hepatic repair system for O^6-methylguanine. *Cancer Res.,* 1983, *43,* 1306–1311.

Bammer, K. Stress, spread and cancer. In K. Bammer & B. H. Newberry (Eds.), *Stress and cancer.* Toronto: C. J. Hogrefe, 1981.

Bartrop, R. W., Lazarus, L., Luckhurst, E., Kiloh, L. G., & Penny, R. Depressed lymphocyte function after bereavement. *Lancet,* 1977, *1,* 834–836.

Becker, F. F. (Ed.). *Cancer: A comprehensive treatise* (4 Vols.). New York: Plenum, 1975.

Bengtsson, M., & Rydström, J. Regulation of carcinogen metabolism in the rat ovary by the estrous cycle and gonadotropin. *Science,* 1983, *219,* 1437–1438.

Bennett, A. Prostaglandins and their synthesis inhibitors in cancer. In S. Iacobelli, R. J. B. King, H. R. Lindner, & M. E. Lippman (Eds.), *Hormones and cancer.* New York: Raven Press, 1980.

Berczi, I., Nagy, E., Kovacs, K., & Horvath, E. Regulation of humoral immunity in rats by pituitary hormones. *Acta Endocrinol.,* 1981, *98,* 506–513.

Besedovsky, H. O., & Sorkin, E. Immunologic-neuroendocrine circuits: Physiological approaches. In R. Ader (Ed.), *Psychoneuroimmunology.* New York: Academic Press, 1981.

Bhattacharyya, A. K., & Pradhan, S. N. Effects of stress on DMBA-induced tumor growth, plasma corticosterone and brain biogenic amines. *Res. Commun. Chem. Pathol. Pharmacol.,* 1979, *23,* 107–116.

Bieliauskas, L. A., & Garron, D. C. Psychological depression and cancer. *Gen. Hosp. Psychiatry,* 1982, *4,* 187–195.

Bishop, J. M. Oncogenes. *Sci. Am.,* 1982, *246* (3), 80–92.

Black, P. H. Shedding from the cell surface of normal and cancer cells. In G. Klein & S. Weinhouse (Eds.), *Advances in cancer research* (Vol. 32). New York: Academic Press, 1980.

Borysenko, J. Z. Behavioral-physiological factors in the development and management of cancer. *Gen. Hosp. Psychiatry,* 1982, *4,* 69–74(a).

Borysenko, J. Z. Higher cortical function and neoplasia: Psychoneuroimmunology. In S. M. Levy (Ed.), *Biological mediators of behavior and disease: Neoplasia.* New York: Elsevier Biomedical, 1982(b).

Borysenko, M., & Borysenko, J. Stress, behavior, and immunity: Animal models and mediating mechanisms. *Gen. Hosp. Psychiatry,* 1982, *4,* 59–67.

Bottazzi, B., Polentarutti, N., Acero, R., Balsari, A., Boraschi, P., Ghezzi, P., Salmona, M., & Mantovani, A. Regulation of the macrophage content of neoplasms by chemoattractants. *Science,* 1983, *220,* 210–212.

Boyd, S. C., Sasame, H. A., & Boyd, M. R. Effects of cold-restraint stress on rat gastric and hepatic glutathione: A potential determinant of response to chemical carcinogens. *Physiol. Behav.,* 1981, *27,* 377–379.

Boyle, D. A. Restraint duration and development of DMBA-induced rat mammary tumor. Unpublished thesis, Kent State University, 1982.

Brady, J. V. Toward a behavioral biology of emotion. In L. Levi (Ed.), *Emotions: Their parameters and measurement.* New York: Raven Press, 1975.

Branceni, D., & Arnason, B. G. Thymic involution and recovery: Immune responsiveness and immunoglobulins after neonatal prednisolone in rats. *Immunology,* 1966, *10,* 35–44.

Brand, K. G. Diversity and complexity of carcinogenic processes: Conceptual inferences from foreign-body tumorigenesis. *J. Natl. Cancer Inst.,* 1976, *57,* 973–976.

Briles, W. E., Briles, R. W., Taffs, R. E., & Stone, H. A. Resistance to a malignant lymphoma in chickens is mapped to subregion of major histocompatibility (B) complex. *Science,* 1983, *219,* 977–979.

Brown, G. W. Meaning, measurement, and stress of life events. In B. P. Dohrenwend & B. S. Dohrenwend (Eds.), *Stressful life events: Their nature and effects.* New York: Wiley, 1974.

Bull, J. M. C. Whole body hyperthermia as an anticancer agent. *CA,* 1982, *32,* 123–128.

Burchfield, S. R., Woods, S. C., & Elich, M. S. Effects of cold stress on tumor growth. *Physiol. Behav.,* 1978, *21,* 537–540.

Burger, J. M., & Arkin, R. M. Prediction, control, and learned helplessness. *J. Pers. Soc. Psychol.,* 1980, *38,* 482–491.

Bürki, K., Liebelt, A. G., & Bresnick, E. Simple vs. complex inheritance of inducible aryl hydrocarbon hydroxylase in mouse tissues. *Biochem. Genet.,* 1975, *13,* 417–433.

Byck, R. Drugs and the treatment of psychiatric disorders. In L. S. Goodman & A. Gilman (Eds.), *The pharmacological basis of theraputics* (5th ed.). New York: Macmillan, 1975.

Cameron, I. L., & Hunter, K. E. Effect of cancer cachexia and amiloride treatment on the intracellular sodium content in tissue cells. *Cancer Res.,* 1983, *43,* 1074–1078.

Cannon, J. G., & Kluger, M. J. Endogenous pyrogen activity in human plasma after exercise. *Science,* 1983, *220,* 617–619.

Chan, P., Ferguson, K. A., & Dao, T. L. Effects of different dietary fats on mammary carcinogenesis. *Cancer Res.,* 1983, *43,* 1079–1083.

Chirigos, M. A., Mitchell, M., Mastrangelo, M. J., & Krim, M. (Eds.). *Mediation of cellular immunity in cancer by immune modifiers.* New York: Raven Press, 1981.

Cho-Chung, Y. S., Clair, T., Bodwin, J. S., & Berghoffer, B. Growth arrest and morphological change of human breast cancer cells by dibutyryl cyclic AMP and L-arginine. *Science,* 1981, *214,* 77–79.

Claman, H. N. Corticosteroids and lymphoid cells. *N. Engl. J. Med.,* 1972, *287,* 388—397.

Cohen, F., & Lazarus, R. S. Coping with the stresses of illness. In G. C. Stone, F. Cohen, & N. Adler (Eds.), *Health psychology.* San Francisco: Jossey Bass, 1979.

Cohen, J., Cullen, J. W., & Martin, L. R. (Eds.), *Psychosocial aspects of cancer.* New York: Raven Press, 1982.

Committee on Diet, Nutrition, and Cancer. *Diet, nutrition, and cancer.* Washington D. C.: National Academy Press, 1982.

Coover, G. D., Sutton, B. R., & Heybach, J. B. Conditioning decreases in plasma corticosterone level in rats by pairing stimuli with daily feedings. *J. Comp. Physiol. Psychol.,* 1977, *91,* 716—726.

Corson, S. A., & Corson, E. O. Constitutional differences in physiologic adaptation to stress. In G. Serban (Ed.), *Psychopathology of human adaptation.* New York: Plenum, 1976.

Cotzias, G. C., & Tang, L. An adenylate cyclase of brain reflects propensity for breast cancer in mice. *Science,* 1977, *197,* 1094—1096.

Cox, T., & Mackay, C. Psychosocial factors and psychophysiological mechanisms in the aetiology and development of cancers. *Soc. Sci. Med.,* 1982, *16,* 381—396.

Cranston, E. M. Effects of some tranquilizers on a mammary adenocarcinoma in mice. *Cancer Res.,* 1958, *18,* 897—899.

Cunningham, A. J. Should we investigate psychotherapy for physical disease, especially cancer? In S. M. Levy (Ed.), *Biological mediators of behavior and disease: Neoplasia.* New York: Elsevier Biomedical, 1982.

Curtis, G. C. Psychoendocrine stress response: Steroid and peptide hormones. In B. A. Stoll (Ed.), *Mind and cancer prognosis.* Chichester, U. K.: Wiley, 1979.

Daniel, P. M., & Prichard, M. L. L. The effect of adrenalectomy on the growth of mammary tumors induced by 3-methylcholanthrene in rats. *Int. J. Cancer,* 1967, *2,* 619—627.

Dannenberg, A. M., Jr. The antiinflammatory effect of glucocorticoids: A brief review of the literature. *Inflammation,* 1979, *3,* 329—343.

Dao, T. L. (Ed.). *Estrogen target tissues and neoplasia.* Chicago: Univ. of Chicago Press, 1972.

Davidson, J. M., Smith, E. R., & Levine, S. Testosterone. In H. Ursin, E. Baade, & S. Levine (Eds.), *Psychobiology of stress: A study of coping men.* New York: Academic Press, 1978.

Dechambre, R. P. Psychosocial stress and cancer in mice. In K. Bammer & B. H. Newberry (Eds.), *Stress and cancer.* Toronto: C. J. Hogrefe, 1981.

Delmonte, L., Liebelt, A. G., & Liebelt, R. A. Granulopoiesis and thrombopoiesis in mice bearing transplanted mammary cancer. *Cancer Res.,* 1966, *26,* 149—159.

de Wied, D., Bohus, B., Gispen, W. H., Urban, I., & van Wimersma Greidanus, T. B. Hormonal influences on motivational, learning, and memory processes. In E. J. Sachar (Ed.), *Hormones, behavior, and psychopathology.* New York: Raven Press, 1976.

De Wys, W. Studies correlating the growth rate of a tumor and its metastases and providing evidence for tumor-related systemic growth-retarding factors. *Cancer Res.,* 1972, *32,* 374—379.

Diamond, L., O'Brien, T., & Baird, W. M. Tumor promoters and the mechanism of tumor promotion. In G. Klein & S. Weinhouse (Eds.), *Advances in cancer research* (Vol 32). New York: Academic Press, 1980.

Donati, M. B., Poggi, A., Mussoni, L., de Gaetano, G., & Garattini, S. Hemostasis and experimental cancer dissemination. In S. B. Day, W. P. L. Myers, P. Stansly, S. Garattini, & M. G. Lewis (Eds.), *Cancer invasion and metastasis: Biologic mechanisms and therapy.* New York: Raven Press, 1977.

Dorian, B. J., Keystone, E., Garfinkel, P. E., & Brown, G. M. Immune mechanisms in acute psychological stress. *Psychosom. Med.,* 1981, *43,* 84. (Abstract)

Dougherty, T. F., & White, A. Influence of adrenal cortical secretion on blood elements. *Science,* 1943, *98,* 367–369.

Duszynski, K. R., Shaffer, J. W., & Thomas, C. B. Neoplasm and traumatic events in childhood: Are they related? *Arch. Gen. Psychiatry,* 1981, *38,* 327–331.

Dworkin, B. R., Filewich, R. J., Miller, N. E., Craigmyle, N., & Pickering, T. G. Baroreceptor activation reduces reactivity to noxious stimulation: Implications for hypertension. *Science,* 1979, *205,* 1299–1301.

Enstrom, J. E. Assessing human epidemiologic data on diet as an etiologic factor in cancer development. *Bull. NY Acad. Med.,* 1982, *58,* 313–322.

Eysenck, H. J. *Smoking, health, and personality.* New York: Basic Books, 1965.

Farber, E. Chemical carcinogenesis. *N. Engl. J. Med.,* 1981, *305,* 1379–1389.

Fidler, I. J. Lymphocytes are not only immunocytes. *Biomedicine,* 1980, *32,* 1–3.

Fidler, I. J., Hart, I. R. Biological diversity in metastatic neoplasms: Origins and implications. *Science,* 1982, *217,* 998–1003.

Fidler, I. J., Kripke, M. L. Tumor cell antigenicity, host immunity, and cancer metastasis. *Cancer Immunol. Immunother.,* 1980, *7,* 201–205.

Fiore, N. Fighting cancer—One patient's perspective. *N. Engl. J. Med.,* 1979, *300,* 284–289.

Foulds, L. *Neoplastic development* (Vol. 1). New York: Academic Press, 1969.

Fox, B. H. Premorbid psychological factors as related to cancer incidence. *J. Behav. Med.,* 1978, *1,* 45–133.

Fox, B. H. Psychosocial factors and the immune system in human cancer. In R. Ader (Ed.), *Psychoneuroimmunology.* New York: Academic Press, 1981.

Fox, B. H. Current theory of psychogenic effects on cancer incidence and prognosis. *J. Psychosoc. Oncol.,* 1983, *1,* 17–31.

Furth, J. Hormones as etiological agents in neoplasia. In F. F. Becker (Ed.), *Cancer: A comprehensive treatise* (Vol. 1). New York: Plenum, 1975.

Garcia, M., & Rochefort, H. Androgen effects mediated by estrogen receptor in 7,12-dimethylbenz(a)anthracene-induced rat mammary tumors. *Cancer Res.,* 1978, *38,* 3922-3929.

Gilman, A. G., Goodman, L. S., & Gilman, A. *The pharmacological basis of theraputics* (6th ed.). New York: Macmillan, 1980.

Goral, J. E., & Wittliff, J. L. Characteristics of progesterone-binding components in neoplastic mammary tissue of the rat. *Cancer Res.,* 1976, *36,* 1886–1893.

Goyette, M., Petropoulos, C. J., Shank, P. R., & Fausto, N. Expression of a cellular oncogene during liver regeneration. *Science,* 1983, *219,* 510–512.

Greene, W. A. The psychological setting of the development of leukemia and lymphoma. *Ann. NY Acad. Sci.,* 1966, *125,* 794–801.

Greer, S., & Morris, T. Psychological attributes of women who develop breast cancer: A controlled study. *J. Psychosom. Res.,* 1975, *19,* 147–153.

Greer, S., & Morris, T. The study of psychological factors in breast cancer: Problems of method. *Soc. Sci. Med.*, 1978, *12*, 129—134.

Greer, S., Morris, T., & Pettingale, K. K. Psychological response to breast cancer: Effect on outcome. *Lancet*, 1979, *2*, 785—787.

Griswold, D. P., & Greene, C. H. Observations on the hormone sensitivity of 7,12-dimethylbenz(a)anthracene-induced mammary tumors in the Sprague-Dawley rat. *Cancer Res.*, 1970, *30*, 819—826.

Gross, J., Azizkhan, R. G., Biswas, C., Bruns, R. R., Hsieh, D., & Folkman, J. Inhibition of tumor growth, vascularization, and collagenolysis in the rabbit cornea by medroxyprogesterone. *Proc. Natl. Acad. Sci. USA*, 1981, *78*, 1176—1180.

Guillemin, R., Vargo, T., Rossier, J., Minick, S., Ling, N., Rivier, C., Vale, W., & Bloom, F. E. β-endorphin and adrenocorticotropin are secreted concomitantly by the pituitary gland. *Science*, 1978, *197*, 1367—1369.

Gupta, P., & Rapp, F. Effect of hormones on Herpes simplex virus type-2-induced transformation. *Nature*, 1977, *267*, 254—255.

Hagnell, O. The premorbid personality of persons who develop cancer in a total population investigated in 1947 and 1957. *Ann. NY Acad. Sci.*, 1966, *125*, 846—855.

Haynes, R. C., & Murad, F. Adrenocorticotropic hormone; adrenocortical steroids and their synthetic analogs; inhibitors of adrenocortical steroid biosynthesis. In A. G. Gilman, L. S. Goodman, & A. Gilman (Eds.), *The pharmacological basis of theraputics* (6th ed.). New York: Macmillan, 1980.

Heise, E., & Gorlich, M. Growth and therapy of mammary tumors induced by 7,12-dimethylbenz(a)anthracene in rats. *Br. J. Cancer*, 1966, *20*, 539—545.

Henry, J. P., Ely, D. L., Watson, F. M. C., & Stephens, P. M. Ethological methods as applied to the measurement of emotion. In L. Levi (Ed.), *Emotions: Their parameters and measurement*. New York: Raven Press, 1975.

Henry, J. P., & Meehan, J. P. Psychosocial stimuli, physiological specificity, and cardiovascular disease. In H. Weiner, M. A. Hofer, & A. J. Stunkard (Eds.), *Brain, behavior, and bodily disease*. New York: Raven Press, 1981.

Henry, J. P., & Stephens, P. M. Caffeine as an intensifier of stress-induced hormonal and pathophysiologic changes in mice. *Pharmacol. Biochem. Behav.*, 1980, *13*, 719—727.

Henry, J. P., Stephens, P. M., & Watson, F. M. Force breeding, social disorder, and mammary tumor formation in CBA/USC mouse colonies: A pilot study. *Psychosom. Med.*, 1975, *37*, 277—283.

Herberman, R. B. Possible effects of central nervous system on natural killer (NK) cell activity. In S. M. Levy (Ed.), *Biological mediators of behavior and disease: Neoplasia*. New York: Elsevier Biomedical, 1982.

Herberman, R. B., & Ortaldo, J. R. Natural killer cells: Their role in defenses against disease. *Science*, 1981, *214*, 24—30.

Hersh, E. M., Reuben, J. M., Bogerd, H., Rosenblum, M., Bielski, M., Mansell, P. W. A., Rios, A., Newell, G. R., & Sonnenfeld, G. Effect of the recreational agent isobutyl nitrite on human peripheral blood leukocytes and on in vitro interferon production. *Cancer Res.*, 1983, *43*, 1365—1371.

Heston, W. E. The genetic aspects of human cancer. In G. Klein & S. Weinhouse (Eds.), *Advances in cancer research* (Vol. 23). New York: Academic Press, 1976.

Heuson, J., & Legros, N. Influence of insulin deprivation on the growth of the 7,12-di-methylbenz(a)anthracene-induced mammary carcinoma in rats subjected to alloxan diabetes and food restriction. *Cancer Res.,* 1972, *32,* 226–232.

Hewitt, H. B. The choice of animal tumors for experimental studies of cancer therapy. In G. Klein & S.Weinhouse (Eds.), *Advances in cancer research.* New York: Academic Press, 1978.

Holland, J. C., & Rowland, J. H. Psychiatric, psychosocial, and behavioral interventions in the treatment of cancer: An historical review. In S. M. Weiss, J. A. Herd, & B. H. Fox (Eds.), *Perspectives on behavioral medicine.* New York: Academic Press, 1981.

Horrobin, D. F., & Trosko, J. E. The possible effect of diazepam on cancer development and growth. *Med. Hypotheses,* 1981, *7,* 133–143.

Huggins, C., Briziarelli, G., & Sutton, H. Rapid induction of mammary carcinoma in the rat and the influence of hormones on the tumors. *J. Exp. Med.,* 1959, *109,* 25–42.

Huggins, C., & Morii, S. Selective adrenal apoplexy and necrosis induced by 7,12-di-methylbenz(a)anthracene. *J. Exp. Med.,* 1961, *114,* 741–761.

Huggins, C., Oka, H., & Fareed, G. Induction of mammary cancer in rats of Long and Evans strain. In T. L. Dao (Ed.), *Estrogen target tissues and neoplasia.* Chicago: Univ. of Chicago Press, 1972.

Iacobelli, S., King, R. J. B., Lindner, H. R., & Lippman, M. E. (Eds.), *Hormones and cancer.* New York: Raven Press, 1980.

Jackson, M. R., & Harris, P. A. Absence of effect of diazepam on tumors. *Lancet,* 1981, *1,* 104.

Jackson, R. L., Maier, S. F., & Coon, D. J. Long-term analgesic effects of inescapable shock and learned helplessness. *Science,* 1979, *206,* 91–93.

Jassem, J., & Serkies, K. Skin reactivity to dinitrochlorobenzene in cancer patients. *Neoplasma,* 1980, *27,* 589–593.

Jensen, M. M. The influence of stress on murine leukemia virus infection. *Proc. Soc. Exp. Biol. Med.,* 1968, *127,* 610–614.

Kavetsky, R. E., Turkevich, N. M., & Balitsky, K. P. On the psychophysiological mechanism of the organism's resistance to tumor growth. *Ann. NY Acad. Sci.,* 1966, *125,* 933–945.

Keast, D. Immune surveillance and cancer. In K. Bammer & B. H. Newberry (Eds.), *Stress and cancer.* Toronto: C. J. Hogrefe, 1981.

Keller, R., & Keist, R. Suppression of growth of P-815 mastocytoma cells *in vitro* by drugs increasing cellular cyclic 3′, 5′-adenosine monophosphate. *Life Sci.,* 1973, *12* (Part II), 97–105.

Keller, S. E., Weiss, J. M., Schleifer, S. J., Miller, N. E., & Stein, M. Suppression of immunity by stress: Effect of a graded series of stressors on lymphocyte stimulation in the rat. *Science,* 1981, *213,* 1397–1400.

Kennett, R. H., Jonak, Z. L., & Byrd, R. Cell surface changes in malignancy. In H. Busch & L. C.Yeoman (Eds.), *Tumor markers.* New York: Academic Press, 1982.

Kiang, D. T., King, M., Zhang, H., Kennedy, B. J., & Wang, N. Cyclic biological expression in mouse mammary tumors. *Science,* 1982, *216,* 68–70.

Kirschbaum, A., & Liebelt, A. G. Thymus and the carcinogenic induction of mouse leukemia. *Cancer Res.,* 1955, *15,* 689–692.

Kirschbaum, A., Liebelt, A. G., & Falls, N. G. Influence of gonadectomy and androgenic hormone on the induction of leukemia by methylcholanthrene in DBA/2 mice. *Cancer Res.,* 1955, *15,* 685–688.

Kissen, D. M., Brown, R., & Kissen, M. A further report on personality and psychosocial factors in lung cancer. *Ann. NY Acad. Sci.,* 1969, *164,* 535—544.

Kobayashi, H. Viral xenogenization of intact tumor cells. In G. Klein & S. Weinhouse (Eds.), *Advances in cancer research* (Vol. 30). New York: Academic Press, 1979.

Konstantinidis, A., Smulow, J. B., & Sonnenschein, C. Tumorigenesis at a predetermined oral site after one intraperitoneal injection of N-nitroso-N-methylurea. *Science,* 1982, *216,* 1235—1237.

Krieger, D. T., & Hughes, J. C. (Eds.). *Neuroendocrinology.* Sunderland, Mass.: Sinauer, 1980.

LaBarba, R. C. Experiential and environmental factors in cancer: A review of research with animals. *Psychosom. Med.,* 1970, *32,* 259—276.

Lahti, R. A., & Barsuhn, C. The effect of minor tranquilizers on stress-induced increases in rat plasma corticosteroids. *Psychopharmacologia,* 1974, *35,* 215—220.

Levine, A. J. Transformation-associated tumor antigens. In G. Klein & S. Weinhouse (Eds.), *Advances in cancer research* (Vol. 37). New York: Academic Press, 1982.

Levy, S. M. (Ed.). *Biological mediators of behavior and disease: Neoplasia.* New York: Elsevier Biomedical, 1982.

Levy, S. M. Host differences in neoplastic risk: Behavioral and social contributors to disease. *Health Psychol.,* 1983, *2,* 21—24.

Lewis, M. G., & Phillips, T. M. The possible effects of emotional stress on cancer mediated through the immune system. In J. Taché, H. Selye, & S. B. Day (Eds.), *Cancer, stress, and death.* New York: Plenum Medical, 1979.

Lewis, M. G., Phillips, T. M., Rowden, G., & Jerry, L. M. Humoral immune factors in metastasis in human cancer. In S. B. Day, W. P. L. Myers, P. Stansly, S. Garattini, & M. G. Lewis (Eds.), *Cancer invasion and metastasis: Biologic mechanisms and therapy.* New York: Raven Press, 1977.

Liebelt, A. G., & Liebelt, R. A. Influence of gonadal hormones and cortisone on spontaneous and methylcholanthrene-induced leukemia in inbred mice. *Cancer Res.,* 1962, *22,* 1180—1187.

Liebelt, A. G., & Liebelt, R. A. Chemical factors in mammary tumorigenesis. In *Carcinogenesis: A broad critique.* (Published for the University of Texas M. D. Anderson Hospital and Tumor Institute.) Baltimore: Williams & Wilkins, 1967 (a).

Liebelt, A. G., & Liebelt, R. A. Transplantation of tumors. In H. Busch (Ed.), *Methods in cancer research* (Vol. 1). New York: Academic Press, 1967 (b).

Liebelt, R. A., Liebelt, A. G., Gulledge, A. A., & Calvert, J. Autoregulation—Normal organ and tumor homeostasis. In *The regulation and spread of neoplastic cells.* (Published for the University of Texas M. D. Anderson Hospital and Tumor Institute.) Baltimore: Williams & Wilkins, 1968.

Liebelt, R. A., Liebelt, A. G., & Lane, M. Hormonal influences on urethan carcinogenesis in C3H/f mice. *Cancer Res.,* 1964, *24,* 1869—1879.

Lippman, M. Interactions of psychic and endocrine factors with progression of neoplastic disease. In S. M. Levy (Ed.), *Biological mediators of behavior and disease: Neoplasia.* New York: Elsevier Biomedical, 1982.

LoBuglio, A. F., Robinson, P., Chirigos, M. A., & Solvay, M. Human monocyte direct cytotoxicity to tumor cells. In M. A. Chirigos, M. Mitchell, M. J. Mastrangelo, & M. Krim (Eds.), *Mediation of cellular immunity in cancer by immune modifiers.* New York: Raven Press, 1981.

Locke, S. E. Stress, adaptation, and immunity: Studies in humans. *Gen. Hosp. Psychiatry,* 1982, *4,* 49—58.

Locke, S., & Kraus, L. Modulation of natural killer cell activity by life stress and coping ability. In S. M. Levy (Ed.), *Biological mediators of behavior and disease: Neoplasia.* New York: Elsevier Biomedical, 1982.

Lubow, R. E., Rosenblatt, R., & Weiner, I. Confounding of controllability in the triadic design for demonstrating learned helplessness. *J. Pers. Soc. Psychol.,* 1981, *41,* 458—468.

Luk, G. D., Civin, C. I., Weissman, R. M., & Baylin, S. B. Ornithine decarboxylase: Essential in proliferation but not differentiation of human promyelocytic leukemia cells. *Science,* 1982, *216,* 75—77.

Lundy, J., Lovett, E. J., Hamilton, S., & Conran, P. Halothane, surgery, immunosuppression and artificial pulmonary metastases. *Cancer,* 1978, *41,* 827—830.

MacLennan, A. J., Drugan, R. C., Hyson, R. L., Maier, S. F., Madden, J., & Barchas, J. D. Corticosterone: A critical factor in an opioid form of stress-induced analgesia. *Science,* 1982, *215,* 1530—1532.

MacLennan, A. J., & Maier, S. F. Coping and stress-induced potentiation of stimulant stereotypy in the rat. *Science,* 1983, *219,* 1091—1093.

Marsh, J. T., Miller, B. E., & Lamson, B. G. Effect of repeated brief stress on growth of Ehrlich carcinoma in mice. *J. Natl. Cancer Inst.,* 1959, *22,* 961—977.

Mason, J. W. A re-evaluation of the concept of "non-specificity" in stress theory. *J. Psychiatr. Res.,* 1971, *8,* 323—333.

Mason, J. W. Emotion as reflected in patterns of endocrine integration. In L. Levi (Ed.), *Emotions: Their parameters and measurement.* New York: Raven Press, 1975.

Matthes, T. Experimental contribution to the question of emotional stress reactions on the growth of tumors in animals. *Proc. Eighth Anti-Cancer Cong.,* 1963, *3,* 471—473.

McCarty, R., Chiueh, C. C., & Kopin, I. J. Spontaneously hypertensive rats: Adrenergic hyperresponsivity to anticipation of electric shock. *Behav. Biol.,* 1978, *23,* 180—188.

Melief, C. J. M., & Schwartz, R. S. Immunocompetence and malignancy. In F. F. Becker (Ed.), *Cancer: A comprehensive treatise* (Vol. 1). New York: Plenum, 1975.

Meltzer, H. Y., & Fang, V. S. Serum prolactin levels in schizophenia — Effect of antipsychotic drugs: A preliminary report. In E. J. Sachar (Ed.), *Hormones, behavior, and psychopathology.* New York: Raven Press, 1976.

Metcalf, D. Adrenal cortical function in high- and low-leukemia strains of mice. *Cancer Res.,* 1960, *20,* 1347—1353.

Miller, E. C., Miller, J. A., & Hartmann, H. A. N-hydroxy-2-acetylaminofluorene: A metabolite of 2-acetylaminofluorene with increased carcinogenic activity in the rat. *Cancer Res.,* 1961, *21,* 815—824.

Miller, N. E. An overview of behavioral medicine: Opportunities and dangers. In S. M. Weiss, J. A. Herd, & B. H. Fox (Eds.), *Perspectives on behavioral medicine.* New York: Academic Press, 1981.

Molomut, N., Lazare, F., & Smith, L. W. Effect of audiogenic stress upon methylcholanthrene-induced carcinogenesis in mice. *Cancer Res.,* 1963, *23,* 1097—1101.

Monaco, M. E., Kidwell, W. R., Kohn, P. H., Strobl, J. S., & Lippman, M. E. Neurohypophyseal hormones and cancer. In S. Iacobelli, R. J. B. King, H. R. Lindner, & M. E. Lippman (Eds.), *Hormones and cancer.* New York: Raven Press, 1980.

Monjan, A. A. Stress and immunologic competence: Studies in animals. In R. Ader (Ed.), *Psychoneuroimmunology.* New York: Academic Press, 1981.

Monjan, A. A., & Collector, M. I. Stress-induced modulation of the immune response. *Science,* 1977, *196,* 307—308.

Moore, D. H. Mammary tumor virus. In F. F. Becker (Ed.), *Cancer: A comprehensive treatise* (Vol. 2). New York: Plenum, 1975.

Morrison, F. R., & Paffenbarger, R. A., Jr. Epidemiological aspects of biobehavior in the etiology of cancer: A critical review. In S. M. Weiss, J. A. Herd, & B. H. Fox (Eds.), *Perspectives on behavioral medicine.* New York: Academic Press, 1981.

Murison, R., Isaksen, E., & Ursin, H. "Coping" and gastric ulceration in rats after prolonged active avoidance performance. *Physiol. Behav.,* 1981, *27,* 345—348.

Muschel, R. J., Khoury, G., Lebowitz, P., Koller, R., & Dhar, R. The human c-ras_1^H oncogene: A mutation in normal and neoplastic tissue from the same patient. *Science,* 1983, *219,* 853—856.

Muslin, H. L., Gyarfas, K., & Pieper, W. J. Separation experience and cancer of the breast. *Ann. NY Acad. Sci.,* 1966, *125,* 802—806.

Nakajima, M., Irimura, T., DiFerrante, D., DiFerrante, N., & Nicolson, G. L., Heparin sulfate degradation: Relation to tumor invasive and metastatic properties of mouse B16 melanoma sublines. *Science,* 1983, *220,* 611—613.

Newberry, B. H. Restraint-induced inhibition of 7,12-dimethylbenz(a)anthracene-induced mammary tumors: Relation to stages of tumor development. *J. Natl. Cancer Inst.,* 1978, *61,* 725—729.

Newberry, B. H. Effects of presumably stressful stimulation (PSS) on the development of animal tumors: Some issues. In S. M. Weiss, J. A. Herd, & B. H. Fox (Eds.), *Perspectives on behavioral medicine.* New York: Academic Press, 1981 (a).

Newberry, B. H. Stress and mammary cancer. In K. Bammer & B. H. Newberry (Eds.), *Stress and cancer.* Toronto: C. J. Hogrefe, 1981 (b).

Newberry, B. H., Frankie, G., Beatty, P. A., Maloney, B. D., & Gilchrist, J. C. Shock stress and DMBA-induced mammary tumors. *Psychosom. Med.,* 1972, *34,* 295—303.

Newberry, B. H., Gildow, J., Wogan, J., & Reese, R. L. Inhibition of Huggins tumors by forced restraint. *Psychosom. Med.,* 1976, *38,* 155—162.

Newberry, B. H., Mactutus, C. F., Boyle, D. A., Gerstenberger, T., & Chambers, L. K. Rodent mammary tumors: Evidence for tumor system specificity in response to presumably stressful conditions. Manuscript submitted for publication.

Nieburgs, H. E., Weiss, J., Navarrete, M., Strax, P., Tierstein, A., Grillone, G., & Siedlecki, B. The role of stress in human and experimental oncogenesis. *Cancer Detect. Prev.,* 1979, *2,* 307—336.

Nimberg, R. B., Glasgow, A. H., Menzoian, J. O., Constantian, M. B., Cooperband, S. R., Mannick, J. A., & Schmid, K. Isolation of an immunosuppressive peptide fraction from the serum of cancer patients. *Cancer Res.,* 1975, *35,* 1489—1494.

Nomura, T. Comparative inhibiting effects of methylxanthines on urethan-induced tumors, malformation, and presumed somatic mutations in mice. *Cancer Res.,* 1983, *43,* 1342—1346.

Novi, A. M. Regression of aflatoxin B_1-induced hepatocellular tumors by reduced glutathione. *Science,* 1981, *212,* 541—542.

Old, L. J. Cancer immunology: The search for specificity. In *Research frontiers in aging and cancer.* (National Cancer Institute Monograph No. 60, NIH Publication No. 82—2436). Washington, D. C.: U. S. Government Printing Office, 1982.

Oppenheimer, S. B. Causes of cancer: Gene alteration versus gene activation. *Am. Lab.,* 1982, *14* (11), 40—46.

Palmblad, J. Stress and immunologic competence: Studies in man. In R. Ader (Ed.), *Psychoneuroimmunology.* New York: Academic Press, 1981.

Parks, W. P., Scolnick, E. M., & Kozikowski, E. H. Dexamethasone stimulation of murine mammary tumor virus replication: A tissue culture source of virus. *Science,* 1974, *184,* 158—160.

Pavlidis, N., & Chirigos, M. Stress-induced impairment of macrophage tumoricidal function. *Psychosom. Med.,* 1980, *42,* 47—54.

Pearson, O. H., Llerena, O., Llerena, L., Molina, A., & Butler, T. Prolactin-dependent rat mammary cancer: A model for man? *Trans. Assoc. Am. Physicians,* 1969, *82,* 225—237.

Perrin, G. M., & Pierce, I. R. Psychosomatic aspects of cancer: A review. *Psychosom. Med.,* 1959, *15,* 397—421.

Peters, L. J., & Kelly, H. The influence of stress and stress hormones on the transplantability of a non-immunogenic syngeneic murine tumor. *Cancer,* 1977, *39,* 1482—1488.

Peters, L. J., & Mason, K. A. Influence of stress on experimental cancer. In B. A. Stoll (Ed.), *Mind and cancer prognosis.* Chichester, U. K.: Wiley, 1979.

Plas-Roser, S., & Aron, C. Stress related effects in the control of sexual receptivity and in the secretion of progesterone by the adrenals in cyclic female rats. *Physiol. Behav.,* 1981, *27,* 261—264.

Popovic, M., Sarin, P. S., Robert-Gurroff, M., Kalyanaraman, V. S., Mann, D., Minowada, J., & Gallo, R. C. Isolation and transmission of human retrovirus (human T-cell leukemia virus). *Science,* 1983, *219,* 856—859.

Poste, G. The cell surface and metastasis. In S. B. Day, W. P. L. Myers, P. Stansly, S. Garattini, & M. G. Lewis (Eds.), *Cancer invasion and metastasis: Biologic mechanisms and therapy.* New York: Raven Press, 1977.

Prehn, R. T. Tumor progression and homeostasis. In G. Klein & S. Weinhouse (Eds.), *Advances in cancer research* (Vol. 23). New York: Academic Press, 1976.

Puckett, C. L., & Shingleton, W. W. The effect of induced diabetes on experimental tumor growth in mice. *Cancer Res.,* 1972, *32,* 789—790.

Ray, P., & Pradhan, S. N. Growth of transplanted and induced tumors in rats under a schedule of punished behavior. *J. Natl. Cancer Inst.,* 1974, *52,* 575—577.

Reif, A. E. Antigenicity of tumors: A comprehensive system of measurement. In H. Busch & L. C. Yeoman (Eds.), *Methods in cancer research* (Vol. XX). New York: Academic Press, 1982.

Riley, V. Spontaneous mammary tumors: Decrease in incidence of mice infected with an enzyme-elevating virus. *Science,* 1966, *153,* 1657—1658.

Riley, V. Mouse mammary tumors: Alteration of incidence as apparent function of stress. *Science,* 1975, *189,* 465—467.

Riley, V. Stress-cancer contradictions: A continuing puzzlement. *Cancer Detect. Prev.,* 1979, *2,* 159—162 (a).

Riley, V. Cancer and stress: Overview and critique. *Cancer Detect. Prev.,* 1979, *2,* 163—195 (b).

Riley, V. Psychoneuroendocrine influences on immunocompetence and neoplasia. *Science,* 1981, *212,* 1100—1109.

Riley, V., Fitzmaurice, M. A., & Spackman, D. H. Psychoneuroimmunologic factors in neoplasia: Studies in animals. In R. Ader (Ed.), *Psychoneuroiummunology.* New York: Academic Press, 1981.

Riley, V., Fitzmaurice, M. A., & Spackman, D. H. Immunocompetence and neoplasia: Role of anxiety stress. In S. M. Levy (Ed.), *Biological mediators of behavior and disease: Neoplasia.* New York: Elsevier Biomedical, 1982.

Rogentine, G. N., van Kammen, D. P., Fox, B. H., Docherty, J. P., Rosenblatt, J. E., Boyd, S. C., & Bunney, W. E. Psychological factors in the prognosis of malignant melanoma: A prospective study. *Psychosom. Med.,* 1979, *41,* 647–655.

Rosch, P. J. Stress and cancer: A disease of adaptation? In J. Taché, H. Selye, & S. B. Day (Eds.), *Cancer, stress, and death.* New York: Plenum Medical, 1979.

Rosellini, R. A., & Seligman, M. E. P. Role of shock intensity in the learned helplessness paradigm. *Anim. Learn. Behav.,* 1978, *6,* 143–146.

Sandberg, G., Ernström, V., Nordlind, K., & Fredholm, B. B. Effect of immunization on the cyclic AMP level and ^{3}H-thymidine incorporation in cultured lymphoid cells. *Int. Arch. Allergy Appl. Immunol.,* 1978, *56,* 449–456.

Sandman, C. A., Kastin, A. J., Schally, A. V., Kendall, J. W., & Miller, L. H. Neuroendocrine responses to physical and psychological stress. *J. Comp. Physiol. Psychol.,* 1973, *81,* 386–390.

Sato, G. H. Towards an endocrine physiology of human cancer. In S. Iacobelli, R. J. B. King, H. R. Lindner, & M. E. Lippman (Eds.), *Hormones and cancer.* New York: Raven Press, 1980.

Schmale, A., & Iker, H. The psychological setting of uterine cervical cancer. *Ann. NY Acad. Sci.,* 1966, *125,* 807–813.

Scott, G. B., Christian, H. J., & Currie, A. R. The Huggins rat mammary tumors: Cellular changes associated with regression. In R. W. Wissler, T. L. Dao, & S. Wood (Eds.), *Endogenous factors influencing host-tumor balance.* Chicago: Univ. of Chicago Press, 1967.

Seifter, E. Of stress, vitamin A, and tumors. *Science,* 1976, *193,* 74–75.

Seligman, M. E. P., Maier, S. F., & Solomon, R. L. Unpredictable and uncontrollable aversive events. In F. R. Brush (Ed.), *Aversive conditioning and learning.* New York: Academic Press, 1971.

Selye, H. *The stress of life* (Rev. ed.). New York: McGraw-Hill, 1976.

Selye, H., & Heuser, G. (Eds.), *Fifth annual report on stress.* Montreal: Acta, 1956.

Senger, D. R., Galli, S. J., Dvorak, A. M., Perruzzi, C. A., Harvey, V. S., & Dvorak, H. F. Tumor cells secrete a vascular permeability factor that promotes accumulation of ascites fluid. *Science,* 1983, *219,* 983–985.

Shapot, V. S. On the multiform relationships between the tumor and the host. In G. Klein & S. Weinhouse (Eds.), *Advances in cancer research* (Vol. 30). New York: Academic Press, 1979.

Shekelle, R. B., Raynor, W. J., Ostfeld, A. M., Garron, D. C., Bieliauskas, L. A., Liu, S. C., Maliza, C., & Paul, O. Psychological depression and 17-year risk of death from cancer. *Psychosom. Med.,* 1981, *43,* 117–125.

Sherwin, S. A., Twardzik, D. R., Bohn, W. H., Cockley, K. D., & Todaro, G. J. High-molecular-weight transforming growth factor activity in the urine of patients with disseminated cancer. *Cancer Res.,* 1983, *43,* 403–407.

Simonton, O. C., & Simonton, S. S. Belief systems and management of the emotional aspects of malignancy. *J. Transpers. Psychol.,* 1975, *7,* 29–47.

Sklar, L. S., & Anisman, H. Stress and coping factors influence tumor growth. *Science,* 1979, *205,* 513—515.

Sklar, L. S., & Anisman, H. Social stress influences tumor growth. *Psychosom. Med.,* 1980, *42,* 347—365.

Sklar, L. S., & Anisman, H. Stress and cancer. *Psychol. Bull.,* 1981, *89,* 369—406 (a).

Sklar, L. S., & Anisman, H. Contributions of stress and coping to cancer development and growth. In K. Bammer & B. H. Newberry (Eds.), *Stress and cancer.* Toronto: C. J. Hogrefe, 1981 (b).

Sklar, L. S., Bruto, V., & Anisman, H. Adaptation to the tumor enhancing effects of stress. *Psychosom. Med.,* 1981, *43,* 331—342.

Smithline, F., Sherman, L., & Kolodny, H. D. Prolactin and breast carcinoma. *N Engl. J. Med.,* 1975, *292,* 784—792.

Snyder, S. H. Brain peptides as neurotransmitters. *Science,* 1980, *209,* 976—983.

Solomon, G. F., Amkraut, A. A., & Rubin, R. T. Stress and psychoimmunological response. In B. A. Stoll (Ed.), *Mind and cancer prognosis.* Chichester, U. K.: Wiley, 1979.

Starzec, J., Hesse, R., Pytko, D., Dewey, L., & Berger, D. Running and response to stress in rats. Paper presented at the meeting of the Midwestern Psychological Association, Chicago, 1979.

Stein, M. Aging and the immune system: Psychosocial perspective. Paper presented at the Meeting of the Academy of Behavioral Medicine Research, Reston, Virginia, 1983.

Stein, M., Schleifer, S. J., & Keller, S. E. Hypothalamic influences on immune responses. In R. Ader (Ed.), *Psychoneuroimmunology.* New York: Academic Press, 1981.

Stone, J. P., Holtzman, S., & Shellabarger, C. J. Neoplastic responses and correlated prolactin levels in diethylstilbestrol-treated ACI and Sprague—Dawley rats. *Cancer Res.,* 1979, *39,* 773—778.

Strupp, H. H. Psychotherapy research and practice: An overview. In A. E. Bergin & S. L. Garfield (Eds.), *Handbook of psychotherapy and behavior change.* New York: Wiley, 1978.

Stutman, O. Immunodepression and malignancy. In G. Klein, S. Weinhouse, & A. Haddow (Eds.), *Advances in cancer research* (Vol. 22). New York: Academic Press, 1975.

Sugarbaker, E. V. The organ selectivity of experimentally induced metastases in rats. *Cancer,* 1952, *5,* 606—612.

Sugarbaker, E. V., Cohen, A. M., & Ketcham, A. S. Facilitated metastatic distribution of the Walker 256 tumor in Sprague-Dawley rats with hydrocortisone and/or cyclophosphamide. *J. Surg. Oncol.,* 1970, *2,* 277—289.

Sugarbaker, E. V., Thornthwaite, J., & Ketcham, A. S. Inhibitory effect of a primary tumor on metastasis. In S. B. Day, W. P. L. Myers, P. Stansly, S. Garattini, & M. G. Lewis (Eds.), *Cancer invasion and metastasis: Biologic mechanisms and therapy.* New York: Raven Press, 1977.

Sunkara, P. S., Prakash, N. J., Mayer, G. D., & Sjoerdsma, A. Tumor suppression with a combination of α-difluoromethyl ornithine and interferon. *Science,* 1983, *219,* 851—853.

Tannenbaum, A. The initiation and growth of tumors. I. Effects of underfeeding. *Am. J. Cancer,* 1940, *38,* 335—350.

Tarlau, M., & Smalheiser, I. Personality patterns in patients with malignant tumors of the breast and cervix. *Psychosom. Med.,* 1951, *13,* 117—121.

Thomas, C. B., Duszynski, K. R., & Shaffer, J. W. Family attitudes reported as potential predictors of cancer. *Psychosom. Med.,* 1979, *41,* 287–302.

Tofilon, P. J., Oredsson, S. M., Deen, D. F., & Marton, L. J. Polyamine depletion influences drug-induced chromosomal damage. *Science,* 1982, *217,* 1044–1046.

Turkevich, N. M. The development of the neoplastic process during functional changes of the higher part of the nervous system. In R. E. Kavetsky (Ed.), *The neoplastic process and the nervous system.* Kiev: The State Medical Publishing House, 1958. (Translated by the Israel Program for Scientific Translations. Published by NSF, Washington, D. C., 1960.)

Van Vugt, D. A., Bruni, J. F., & Meites, J. Naloxone inhibition of stress-induced increases in prolactin secretion. *Life Sci.,* 1978, *22,* 85–89.

Visintainer, M. A., Volpicelli, J. R., & Seligman, M. E. P. Tumor rejection in rats after inescapable or escapable shock. *Science,* 1982, *216,* 437–439.

Watkins, L. R., & Mayer, D. J. Organization of endogenous opiate and nonopiate pain control systems. *Science,* 1982, *216,* 1185–1192.

Weinshilboum, R. M. Biochemical genetics of catecholamines in humans. *Mayo Clin. Proc.,* 1983, *58,* 319–330.

Welker, R. L., Garber, J., & Brooks, F. Stress as a function of irregular feeding of food deprived rats. *Physiol. Behav.,* 1977, *18,* 639–645.

Wellisch, D. K. Intervention with the cancer patient. In C. K. Prokop & L. A. Bradley (Eds.), *Medical psychology: Contributions to behavioral medicine.* New York: Academic Press, 1981.

Wunderlich, J. Behavioral regulation of immunity: Implications for human cancer. In S. M. Levy (Ed.), *Biological mediators of behavior and disease: Neoplasia.* New York: Elsevier Biomedical, 1982.

Wurtman, R. J., & Fernstrom, J. D. Neuroendocrine effects of psychotropic drugs. In E. J. Sachar (Ed.), *Hormones, behavior, and psychopathology.* New York: Raven Press, 1976.

Yates, J., Couchman, J. R., & King, R. J. B. Androgen effects on growth, morphology, and sensitivity of S 115 mouse mammary tumor cells in culture. In S. Iacobelli, R. J. B. King, H. R. Lindner, & M. E. Lippman (Eds.), *Hormones and cancer.* New York: Raven Press, 1980.

Zbar, B., Nagai, A., Terata, N., & Hovis, J. Tumor rejection mediated by an amphotropic murine leukemia virus. *Cancer Res.,* 1983, *43,* 46–53.

Zimbardo, P. G. (Ed.), *The cognitive control of motivation.* Glenview, Ill.: Scott, Foresman, 1969.

Conditioned Responses to Cancer Chemotherapy: Etiology and Treatment

Thomas G. Burish and Michael P. Carey[1]

Since chemotherapeutic agents were first systematically prescribed for the treatment of cancer approximately 40 years ago, the use of these drugs has increased dramatically. In contrast to the early prescription of chemotherapy primarily as a last-resort treatment for cancers that could not be treated with or did not respond to other approaches, chemotherapy is now considered the treatment of choice for several types of cancers. Moreover, rather than using chemotherapy primarily as a means of causing remissions in patients, it is now often used with the intent of cure (Laszlo, 1983b). Clearly, in dealing with the *physical* progression of the disease, cancer chemotherapies have made considerable gains.

Unfortunately, these gains have not come without costs. As has been pointed out by physicians (e.g., Harris, 1978; Laszlo & Lucas, 1981; Siegal & Longo, 1981), nurses (e.g., Oberst, 1978), and cancer patients themselves (e.g., Cohn, 1982; Rosenthal, 1973), chemotherapy can produce some of the most adverse side effects of any cancer treatment. One particular cancer patient that we treated conveyed to us the horrors she experienced as follows: "The best way I can describe to you my chemotherapy experience is to ask you to recall the last time you had the flu. Remember especially the worst 10 minutes of that flu episode, when you were hovering over a toilet or basket as you threw up whatever was in your stomach; after that was gone, you just continued to retch without control. You felt tired. Your muscles ached. You were always cold and shivering. You did not like how you felt, the way you looked, or the putrid odor of vomit you could never get rid of. Then, multiply that experience by 50 or 100 times so that it lasts 8 to 16 hours

[1] The writing of this chapter was supported in part by a grant from the National Cancer Institute (CA25516). The authors thank William H. Redd, Beth E. Meyerowitz, and Gary R. Morrow for their helpful comments on an earlier draft of the manuscript.

in a row, without much let-up. Finally, to all of this, add the fear—a real honest-to-God fear—that you may never wake up from this nightmare, that you may die."

As a result of the aversiveness of cancer chemotherapy, some patients become severely depressed and even suicidal, while many others refuse to continue treatment, well aware that a hastened death is the probable consequence of their decision. This sequence of events has led some oncologists to suggest that the side effects of chemotherapy are not only aversive, but can in effect be considered fatal (e.g., Penta, Poster, & Bruno, 1983), and has led many physicians to join with distressed cancer patients in pleading for the development of agents effective in counteracting these side effects (e.g., Whitehead, 1975).

There are basically two types of side effects associated with cancer chemotherapy. The most widely acknowledged and thoroughly researched type of side effect is *pharmacological* in nature. Pharmacological side effects result from the fact that the cytotoxic drugs used in cancer chemotherapy do not limit their action to cancerous tissue but rather affect virtually every cell in the body. The damage caused to noncancerous tissue by these drugs often results in a number of noxious side effects, with gastrointestinal problems such as nausea and vomiting probably being the most severe (Golden, 1975; Greer, 1979). These pharmacological side effects usually occur one to two hours following chemotherapy administration and can last for as long as several days (Frytak & Moertel, 1981). They are generally treated with some type of antianxiety or antiemetic medication, for example, proclorperazine, metoclopramide, or delta-9-tetrahydrocannabinol (THC). Unfortunately, none of the currently used antianxiety or antiemetic medications is both nontoxic and completely effective in reducing pharmacologically based chemotherapy side effects (see Laszlo, 1983a).

The second type of side effects, most commonly referred to as *conditioned* side effects, are psychological rather than pharmacological in nature, and are the focus of the present chapter. Although conditioned side effects can be as aversive as or more aversive than pharmacological side effects, they have only recently been the object of systematic empirical investigation. In contrast to pharmacological side effects, little research has been carried out to assess the effectiveness of antiemetic medications in alleviating these symptoms. However, several increasingly well-designed investigations suggest that behavioral relaxation techniques may be very effective in this regard. If that is so, behavioral interventions may hold promise for increasing the quality and perhaps length of life for many cancer patients.

The present chapter is divided into four major sections. The first section focuses on the nature, etiology, and prevalence of conditioned side effects, while the second section focuses on their treatment with pharmacological and especially behavioral techniques. The next section of the paper is devoted to issues relevant to the clinical application of behavioral techniques on a large scale basis. The final section provides a brief summary and a discussion of conclusions that can be drawn about the etiology and treatment of conditioned side effects associated with cancer chemotherapy.

Nature and Development of Nonpharmacological Side Effects

It has been commonly noted that many patients who undergo cancer chemotherapy display nausea, vomiting, and increased levels of negative emotions such as anxiety not only after they receive their chemotherapy treatment but also before. For example, Redd and Andresen (1981) reported that they have had patients vomit as they dressed at home in preparation for their chemotherapy clinic visit, and we have had a patient vomit in a drugstore when she recognized that the nurse who administered her chemotherapy was standing in the same aisle (Lyles, Burish, Krozely, & Oldham, 1982). Additionally, it has been commonly noted that the intensity of postchemotherapy side effects in some patients seems to be much greater than what one would expect based upon the emetic potential of the antineoplastic drugs they are receiving. Such observations have led many clinicians and researchers to hypothesize that psychological factors ranging from unconscious conflicts to classically conditioned associations might be responsible for some of the side effects of chemotherapy. That is, while chemotherapy drugs are clearly toxic agents that can cause a variety of adverse side effects in addition to their antineoplastic effects, other factors must clearly be present to account for prechemotherapy symptoms or unusually high levels of postchemotherapy symptoms. Unfortunately, these nonpharmacological side effects can be very intense, and in some patients can be more aversive than the pharmacological side effects. Moreover, because they can occur before and during chemotherapy, they can also be particularly problematic for the medical staff involved in administering the chemotherapy. For example, with some patients chemotherapy treatments must be interrupted several times because of the patients' crying and shaking or frequent vomiting.

While the presence of nonpharmacological nausea, vomiting, and other side effects in some chemotherapy patients is widely acknowledged, the cause of these side effects is controversial. At least five hypotheses have been offered to explain these symptoms. First, Redd and Andrykowski (1982) have suggested that it is conceivable that an operant learning mechanism might be able to account in part for these symptoms in some patients. That is, the secondary gains (e.g., sympathy, attention) accrued from these illness behaviors might be sufficient to maintain their expression. While research on operantly determined illness behavior in other chronic disease areas (e.g., pain, Fordyce, 1978; diabetes, Turkat, 1982) has implicated this mechanism, few data exist to support the notion that nonpharmacological nausea, vomiting, and other side effects develop in patients because of the attention or other reinforcement they may produce. It is likely that many chemotherapy patients receive attention and other secondary gains simply because they have cancer, and additional attention because of their pharmacologically produced side effects. As a result there would appear to be little additional reinforcement value, but a considerable cost, to developing nonpharmacological nausea, vomiting, anxiety, and other symptoms.

Second, Chang (1981, 1982) has suggested a psychodynamic interpretation of anticipatory nausea and vomiting. Chang hypothesized that nonpharmacological side effects "may be surfacing manifestations of underlying psychological readjustment problems associated with life-threatening illnes" (1981, p.707). Chang suggested further that nonpharmacological side effects develop in those patients who cannot fully accept the diagnosis of cancer and the treatment it requires. Consequently, these patients become angry, anxious, and/or frustrated with no target for these negative affects, and therefore, they direct these emotions toward the chemotherapy treatment by exhibiting "psychological" side effects. To date, there are no data to support this hypothesis.

Third, it has been suggested (Redd & Andrykowski, 1982) that anxiety might be the mediating factor in the development of nonpharmacological side effects. That is, nausea and vomiting might be the consequence of an extreme anxiety reaction. Although similar mechanisms have been suggested to account for the nausea and vomiting observed in psychiatric patients (e.g., Swanson, Swenson, Huizenga, & Melson, 1976), no direct evidence exists for this mode of development in chemotherapy patients. Nerenz, Leventhal, and Love (1982) reported that patients who developed nonpharmacological side effects reported higher anxiety levels than those who did not develop nonpharmacological side effects; however, it is not clear from these data whether the anxiety was a cause or result of the increased side effects. Moreover, if high levels of anxiety were the causes of the nausea and vomiting, one might expect that these patients would have displayed nausea and vomiting in at least some other high anxiety situations. However, apparently this has not been the case (e.g., Morrow, 1982; Nesse, Carli, Curtis, & Kleinman, 1980). Thus, although anxiety may be associated with the presence of conditioned nausea and vomiting, and may play a role in exacerbating these symptoms, it is unlikely that with most cancer patients high levels of anxiety alone are responsible for the development of nonpharmacological side effects.

Fourth, a physiological mechanism has been proposed to account for the development of nonpharmacological side effects. Specifically, it has been hypothesized that anticipatory symptoms may "be produced by brain metastasis or local cancer involvement of the gastrointestinal tract" (Chang, 1981, p.707). While this explanation may be correct for a few patients, it is highly improbable that it can account for the development of nonpharmacological symptoms in most patients. For example, Morrow (1982) reported screening his patients for brain metastases and gastrointestinal tumors that might cause nausea or vomiting and found that none of the 47 patients in his study who developed nonpharmacological side effects had such problems.

A fifth hypothesis, and the one with appears to have the most empirical support, suggests that nonpharmacological side effects represent classically conditioned responses (Andrykowski, Redd, & Hatfield, 1982; Burish & Lyles, 1979, 1981; Katz, 1982; Nesse et al., 1980; Redd & Andresen, 1981). This hypothesis states that after several courses of chemotherapy an association is established between the pharmacological side effects caused by chemotherapy and the various sights, smells, and even thoughts associated with the chemotherapy setting (see Figure 1). As a result of this association, the neutral stimuli

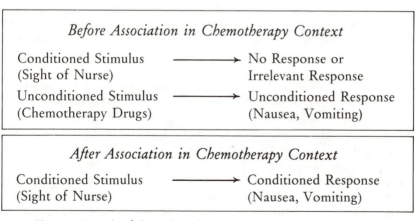

Figure 1. Example of classical conditioning in the chemotherapy context.

themselves begin to elicit the side effects. Thus, the sight of a syringe, the odor of alcohol, or even the thought of receiving chemotherapy can come to elicit nausea, retching, and vomiting. Support for the classical conditioning hypothesis comes from a variety of *indirect* sources. First, experimental laboratory research has clearly demonstrated that animals that ingest drugs that cause vomiting, even if the vomiting occurs hours after drug ingestion, quickly develop conditioned responses to stimuli associated with the drug injection experience, including the development of conditioned emesis (see Redd & Andrykowski, 1982). Second, Bernstein and her colleagues (e.g., Bernstein, 1978; Bernstein & Webster, 1980) have demonstrated that both children and adults receiving chemotherapy develop conditioned taste aversions to foods associated with the chemotherapy treatment, illustrating that the chemotherapy situation can become a conditioned stimulus. Third, as is discussed at length later in the chapter, behavioral approaches predicated upon the hypothesis that anticipatory nausea and vomiting are conditioned responses have been found to be highly effective in reducing these responses. Finally, the nature and development of anticipatory responses in cancer chemotherapy patients appear to correspond closely with what would be expected on the basis of a classical conditioning model.

Obviously, each of the four lines of reasoning described above is indirect, and none of them scientifically and conclusively establishes that the anticipatory responses displayed by cancer patients are classically conditioned in nature. However, the fact that the only evidence of any kind available concerning the origin of these responses is indirect, and that most if not all of this evidence supports a conditioning model has led the large majority of researchers in the area (e.g., Moore & Altmaier, 1981; Morrow, 1982; Nesse et al., 1980; Redd & Andrykowski, 1982), including ourselves (e.g., Burish & Lyles, 1981; Burish, Carey, Redd, & Krozely, 1983) to endorse this explanation. Consistent with this orientation, throughout the remainder of the chapter we will frequently refer to nonpharmacological side effects as conditioned side effects.

Finally, it is possible that nonpharmacological side effects might develop when several of the mechanisms reviewed above operate together. For example, it is conceivable that anticipatory side effects are developed through classical conditioning and are maintained partially by operant mechanisms (e.g., secondary gains). Additionally, the presence of "psychological readjustment problems" or anxiety might make a patient more susceptible to the conditioning process. This vulnerability might be conceptualized as a kind of "preparedness" (Seligman, 1971) which predisposes certain individuals to learn more quickly the association between chemotherapy-related stimuli and the drug-induced side effects.

Hopefully, future research will explore the possible interaction of several factors in the development and maintenance of nonpharmacological side effects.

Prevalence of Conditioned Side Effects

One difficulty in obtaining a valid and reliable estimate of the prevalence of conditioned side effects is that these symptoms can occur in combination with the pharmacological symptoms following chemotherapy treatment. Because it is very difficult to disentangle these two components of postchemotherapy symptoms, most researchers interested in the prevalence of conditioned side effects have focused on anticipatory side effects, i.e., side effects occurring before the chemotherapy is actually administered. Moreover, because almost all patients show an increase in anxiety and other negative emotions as treatment times approach, most researchers have not focused on these symptoms but rather on the presence of anticipatory nausea and vomiting.

At least ten investigations have been reported to date on the prevalence of anticipatory nausea and vomiting (Coons, 1981; Morrow, 1982; Morrow, Arseneau, Asbury, Bennett, & Boros, 1982; Nerenz et al., 1982; Nesse et al., 1980; Nicholas, 1982; Scogna & Smalley, 1979; Wilcox, Fetting, Nettesheim, & Abeloff, 1982; Cohen, Sheehan, Ruckdeschel, & Blanchard, 1982; Nerenz, Leventhal, Love et al., 1982). These 10 reports have differed widely in their estimates of the number of chemotherapy patients who develop anticipatory side effects. For example, Coons (1981) reported that 65% of the patients she observed exhibited anticipatory side effects, while Nicholas (1982) reported that only 18.3% of his patients experienced these side effects. The apparent discrepancy between the reported rates can be resolved partially by examining several of the more important methodological differences among the studies.

First, the criteria which have been used to identify a patient as experiencing anticipatory side effects have not been consistent across studies. Some studies have defined anticipatory side effects as the presence of either anticipatory nausea or anticipatory vomiting, whereas other studies have required the presence of both anticipatory nausea and vomiting to classify a patient as having anticipatory side effects. A recent report by Morrow et al. (1982) illustrates this assessment problem clearly: when the presence of anticipatory vomiting was necessary to meet the criterion, only 9% of the patients were identified as experiencing anticipatory side effects, whereas when anticipatory nausea only was used, 24% of the patients were found to have anticipatory side effects. Thus, to a limited extent, the different prevalence rates reported are the product of differing assessment criteria. Future investigators would do well to present data for anticipatory nausea and vomiting separately (e.g., Morrow et al., 1982; Cohen et al., 1982).

A second methodological difference which might account for different prevalence rates is that time of assessment has varied across the reported studies. For example, Morrow (1982) assessed all patients during their fourth treatment cycle while Scogna and Smalley (1979) questioned patients after their third course of chemotherapy. In other studies patients are not equated on number of cycles of treatment, leaving this factor completely confounded (e.g., Nicholas, 1982). It is likely that for many patients the prevalence of anticipatory side effects increases as the number of chemotherapy treatments received increases. For example, Nerenz et al. (1982) reported that the proportion of patients reporting anticipatory nausea increased from 14% during cycle 1 to 35% during cycles 4–6. Therefore, differences in reported prevalence rates may to some extent be a reflection of the point in the treatment cycle when the anticipatory side effects are assessed.

Finally, differences in reported prevalence rates may reflect to a large degree the specific antineoplastic drugs that the patients on a particular study were receiving. For example, Nerenz et al. (1982) have reported that 65% of their patients receiving Cis-platinum exhibited anticipatory side effects whereas only 15% of their patients receiving Cytoxan, Methotrexate and 5-FU (CMF) exhibited these side effects. Morrow (1982) also reported that patients taking Cis-platinum were more likely to exhibit anticipatory side effects than patients receiving other chemotherapeutic agents.

Because of methodological problems such as those discussed above, it is difficult to identify with certainty the prevalence of anticipatory side effects. However, it is possible to estimate this figure by combining the data across all studies to get a composite index of the prevalence of anticipatory side effects in the general population of cancer chemotherapy patients. In the 10 studies cited above, a total of 880 patients were evaluated. Using the criteria of anticipatory nausea and/or anticipatory vomiting as indicating the presence of anticipatory side effects, approximately 329 or 37% of the patients can be identified as experiencing anticipatory side effects.

Prediction of Conditioned Side Effects

Because not all chemotherapy patients experience conditioned side effects, several investigators have attempted to determine which patients are and are not likely to develop these symptoms. Identifying patients who are likely to develop conditioned side effects might make possible the efficient use of intervention aimed at preventing or weakening the development of these side effects.

At least eight different characteristics have been identified as potential predictors of the development of conditioned side effects: high levels of frequency, severity, and duration of posttreatment nausea and vomiting (Cohen et al., 1982; Morrow, 1982; Nesse et al., 1980; Nicholas, 1982; Scogna & Smalley, 1979; Wilcox et al., 1982); comparatively young (e.g., less than 60) as opposed to old (e.g., greater than 60) age (Cohen et al., 1982; Morrow, 1982); high levels of anxiety (Altmaier, Ross, & Moore, 1982; Coons, 1981; Love, Nerenz, & Leventhal, in press; Nerenz, Leventhal, Love, et al., 1982); strong sensations of taste or smell during chemotherapy (Coons, 1981; Love et al., in press; Nerenz, Leventhal, & Love, 1982; Nerenz, Leventhal, Love et al., 1982); high as opposed to low numbers of previous chemotherapy treatments (Nesse et al., 1980); multi-drug as opposed to single drug chemotherapy regimens (Morrow, 1982); high as opposed to low emetic potential of the chemotherapy regimen (Morrow, 1982; Nerenz, Leventhal, Love et al., 1982); and an inhibitive rather than a facilitative coping style (Altmaier et al., 1982). While the number of possible predictors which have been identified is large, it may be possible for heuristic purposes to condense these variables into three factors: (1) emetic potential of the chemotherapy agent; (2) strength of the conditioning experience; and (3) individual differences.

The emetic potential of the chemotherapy agent can account, in large part, for the frequency, severity, and duration of posttreatment nausea and vomiting (Rozencweig, Von Hoff, Slavik, & Muggia, 1977). Similarly, patients who are younger are more likely to have certain forms of cancer, such as testicular cancer, which require chemotherapy agents that tend to have a greater emetic potential (Laszlo, 1983b). Finally, an increase in the number of drugs in the chemotherapy regimen typically indicates an increase in the emetic potential of the regimen (Laszlo, 1983b). Overall, the variables we believe contribute to the emetic potential of a chemotherapy treatment have been cited as important factors in virtually every investigation on the development of conditioned side effects to chemotherapy. This fact suggests that if the chemotherapy agent has a strong enough emetic potential, it alone may be sufficient to produce anticipatory side effects.

A second and related factor that might also predict conditioned side effects is the strength of the conditioning experience. Specifically, an increase in the number of exposures as well as an increase in the salience of the conditioned stimuli are likely to result in a stronger conditioned response. Therefore, as the number of chemotherapy treatments (i.e., the number of conditioning trials) increases, it is likely that the development of classically conditioned responses (i.e., conditioned side effects such as nausea and vomiting) will be strengthened. Similarly, conditioned stimuli which are very salient (e.g., strong sensations of taste or smell associated with chemotherapy drugs) are likely to increase the strength of the conditioned response. As mentioned above, however, if chemotherapy agents have a sufficiently strong emetic potential, only one treatment may be needed for the development of conditioned side effects.

A third factor which might be predictive of the development of conditioned side effects consists of individual differences such as the effectiveness of one's coping skills. These individual difference factors may in turn affect the strength of the conditioning experience, and as a result affect the development of conditioned responses. For example, high anxiety levels generally produce more rapid conditioning. Patients who do not possess an effective coping style and therefore experience high levels of anxiety during the chemotherapy treatment may be more likely to develop stronger conditioned side effects than patients who are able to cope effectively and, therefore, experience less anxiety. In those patients who are receiving chemotherapy agents which are relatively weak in their emetic potential, the presence or absence of coping skills thus may be a critical factor in determining whether or not anticipatory side effects develop. However, even when the presence of strong coping skills may not be sufficient to prevent the occurrence of anticipatory side effects, for example, when the emetic potential of the chemotherapy agent is great, these skills may nonetheless be useful in reducing the perceived aversiveness of the conditioned (and pharmacological) symptoms.

Additional individual differences that might be important include a patient's personal (e.g., family and friends) and medical (e.g., nurses and physicians) support system, previous coping history, and perceived self-efficacy. These and other individual differences will affect the chemotherapy experience of each patient differently.

In summary, we suggest that an assessment of the emetic potential of the chemotherapy drugs, the strength of the conditioning experience, and individual differences in coping skills may allow a fairly accurate prediction of which patients will develop conditioned side effects. In this assessment, it will be necessary to weigh each of the factors differently, for although each factor will be present to some degree in each patient, the factors will not be equal in their influence. As suggested previously, for example, a high emetic potential of the chemotherapy drugs may be sufficient for the development of conditioned responses regardless of the strength of the other two factors. Future research is needed to determine the validity and importance of these hypothesized factors and the nature of their interactions.

Summary

Many cancer patients display nonpharmacologically based as well as pharmacologically based side effects to their chemotherapy treatment. Of the several hypotheses that have been proferred for the etiology of nonpharmacological side effects, the one that appears the most valid is that they result from a classical conditioning process through which sights, smells, tastes, and even thoughts associated with the chemotherapy process become able to elicit by themselves responses such as nausea, vomiting, and increased levels of anxiety and other negative emotions. Studies of the prevalence of conditioned side effects indicates that approximately one-third of all chemotherapy patients experience anticipatory nausea and/or emesis. Three factors have been proposed that might predict which patients are most likely to develop conditioned side effects: the emetic potential of the chemotherapy agent, the strength of the conditioning experience, and individual differences in coping skills and available support systems.

Interventions for Treating Conditioned Side Effects

Pharmacological Interventions

The vast majority of studies assessing the effectiveness of various antianxiety and antiemetic medications have focused on those side effects that appear during or after chemotherapy (see Poster, Penta, & Bruno, 1981). For the most part, these side effects have been considered pharmacological in nature, though in actuality they probably reflect a combination of both pharmacological and conditioned responses. For example, Chang and his colleagues, in a report on the effectivness of THC in reducing nausea and vomiting, observed a decrease in the effectiveness of THC over time and suggested that this decrease may have been due to "the development of anticipatory or conditioned nausea and vomiting, which commonly occurs in patients receiving repeated courses of chemotherapy" (Chang et al., 1979, p. 823). However, Chang et al.'s study "was not designed to assess the ability of THC to prevent or reduce anticipatory nausea or vomiting" (p. 823). Unfortunately, the same design limitation applies to most if not all of the other pharmacologically oriented treatment studies published to date. Thus, the effectiveness of antiemetic medications on conditioned side effects is essentially unknown.

Although no research has been carried out to assess the specific effects of antiemetic medication on conditioned nausea and vomiting, two general points should be made in regard to the use of antiemetics to treat these symptoms. First, the fact that researchers have not addressed the impact of pharmacologic agents on conditioned side effects does not imply that these agents are ineffective in this regard. It may be that if antiemetic medications are given during the hours or days before chemotherapy, as some oncologists have suggested (e. g., Lucas & Laszlo, 1980), anticipatory symptoms could be significantly reduced. Moreover, it is possible and perhaps likely that the reductions in postchemotherapy nausea and vomiting caused by some antiemetics are in part due to a reduction of conditioned as well as pharmacological side effects. Clearly, carefully designed research is needed to determine the impact of pharmacological treatments on conditioned symptoms.

Second, it should be noted that even if various drugs prove to be strikingly effective in reducing chemotherapy-associated nausea and vomiting, most of these drugs appear to produce several side effects, for example, tiredness, loss of muscle coordination, hallucinations, psychological highs and lows, and various organ toxicities. For some patients, these side effects can outweigh potential benefits. For instance, although some patients admit that THC helps to control emesis, they refuse to continue taking the drug because it can cause hallucinations, concentration difficulties, tachycardia, and usually results in a perceived loss of muscle coordination (Frytak et al., 1979). Thus, while the search for effective pharmacological treatments should continue, this search should not dampen present enthusiasm for or acceptance of the pursuit of alternate approaches to controlling the side effects of chemotherapy, including behavioral approaches. Of course, if a completely effective and nontoxic antiemetic drug were developed, pharmacologically caused nausea and vomiting would be eliminated, and therefore conditioned nausea and vomiting would not develop. In such a situation, there would be no need of additional antiemetic treatment, including behavioral treatment. As the data reviewed in the next sections show, however, behavioral interventions may have benefits beyond the reduction of nausea and vomiting, and therefore their usefulness must be evaluated in this broader context.

Behavioral Interventions

Most behavioral reseachers interested in reducing the adverse side effects of chemotherapy have focused on conditioned nausea and vomiting, and on the negative affective states such as anxiety, anger, and depression that frequently accompany these conditioned responses. Some researchers have been concerned exclusively with symptoms that occur before the chemotherapy session commences, while other reseachers have focused primarily on postchemotherapy nausea and vomiting. Overall, five different types of behavioral interventions have been reported in the literature: hypnosis, progressive muscle relaxation training, systematic desensitization, EMG biofeedback, and stress inoculation training.

Hypnosis. Hypnosis was perhaps the first behavioral technique to be used to help control the nausea and vomiting associated with chemotherapy. Interestingly, many of the studies investigating hypnosis have been carried out on children and adolescents with cancer, perhaps because children and adolescents are generally considered to be very good hypnotic candidates (e. g., Dash, 1980). The early research on hypnosis with children (e. g., LaBaw, Holton, Tewell, & Eccles, 1975), adolescents (e. g., Ellenberg et al., 1980), and adults (e. g., Dempster, Balson, & Whalen, 1976) consistently suggested that hypnosis could effectively reduce nausea, vomiting, pain, and to a large extent the negative emotions associated with chemotherapy. Though encouraging, this early research is more heuristically than empirically valuable since it did not report objective data, use statistical analyses, or employ adequate methodological controls.

Kellerman et al. (1982) completed the first quasi-experimental test of hypnosis with cancer patients. These researchers gave one to three standard hypnotic training sessions, most frequently using the eye fixation technique, to eight adolescent cancer chemotherapy patients referred for problems with nausea and vomiting. Guided relaxation imagery was also used during the hypnotic sessions. Patients' nausea and vomiting were assessed by self-report scales during one chemotherapy session before hypnotic training and one chemotherapy session after hypnotic training.[2] Analysis of pre-post difference scores revealed a significant reduction in the frequency and intensity, but not duration, of vomiting following training. No data were reported regarding

---

[2] The authors also reported that two patients revealed additional posthypnotic training chemotherapy sessions, and that "data from these adolescents indicated longitudinal maintenance of symptom reduction" (p. 5). However, no numerical data were reported to support this conclusion.

changes in nausea ratings. Although this study provides the first quantifiable data on the effectiveness of hypnosis in reducing chemotherapy-related nausea and vomiting, the small sample size and lack of experimental controls hampers the confidence that can be placed in its findings.

The only experimentally rigorous test of the effectiveness of hypnosis in reducing nausea and vomiting was reported by Redd, Andresen, and Minagawa (1982). Using a multiple baseline design, Redd et al. individually hypnotized and provided relaxation imagery to six chemotherapy patients who had displayed anticipatory nausea and vomiting during at least three consecutive chemotherapy treatments. Patients' ratings of nausea and vomiting were recorded during 7 to 14 prehypnosis chemotherapy sessions, and from 2 to 5 chemotherapy sessions. In these sessions hypnosis was provided immediately before and during the injections. Results indicated that the hypnosis produced a reduction in nausea ratings prior to and during chemotherapy, and a complete elimination of anticipatory vomiting. When three patients missed their hypnosis training prior to a chemotherapy session, anticipatory nausea and vomiting returned. However, these anticipatory side effects were again controlled during subsequent sessions when hypnosis and relaxation imagery were reintroduced.

Overall, the research regarding the use of hypnosis to reduce chemotherapy-related nausea and vomiting is uniformly positive. Moreover, these positive results have withstood progressively more rigorous experimental tests, and have been obtained in spite of the fact that the various investigators have used different types of induction procedures and assessment instruments. It should be noted, however, that two groups of investigators (Kellerman et al., 1982; Redd et al., 1982, as described in Redd & Andrykowski, 1982) reported that up to 25% of the patients they approached were unwilling to attempt hypnosis training, probably because of misperceptions about the effects of hypnosis. If a patient is willing to undertake hypnosis, however, the data clearly indicate that the procedure is likely to result in a reduction of nausea and vomiting.

Progressive muscle relaxation training. While hypnosis was probably the first behavioral technique to be used in the chemotherapy context, progressive muscle relaxation training followed by guided relaxation imagery is probably the most widely used technique. The most commonly employed type of muscle relaxation training program is based on a series of muscle tensing and relaxing exercises developed by Jacobson (1938) and later modified by Bernstein and Borkovec (1973). This procedure is sometimes referred to as active relaxation training because it includes a muscle tensing component. Relaxation training procedures which do not include a tensing component have also been used in the chemotherapy context and are generally referred to as *passive* relaxation procedures.

Perhaps the most systematic series of studies employing progressive muscle relaxation training and guided relaxation imagery have been carried out in our clinic (Burish & Lyles, 1979; Burish & Lyles, 1981; Lyles et al., 1982). The first investigation (Burish & Lyles, 1979) was a case study report that included baseline, treatment, and follow-up sessions conducted on a woman who had displayed anticipatory nausea and vomiting to her chemotherapy sessions. Relaxation training and guided relaxation imagery were given immediately before and during the chemotherapy infusion, and the patient was asked to practice the relaxation procedure daily at home. Results suggested that the relaxation procedure was effective in reducing the patient's anxiety, depression, nausea, vomiting, and physiological arousal (pulse rate and blood pressure) during and following chemotherapy treatment. Independent ratings of the patient's anxiety and nausea by the attending nurse corroborated the patient's report. These effects were found during both the relaxation training and follow-up sessions. In the second study (Burish & Lyles, 1981) 16 patients equated for type of cancer and chemotherapy protocol were randomly assigned to either a relaxation training plus guided imagery or no-treatment control condition. One baseline, two treatment, and two follow-up sessions were conducted using procedures very similar to those used in the former case study report. The results were also similar: during both the training and follow-up sessions, patients in the relaxation condition generally reported feeling significantly less nausea during chemotherapy and were less anxious, angry, depressed, and physiologically aroused (as indicated by pulse rate and blood pressure) following chemotherapy than patients in the no-treatment control condition. In the most recently published project in this line of investigation (Lyles et al., 1982), 50 patients equated for type of cancer and chemotherapy protocol were randomly assigned to one of three conditions: (1) relaxation training plus guided relaxation imagery; (2) therapist control, in which a therapist spent an amount of time with each patient equal to that spent with a yoked patient in the relaxation training condition; and (3) no-treatment control. Results indicated that during both the treatment and follow-up sessions, patients in the relaxation training condition generally showed significantly lower physiological arousal (pulse rate and blood pressure), nausea, anxiety, depression, and anger during and/or immediately after the chemotherapy infusion than patients in the other two conditions, who in general did not significantly differ from each other. Moreover, patients in the relaxation training condition reported significantly less nausea at home during the 36 hours following chemotherapy than did patients in the other two conditions.

Two relaxation training investigations with similarly positive results have been reported by Cotanch (1983b; in press). The first investigation (Cotanch, in press) employed a single group design and included 12 patients who had showed severe nausea and vomiting during at least two consecutive chemotherapy treatments prior to participating in the study. After an initial baseline chemotherapy session during which no behavioral intervention was provided, patients were taught relaxation training *in vivo* and then given an audiotape of the relaxation training procedure and told to use the tape daily and during subsequent chemotherapy sessions. Results tabulated over two to six subsequent chemotherapy treatments indicated a 50% average reduction in nausea and vomiting. Moreover, this reduction in nausea and vomiting apparently allowed patients to ingest more nutrients as all patients showed an increase over baseline in caloric intake at 48 hours postchemotherapy. The second study carried out by Cotanch (1983b) is especially interesting because it included new patients who were scheduled for but had not yet received chemotherapy treatments, and whose prescribed chemotherapy protocols were such that the patients had a strong likelihood of developing severe nausea and vomiting. Forty-three patients were randomly assigned to one of three conditions: (1) progressive muscle relaxation training provided via audiotape; (2) tape control, in which patients listened to a tape of soothing music and were asked to think pleasant thoughts; and (3) no-treatment control. Patients participated in one baseline session (their first chemotherapy session) and varying numbers of postrelaxation training sessions. Preliminary analyses of the data indicated that, as expected, more than 85% of the patients in the tape control and no-treatment control conditions showed progressive increases in nausea and vomiting as the chemotherapy treatments continued. In contrast, approximately 67% of the patients in the relaxation training condition also showed significantly greater post chemotherapy sea and vomiting during subsequent treatments as compared to their first (baseline) chemotherapy treatment. Apparently as a result of these relatively low levels of nausea and vomiting, patients in the relaxation training condition also showed significantly greater postchemotherapy caloric intake than patients in the other two conditions.

Two other studies have reported using relaxation training procedures. The first (Hamberger, 1982) was a single case study carried out on a postradiotherapy patient. However, this study is relevant to the present discussion since the relaxation training procedure was used to treat nausea and vomiting. The patient reported considerable stomach pain, nausea, and vomiting during the course of the radiation treatments. Several months after the radiation treatments were completed, he began to re-experience these symptoms, suggesting to the author some type of conditioning process. The patient was given one relaxation training session in the therapist's office and was asked to practice relaxation regularly at home. The patient's and his spouse's reports indicated that relaxation training produced immediate cessation of the gastric attacks, and that this improvement was still present at a one-year follow-up.

In the only other study published in this area (Kaempfer, 1982), five cancer patients were given an unspecified number of 20-minute relaxation training sessions "at a time and place suitable to each patient's situation" (p. 16). Frontal EMG ratings and scores from three self-report scales were taken before and after the training sessions. Kaempfer concluded that relaxation training had little effect in ameliorating patients' distress. However, a host of methodological difficulties, including sampling problems (fewer than half of the patients referred to the study agreed to participate), reporting omissions (none of the objective data were reported), and the lack of experimental control procedures, makes it impossible to draw conclusions from this study.

Overall, the data suggest that progressive muscle relaxation training, generally in combination with guided relaxation imagery, can be a very effective procedure for reducing the nausea and emesis associated with chemotherapy. Interestingly, however, most of the research using relaxation training has focused on nausea and emesis present during or after chemotherapy rather than before chemotherapy. Thus, although there is every reason to suspect that relaxation training can also be used effectively to control anticipatory nausea and vomiting, extant data do not establish this fact. The finding that nausea and vomiting during and after chemotherapy can be helped by behavioral techniques is consistent with the view that these symptoms probably result from an interaction or addition of both pharmacological and conditioning factors. Finally, the research in this area demonstrates that in addition to reducing nausea and vomiting, relaxation training can improve affective state, reduce physiological arousal, and increase caloric intake.

EMG biofeedback combined with relaxation training. In a single case report, we described the combined use of progressive muscle relaxation training and EMG biofeedback training to reduce the distress of a hospitalized cancer chemotherapy patient (Burish, Shartner, & Lyles, 1981). The patient participated in three baseline, four training, and three followup sessions. During training sessions the patient was given progressive muscle relaxation training followed by auditory biofeedback reflecting the integrated average EMG activity of four different muscle sites. Results indicated that in the training and follow-up sessions, the patient generally reported feeling less anxious and nauseated during chemotherapy than during the baseline sessions, and showed reductions in physiological arousal (EMG, pulse rate, and blood pressure) during and after chemotherapy. Although encouraging, these results must be interpreted cautiously until replicated in experimental investigations employing larger numbers of patients.

Systematic desensitization. Systematic desensitization is a counter-conditioning procedure that has been used widely in the treatment of phobias and other anxiety disorders. The procedure basically consists of teaching a patient a relaxation skill, commonly some form of progressive muscle relaxation training, and then exposing the patient to progressively more anxiety-provoking stimuli. The goal is to counter-condition a relaxation response to the stimuli in place of the anxiety response heretofore elicited by them. In the only application of this procedure to the chemotherapy context, Morrow and Morrel (1982) randomly assigned 60 cancer patients to one of three conditions: (1) systematic desensitization, in which patients received an abbreviated form of progressive muscle relaxation training and then were exposed in imagination to gradually more anxiety-provoking chemotherapy related stimuli (e.g., coming to the clinic, seeing the drugs, feeling the needle stick, etc.); (2) Rogerian-oriented counseling, an individual supportive therapy procedure intended to control for therapist attention, expectancy effects, and other nonspecific factors; and (3) no-treatment control. All patients were asked to rate the frequency, severity, and duration of their anticipatory nausea and vomiting during two baseline and two follow-up chemotherapy treatments. Between the baseline and follow-up treatments patients received two one-hour sessions of the systematic desensitization or counseling procedure. Thus, unlike most investigators, Morrow and Morrell administered their behavioral interventions between chemotherapy treatments rather than immediately before and/or during these treatments, and in a setting geographically separate from the chemotherapy clinic. Results indicated that patients in the systematic desensitization condition, contrary to patients in the counseling and no-treatment control conditions, reported significant reductions in the frequency, severity, and duration of anticipatory nausea, and in the frequency and severity of anticipatory vomiting. No significant differences were found between the counseling and no-treatment control groups. Overall, this well-designed investigation suggests that systematic desensitization can provide an effective self-control procedure for reducing anticipatory nausea and vomiting to cancer chemotherapy.

Stress inoculation training. The last of the five behavioral techniques reported in this area is stress inoculation training. This procedure was originally designed by Meichenbaum (1977) and others as a broad-based technique for helping individuals to cope better with or "inoculate" themselves against stressful situations they routinely encounter. Basically, patients are taught an antianxiety technique such as progressive muscle relaxation training and, after becoming proficient in this skill, they are then taught to apply this procedure in anxiety-related situations, initially through cognitive rehearsal and eventually during *in vivo* exposure. Moore and Altmeier (1981) taught this technique to 9 chemotherapy patients during 6 training sessions. The authors reported no objective data, but suggested that the patients exhibited fewer anxiety-related behaviors following the training sessions. This pilot investigation suggests that the stress inoculation procedure can be taught to chemotherapy patients and it may have a beneficial effect. More research is clearly needed on this technique before conclusions can be drawn regarding its effectiveness in a chemotherapy context.

Summary

While little if any research has been conducted to assess the effectiveness of pharamcological treatments in reducing conditioned nausea and vomiting, a number of studies have assessed the effectiveness of behavioral techniques in this regard. The use of five behavioral procedures has thus far been reported in the literature: hypnosis, progressive muscle relaxation training, EMG biofeedback, systematic desensitization, and stress inoculation training. In most cases, guided relaxation imagery has also been included in the treatment package. Well controlled research suggests that hypnosis, progressive muscle relaxation training, and systematic desensitization can successfully reduce conditioned side effects, including nausea, vomiting, and negative affect, and perhaps can also increase caloric intake. The studies on EMG biofeedback and stress inoculation training are also positive in outcome, but because of their small number of subjects and nonexperimental designs these studies are only suggestive in nature. Overall, the data strongly suggest that behavioral interventions can effectively reduce much of the distress associated with cancer chemotherapy treatments.

Behavioral Interventions:
Proposed Mechanisms of Action

Most of the behavioral research carried out to date has assessed *whether* a given treatment procedure is effective in reducing the distress of chemotherapy, but not *why* it is effective. However, by examining closely the methodologies and results of the studies reported thus far, at least five hypotheses can be offered regarding factors that may be responsible for the effectiveness of behavioral interventions. These factors are not to be viewed as mutually exclusive but rather as mechanisms which may act alone or in combination with other mechanisms to produce the observed treatment effects.

Relaxation

A common element in each of the behavioral procedures reported to date is the induction of a state of relaxation. This relaxation can be achieved by active patient participation, as in the studies by Burish and his colleagues, Cotanch, and Morrow and Morrell, or through passive patient participation, as in the work of Redd and his associates. In either case, by helping the patient to relax, thes techniques may help to reduce anxiety and physiological arousal, thereby also reducing side effects such as gastrointestinal upset that are due to or more likely exacerbated by high levels of anxiety or arousal. Three specific hypotheses have been made in this regard. First, Nerenz, Leventhal, Love et al. (1982) have suggested that at least for some patients a series of conditioning experiences apparently occurs, whereby the chemotherapy context elicits a negative emotional state (e.g., anxiety), which in turn elicits nausea and vomiting. A reduction of this anxiety may therefore also result in a reduction in nausea and vomiting. Second, it has also been suggested that deep muscular relaxation, especially in the gastrointestinal area, may directly inhibit the characteristic sequence of muscular contractions that generally precede vomiting, thereby essentially decreasing or delaying the onset and/or severity of vomiting (Redd & Andrykowski, 1982). Finally, Cotanch (1983a) has suggested that techniques such as relaxation training or biofeedback may increase both patients' awareness of and sensitivity to the somatic changes that accompany nausea and vomiting on the one hand, and on the other their ability to self-regulate these sensations and thereby to decrease their frequency or intensity.

Although a speculative idea, we suggest that in some cases part of the antiemetic effectiveness of behavioral relaxation procedures may be due to the physiological and/or neurochemical sedation effects associated with it. It is well documented, both in the noncancer (e.g., Borkovec & Sides, 1979; Burish, Hendrix & Frost, 1981) and cancer chemotherapy (e.g., Lyles et al., 1982; Cotanch, 1983b) literature, that relaxation training techniques produce a general decrease in sympathetic indices of arousal. It has also recently been demonstrated that a behaviorally induced relaxation response can result in augmented plasma norepinephrine levels under high stress conditions (Hoffman et al., 1982). Interestingly, one of the principal ingredients of most if not all antiemetic drugs that have shown promise in relieving the side effects of chemotherapy is the production of a physiological relaxation effect similar to that produced by behavioral techniques. Borison has noted the potential importance of the relaxation effect of antiemetic therapies: "A common feature of antiemetic therapies is the accompanying sedation, and for practical purposes it is usually impossible to determine whether it is the nonspecific depression [i.e., the sedation] or antiemetic activity per se which accounts for the therapeutic benefit..." (Borison & McCarthy, 1983, p. 15). The law of parsimony would suggest that perhaps it is the sedation effect.

While it seems plausible to us that the physiological and/or neurochemical concomitants of relaxation may be an important ingredient of most effective antiemetic treatments, it is unlikely to be a sufficient ingredient in all cases. For example, most therapies, behavioral as well as pharmacological, have been relatively ineffective in treating the nausea and vomiting caused by some types of cytotoxic drugs, notably Cisplatin. It may be that the pathway through which Cis-platin causes nausea and vomiting is different from the pathways through which many other types of chemotherapy drugs cause nausea and vomiting, and that this pathway is not affected by or only modestly affected by the mechanisms operating when one experiences relaxation. Undoubtedly, different drugs cause nausea and vomiting for different reasons (Borison & McCarthy, 1983), and therefore it is unlikely that any specific antiemetic approach will be effective in all cases.

In summary, while there is some disagreement about the specific manner in which relaxation contributes to the reduction of chemotherapy-related distress, there appears to be considerable agreement that it does play an essential role.

Attentional Diversion

A second commonly suggested mechanism by which behavioral treatments accomplish their effect is distraction or attentional diversion (e.g., Lyles et al., 1982; Redd & Andrykowski, 1982). This hypothesis holds that behavioral techniques serve to distract patients' attention away from the chemotherapy context and onto more pleasant and relaxing stimuli and sensations. To the extent that a patient's attention is distracted away from stress-related stimuli, there should be a corresponding decrease in the number and severity of side effects that have become associated with these stimuli. Simply stated, by removing (through cognitive distraction) conditioned stimuli that have developed in the chemotherapy context, one should be able to remove the conditioned responses that are elicited by these stimuli.

While the attentional diversion (or conditioned stimulus removal) hypothesis is attractive theoretically, there are data which suggest that it is probably not the major explanation for behavioral treatment outcome. For example, the standard "no-intervention" procedures used in our clinic and elsewhere are purposefully replete with cognitive distractors, including television, music, magazines, and having family members present during chemotherapy. Also, several of the control conditions used in various studies reported previously provided cognitive distractors, for example, the tape control procedure used by Cotanch (1983b). Thus, although part of the effect of relaxation procedures may be due to the fact that they are good cognitive distractors, perhaps better than television, music, or other "standard" distractors, it is nevertheless unlikely that their total impact can be accounted for by this explanation.

Increased Feelings of Control

A third hypothesis for the effectiveness of behavioral strategies is that the procedures increase in many patients the belief that they once again have some control over their disease and its impact upon them (e.g., Cotanch, in press; Morrow & Morrell, 1982; Redd et al., 1982). These feelings of self-control may decrease feelings of helplessness and promote an overall more positive psychological state, which in turn helps patients to view their treatment as a less negative and stressful experience. This improvement in patients' general affective state and outlook regarding chemotherapy may result in a corresponding reduction in other symptoms associated with their previously high levels of anxiety and feelings of hopelessness, for example, nausea, vomiting, and decreased motivation for good nutritional care. Although appealing from a holistic perspective, there are unfortunately no data to support this hypothesis. Further, in the only study to assess patients' feelings of control (Morrow & Morrell, 1982), reductions in anticipatory nausea and emesis were not accompanied by corresponding changes in feelings of control as indicated by scores on the Health Locus of Control Scale (Wallston, Wallston & DeVillis, 1978), although admittedly the Health

Locus of Control Scale is a global measure of control and is not specific to feelings of control over chemotherapy-related factors. Overall, therefore, at the present time, the perceived control hypothesis must be considered highly speculative.

Counterconditioning

A fourth explanation for the outcome of at least one of the behavioral procedures, namely, systematic desensitization (Morrow & Morrell, 1982), is that the desensitization procedure produces a situation in which the paired association of chemotherapy-related stimuli with feelings of relaxation counterconditions these stimuli to elicit relaxation rather than anxiety, nausea, vomiting, and the other negative reactions that were formerly associated with them. While this counterconditioning rationale has been demonstrated to be appropriate for explaining the success of systematic desensitization in traditional phobic situations, its application to the chemotherapy context is precarious. It may be possible to eliminate the associative bond between chemotherapy-related stimuli and responses such as nausea and vomiting by establishing a new bond between these stimuli and a relaxation response; however, it would seem to be very difficult to have this new associative bond remain in place because with each actual chemotherapy treatment the chemotherapy-related stimuli (i.e., the conditioned stimuli) are again paired with the chemotherapy drugs (i.e., the unconditioned stimuli) and the adverse drug-induced responses such as nausea, vomiting, and negative affect (i.e., the unconditioned responses). Therefore, the association of the chemotherapy-related stimuli with the adverse side effects is reestablished during every chemotherapy treatment.

Finally, besides being unlikely on theoretical grounds, the counterconditioning explanation lacks parsimony in that it cannot explain the success of other behavioral techniques that did not use counterconditioning principles. In fact, many behavioral investigators have suggested that behavioral relaxation procedures divert subjects' attention away from chemotherapy-related stimuli rather than pair them with the relaxation. Of course, since in most studies the relaxation procedures were carried out in the actual chemotherapy context, it is possible that pairing did occur between chemotherapy-related stimuli and relaxation, and hence some counterconditioning could have taken place. Overall, although the counterconditioning explanation appears to have little support as a general explanation for the effectiveness of behavioral procedures in reducing conditioned responses to chemotherapy, adequate data to rule it out conclusively have not yet been reported.

Nonspecific Factors

Finally, it has been pointed out that nonspecific factors such as patient expectancy, placebo effects, and demand characteristics may explain to some extent the effectiveness of behavioral techniques in reducing the distress of chemotherapy (e.g., Redd & Andrykowski, 1982). Indirect support for the nonspecific factors hypothesis comes from observations by several researchers and clinicians of patients' desire to please the therapist, and from the fact that many behavioral investigations rely totally on self-report measures that could be readily faked by a patient who wanted to appear improved. However, at least four arguments against the nonspecific factors have been voiced. First, several investigators (e.g., Kellerman et al., 1982) have noted that most patients who participate in behavioral studies have already received a number of prior antiemetic medications from their physicians, often with considerable positive expectancy, and that there are abundant data to suggest that many and perhaps most cancer patients view their physicians as important and powerful figures whom they respect and try to please. If factors such as social desirability and placebo effects were sufficient to reduce the side effects to chemotherapy, they therefore should have exerted an observable effect when antiemetic medications were prescribed prior to the delivery of the behavioral interventions. Second, while it is true that the delivery of a behavioral relaxation treatment requires considerably more time and attention than does the prescription of a pill and that this time and attention may result in stronger placebo effects or positive expectancies for change, it is also true that in most clinics and hospitals the nursing staff spends an equally large amount of time with the patient. For example, Lyles et al. (1982) and Cotanch (in press) have observed that their patients had developed close interpersonal and supportive relationships with the clinic and ward nurses before the behavioral interventions were introduced. Thus, attention and social support alone do not appear to be able to reduce nausea, vomiting and many of the other side effects of cancer chemotherapy. Third, while self-report measures capable of being faked were the sole outcome measures used in some studies, objective physiological indices that are difficult to fake (see Houston & Holmes, 1975) were used in others (e.g., Burish & Lyles, 1981; Burish et al., 1981; Lyles et al., 1982). Moreover, although self-report measures can be faked, there is little reason to suspect that cancer chemotherapy patients who have been given prior antiemetic treatments without success would feel a need to begin faking them when they received a behavioral treatment. Finally, in at least three studies (Lyles et al., 1982; Morrow & Morrell, 1982; Cotanch, 1983b) credible attention-placebo procedures were employed, and in each case the behavioral treatment was clearly superior to the placebo condition, which in turn did not differ from the no-treatment control condition. Overall, therefore, while nonspecific factors such as positive expectancies and increased attention may account for some of the impact of behavioral interventions, it is unlikely that they account for most and certainly not for all of the treatment effect.

Summary

While the potential effectiveness of behavioral interventions in reducing the distress of chemotherapy has been well documented, the mechanism(s) by which behavioral treatments exert their effects is unknown. Five hypotheses have been offered to account for these effects, including the notions that they result from relaxation, attentional diversion, increased feelings of control, counterconditioning, and nonspecific factors such as increased attention and placebo effects. None of these hypotheses has been well investigated to date, though the relaxation hypothesis appears to have the most indirect support. It is likely that future research will find that many of these potential causative mechanisms, and perhaps others, operate together to produce the effects observed after the application of behavioral treatments.

Clinical Issues

Although the behavioral intervention research reviewed above is very promising, several issues critical to the clinical application of behavioral techniques remain to be addressed. Three issues in particular can be identified that have been inadequately studied but which are important to the large-scale clinical application of behavioral procedures.

First, little research has been carried out to ensure that the patient eventually is able to relax and reduce conditioned responses without continued intervention by a therapist. In much of the research completed thus far (e.g., Lyles et al., 1982; Redd et al., 1982), therapists have spent upwards of an hour per patient per chemotherapy session administering the behavioral intervention. Obviously, on a large-scale clinical basis this is an expensive and impractical approach considering the number of therapists available, the number of chemotherapy patients that could benefit from behavioral interventions, and the potential monetary costs involved. Unfortunately, however, in much of the research reported, the treatment effects disappeared completely (e.g., Redd et al., 1982) or declined in many patients (e.g., Lyles et al., 1982) when therapist direction was terminated.

Several potentially effective procedures for decreasing therapist time and involvement merit investigation. First, patients receiving systematic desensitization in the Morrow and Morrell (1982) study evidenced treatment maintenance on their own following only two therapist-directed treatment sessions. However, patients were studied for only two sessions following the termination of therapist training, and thus it is not known whether systematic desensitization would produce long-term maintenance. Second, the use of audiotapes to provide relaxation training, as described by Cotanch (1983 b), may be an effective strategy for maintaining treatment effects with little therapist intervention. Third, it may be possible to teach a spouse or hospital volunteer the relaxation procedure at the same time it is taught to the patient, and then let this other person direct the relaxation technique in future sessions. Finally, after sufficient training in any of the behavioral procedures used this far, many patients should be able to relax on their own without the need of further intervention. Self-control relaxation is especially likely to develop if patients practice the relaxation procedure on their own and if they are taught a cue-controlled procedure training such that feelings of anxiety or nausea become cues automatically eliciting the behavioral relaxation strategy. Of course, some patients, including those who receive several courses of chemotherapy over successive days, may not have the strength to practice on their own between chemotherapy sessions. For these patients, the use of audiotapes or spouse-therapists may be the most economical and effective procedure.

A second clinically important issue is deciding which behavioral treatment to give a patient. Obviously, treatment and patient variables as well as their interaction must be considered in choosing an optimal behavioral strategy. Regarding treatment variables, no research has been conducted that directly compared two or more of the behavioral techniques that have been used with cancer patients. Until data on the comparative effectiveness of these techniques are available, decisions regarding which technique to use must be based on less empirical guidelines. For example, since the best supported causal mechanism for the effectiveness of behavioral strategies is the induction of a relaxed state, the technique selected should be one which can maximize this outcome. For instance, if a physically handicapped patient who has difficulty tensing his/her muscles is being treated, a passive rather than an active form of relaxation (e.g., hypnosis) might be preferable. Conversely, if a physically tense patient is being treated, an active treatment (e.g., progressive muscle relaxation training) might be more effective. Another guideline useful in choosing a treatment strategy might be matching the treatment with the patient's preference. The labels and/or nature of various behavioral techniques may be construed by patients as falling along a continuum from "desirable" to "threatening". If a particular treatment is evaluated by a patient as more desirable and potentially more efficacious than another, it may be preferable to use that treatment in order to maximize patient compliance and any nonspecific or placebo factors that may be able to enhance treatment effectiveness. Finally, the skills and experience of the therapist should clearly play a role in deciding which procedure to use. It is unlikely that any procedure will be effective if it is not skilfully presented, and it is less likely to be effective if it is not confidently presented.

Regarding the role of patient variables in determining treatment effectiveness, no research has yet been reported that identifies which types of patients are most likely to benefit from behavioral interventions. However, the fact that there are individual differences in response to behavioral interventions has been documented. For example, Lyles et al. (1982) reported that the majority of patients in their study who received relaxation training showed clinically significant decreases on a number of outcome variables, including systolic blood pressure, nausea, and anxiety. However, as many as one-third of the treated patients evidenced either no change or a worsening on one or more of these outcome measures. Results such as these suggest that individual difference variables may be very important in determining which patients are most likely to benefit from treatment efforts. Research aimed at identifying such variables is clearly warranted.

More important than either treatment variables alone or individual difference variables alone is their interaction. While some clinical impressions regarding this interaction are available (e.g., Kellerman et al., 1982, have suggested that patients who are highly anxious may be less likely to profit from hypnosis training), no relevant empirical data have been reported. Again, research on this topic is needed and warranted.

Finally, it has been noted by several investigators that for a small minority of chemotherapy patients (perhaps 5 to 10 percent overall), the behavioral interventions (especially if they involve the use of audiotapes) actually develop into conditioned stimuli that elicit increased anxiety, nausea, and vomiting, and as a result exacerbate rather than ameliorate the problem. For example, Redd, Rosenberger, and Hendler (1982-1983) reported that several patients who were using audiotapes to induce self-hypnosis began to become nauseated to the sound of the therapist's voice. Interestingly, similar observations have been made regarding antiemetic medications (e.g., Kutz, Borysenko, Come, & Benson, 1980). It is unclear why such conditioning occurs in some patients, but obviously this is a question that deserves further study.

Summary and Conclusions

The chemotherapeutic treatment of cancer has made remarkable advances during the past several decades. Chemotherapy is now used with curative intent as the treatment of choice for several types of cancer. The appeal of chemotherapy has been attenuated, however, by the presence of several side effects, especially nausea, vomiting, anxiety, and depression. When experienced together, these symptoms can be so severe that patients chose a hastened death rather than continue their treatment. These side effects appear to be of two types: those which are pharmacologically caused by the action of the antineoplastic drugs and those which are psychological in nature. Of the two, the psychological side effects are the least understood and have been the least investigated. This chapter has attempted to review what data are available on the nature, etiology, prevalence, and treatment of these psychological side effects.

Probably the most solid conclusions that can be drawn from the data published thus far in this area are that nonpharmacologically caused nausea, vomiting, and other negative side effects (a) are exhibited by approximately one-third of all cancer patients receiving chemotherapy; (b) develop, at least to some extent, through a classical conditioning process; and (c) can be ameliorated through a variety of behavioral relaxation procedures. Why conditioned side effects develop in some cancer patients but not in others; why they respond to behavioral intervention in some patients but not in others; and what the nature of the active mechanism(s) is through which behavioral interventions exert their effect are questions that are not only unanswered but have been barely investigated. Moreover, even though behavioral interventions have been shown to be effective in controlled research investigations, their practicality for large-scale clinical trials has yet to be demonstrated. Additional research aimed at reducing therapist involvement and promoting the acquisition of relaxation as a learned self-control technique is needed before the clinical application of these techniques can be undertaken on a cost-effective basis.

Although this review has emphasized the nonpharmacological etiology of conditioned side effects and their treatment with behavioral interventions, it should not be concluded that conditioned side effects and their treatment are best considered completely independent of pharmacological side effects or medically oriented attempts at symptom reduction. Chemotherapy patients who exhibit conditioned side effects also suffer from pharmacologically caused nausea and vomiting, and hence the separation of conditioned from pharmacological symptoms, especially during the postchemotherapy period, may be more academically interesting than clinically useful. At present, the combined use of the best behavioral and antiemetic treatments available is most likely to produce the greatest overall symptom relief.

In summary, the study of the etiology, nature, prevalence, and treatment of conditioned side effects resulting from cancer chemotherapy is a very young area of investigation, with approximately 90% of the research in the area being published within the last five years. The data generated thus far have indicated the potential importance of conditioning in the chemotherapy context, and have helped investigators to begin to formulate productive questions guiding further research. The continued formulation of these questions and the eventual discovery of their answers promises to help reduce the distress of chemotherapy and further the acceptance of this potentially curative treatment among cancer patients.

References

Altmaier, E. M., Ross, W. E., & Moore, K. A pilot investigation of the psychologic function of patients with anticipatory vomiting. *Cancer,* 1982, *49,* 201–204.

Andrykowski, M. A., Redd, W. H., & Hatfield, A. K. Nausea and vomiting in cancer patients: A reply to Chang. *Psychosomatics,* 1983, *24,* 213–215.

Bernstein, D. A., & Borkovec, T. D. *Progressive relaxation training: A manual for the helping professions.* Champaign, Illinois: Research Press, 1973.

Bernstein, I. L. Learned taste aversions in children receiving chemotherapy. *Science,* 1978, *200,* 1302–1303.

Bernstein, I. L., & Webster, M. M. Learned taste aversions in humans. *Physiol. Behav.,* 1980, *25,* 363–366.

Borison, H. L., & McCarthy, L. E. Neuropharmacologic mechanisms of emesis. In J. Laszlo (Ed.), *Antiemetics and cancer chemotherapy.* Baltimore: Williams & Wilkins, 1983.

Borkovec, T. D., & Sides, J. K. Critical procedural variables related to the physiological effects of progressive relaxation: A review. *Behav. Res. Ther.,* 1979, *17,* 119–125.

Burish, T. G., Carey, M. P., Redd, W. H., & Krozely, M. G. Efficacy of behavioral relaxation techniques in reducing the distress of cancer chemotherapy patients. *Oncol. Nurs. Forum,* 1983, *10(3),* 32–35.

Burish, T. G., Hendrix, E. M., & Frost, R. O. Comparison of frontal EMG biofeedback and several types of relaxation instructions in reducing multiple indices of arousal. *Psychophysiology,* 1981, *18,* 594–602.

Burish, T. G., & Lyles, J. N. Effectiveness of relaxation training in reducing adverse reactions to cancer chemotherapy. *J. Behav. Med.,* 1981, *4,* 65–78.

Burish, T. G., & Lyles, J. N. Effectiveness of relaxation training in reducing the aversiveness of chemotherapy in the treatment of cancer. *Behav. Ther. Exp. Psychiat,* 1979, *10,* 357–361.

Burish, T. G., Shartner, C. D., & Lyles, J. N. Effectiveness of multiple-site EMG biofeedback and relaxation in reducing the aversiveness of cancer chemotherapy. *Biofeedback Self Regul.,* 1981, *6,* 523–535.

Chang, A. E., Shiling, D. J., Stillman, R. C., Goldberg, N. H., Seipp, C. A., Barofsky, I., Simon, R. M., & Rosenberg, S. A. Delta-9-tetrahydrocannabinol as an antiemetic in cancer patients receiving high-dose methotrexate: A prospective, randomized evalution. *Ann. Intern. Med.,* 1979, *91,* 819–824.

Chang, J. C. More on psychological mechanisms in patients with nausea and vomiting following chemotherapy. *Psychosomatics,* 1982, *23,* 651.

Chang, J. C. Nausea and vomiting in cancer patients: An expression of psychological mechanisms? *Psychosomatics,* 1981, *22,* 707–709.

Cohen, R. E., Sheehan, A., Ruckdeschel, J. C., & Blanchard, E. G. *The prediction of post-treatment and anticipatory nausea and vomiting associated with antineoplastic chemotherapy.* Paper presented at the Meeting of the Society of Behavioral Medicine, Chicago, 1982.

Cohn, K. H. Chemotherapy from an insider's perspective. *Lancet,* 1982, *1,* 1006–1009.

Coons, H. L. *Conditioned nausea in cancer patients receiving Cis-platinum chemotherapy.* Unpublished manuscript, University of Wisconsin-Madison, 1981.

Cotanch, P. H. Relaxation techniques as antiemetic therapy. In J. Laszlo (Ed.), *Antiemetics and cancer chemotherapy.* Baltimore, Md.: Williams & Wilkins, 1983 (a).

Cotanch, P. H. *Muscle relaxation versus 'attention placebo' in decreasing the adversiveness of chemotherapy.* Manuscript in preparation, Duke University, 1983 (b).

Cotanch, P. H. Relaxation training for control of nausea and vomiting in refractory patients receiving chemotherapy. *Cancer Nurs.,* in press.

Dash, J. G. Hypnosis for symptom amelioration. In J. Kellerman (Ed.), *Psychological aspects of childhood cancer.* Springfield, Illinois: Charles C. Thomas, Publisher, 1980.

Dempster, C. R., Balson, P., & Whalen, B. T. Supportive hypnotherapy during the radical treatment of malignancies. *Int. J. Clin. Exp. Hypn.,* 1976, *24,* 1–9.

Dennis, V. W. Fluid and electrolyte changes after vomiting. In J. Laszlo (Ed.), *Antiemetics and cancer chemotherapy.* Baltimore, Md.: Williams & Wilkins, 1983.

Ellenberg, L., Kellerman, J., Dash, J., Higgins, G., & Zeltzer, L. Use of hypnosis for multiple symptoms in an adolescent girl with leukemia. *J. Adolesc. Health Care,* 1980, *1,* 132–136.

Fordyce, W. E. Learning processes in pain. In R. A. Sternback (Ed.), *The psychology of pain.* New York: Raven Press, 1978.

Frytak, S., & Moertel, C. G. Management of nausea and vomiting in the cancer patient. *J. Am. Med. Ass.,* 1981, *245,* 393–396.

Frytak, S., Moertel, C. G., O'Fallon, J. R., Rubin, J., Creagan, E. T., O'Connell, M. J., Schutt, A. J., & Schwartau, N. W. Delta-9-tetrahydrocannabinol as an antiemetic for patients receiving cancer chemotherapy. A comparison with prochlorperazine and a placebo. *Ann. Intern. Med.,* 1979, *91,* 825–830.

Garcia, J., Hankins, W. G., & Rusiniak, K. W. Behavioral regulation of the milieu interne in man and rat. *Science,* 1974, *185,* 824–831.

Golden, S. Cancer chemotherapy and management of patient problems. *Nurs. Forum,* 1975, *12,* 279–303.

Greer, S. Psychological inquiry: A contribution to cancer research. *Psychol. Med.,* 1979, *9,* 81–89.

Hamberger, L. K. Reduction of generalized aversive responding in a posttreatment cancer patient: Relaxation as an active coping skill. *J. Behav. Ther. Exp. Psychiat.,* 1982, *13,* 229–233.

Harris, J. G. Nausea, vomiting and cancer treatment. *CA,* 1978, *28,* 194–201.

Hoffman, J. W., Benson, H., Arns, P. A., Stainbrook, G. L., Landsberg, L., Young, J. B., & Gill, A. Reduced sympathetic nervous system responsivity associated with the relaxation response. *Science,* 1982, *215,* 190–192.

Houston, B. K., & Holmes, D. S. Role playing versus deception: The ability of subjects to simulate self-report and physiological responses. *J. Soc. Psychol.,* 1975, *96,* 91–98.

Jacobson, E. *Progressive relaxation.* Chicago: University of Chicago Press, 1938.

Kaempfer, S. H. Relaxation training reconsidered. *Oncol. Nurs. Forum,* 1982, *9,* 15–18.

Katz, E. R. Behavioral conditioning in the development and maintenance of vomiting in cancer patients. *Psychosomatics,* 1982, *23,* 650–651.

Kellerman, J., Zeltzer, L., Ellenberg, L., & Dash, J. *Hypnotic reduction of distress associated with adolescent cancer and treatment. Part II: Nausea and emesis.* Unpublished manuscript, University of Southern California, 1982.

Kutz, I., Borysenko, J., Come, S., & Benson, H. Paradoxical emetic response to antiemetic treatment in cancer patients. *N. Engl. J. Med.,* 1980, *303,* 1480.

LaBaw, W., Holton, C., Tewell, K., & Eccles, D. The use of self-hypnosis by children with cancer. *Am. J. Clin. Hypn.,* 1975, *17,* 233–238.

Laszlo, J. (Ed.), *Antiemetics and cancer chemotherapy.* Baltimore, Md.: Williams & Wilkins, 1983 (a).

Laszlo, J. Emesis as limiting toxicity in cancer chemotherapy. In J. Laszlo (Ed.), *Antiemetics and cancer chemotherapy.* Baltimore, Md.: Williams & Wilkins, 1983 (b).

Laszlo, J. Methods for measuring clinical effectiveness of antiemetics. In J. Laszlo (Ed.), *Antiemetics and cancer chemotherapy.* Baltimore, Md.: Williams & Wilkins, 1983 (c).

Laszlo, J. & Lucas, V. S. Emesis as a critical problem in chemotherapy. *N. Engl. J. Med.,* 1981, *305,* 948–949.

Love, R. R., Nerenz, D. R., & Leventhal, H. The development of anticipatory nausea during cancer chemotherapy. *Proc. Am. Assoc. Cancer Res. – Am. Soc. Clin. Oncol.,* in press.

Lucas, V. S., & Laszlo, J. Delta-9-tetrahydrocannabinol for refractory vomiting induced by cancer chemotherapy. *J. Am. Med. Assoc.,* 1980, *243,* 1241–1243.

Lyles, J. N., Burish, T. G., Krozely, M. G., & Oldham, R. K. Efficacy of relaxation training and guided imagery in reducing the adversiveness of cancer chemotherapy. *J. Consult. Clin. Psychol.,* 1982, *50,* 509–524.

Meichenbaum, D. *Cognitive behavior modification: An integrative approach.* New York: Plenum, 1977.

Moore, K., & Altmaier, E. M. Stress inoculation training with cancer patients. *Cancer Nurs.,* 1981, *4,* 389–393.

Morrow, G. R. Prevalence and correlates of anticipatory nausea and vomiting in chemotherapy patients. *J. Nat. Cancer Inst.,* 1982, *68,* 585–588.

Morrow, G. R., Arseneau, J. C., Asbury, R. F., Bennett, J. M., & Boros, L. Anticipatory nausea and vomiting with chemotherapy. *N. Engl. J. Med.,* 1982, *306,* 431–432.

Morrow, G. R., & Morrell, C. Behavioral treatment for the anticipatory nausea and vomiting induced by cancer chemotherapy. *N. Engl. J. Med.,* 1982, *307,* 1476–1480.

Nerenz, D. R., Leventhal, H., & Love, R. R. Factors contributing to emotional distress during cancer chemotherapy. *Cancer,* 1982, *50,* 1020–1027.

Nerenz, D. R., Leventhal, H., Love, R. R., Coons, H., & Ringler, K. *Anxiety and taste of drugs during injections as predictors of anticipatory nausea in cancer chemotherapy.* Unpublished manuscript, University of Wisconsin-Madison, 1982.

Nesse, R. M., Carli, T., Curtis, G. C., & Kleinman, P. D. Pretreatment nausea in cancer chemotherapy: A conditioned response? *Psychosom. Med.,* 1980, *42,* 33–36.

Nicholas, D. R. Prevalence of anticipatory nausea and emesis in cancer chemotherapy patients. *J. Behav. Med.,* 1982, *5,* 461–463.

Oberst, M. T. Priorities in cancer nursing research. *Cancer Nurs.,* 1978, *1,* 281.

Penta, J., Poster, D., & Bruno, S. The pharmacologic treatment of nausea and vomiting caused by chemotherapy: A review. In J. Laszlo (Ed.), *Antiemetics and cancer chemotherapy.* Baltimore, Md.: Williams & Wilkins, 1983.

Poster, D. S., Penta, J. S., & Bruno, S. *Treatment of cancer chemotherapy-induced nausea and vomiting.* New York: Masson Publishing, Inc., 1981.

Redd, W. H. Behavioral analysis and control of psychosomatic symptoms of patients receiving intensive cancer treatment. *Br. J. Clin. Psychol.,* 1982, *21,* 351–358.

Redd, W. H., & Andresen, G. V. Conditioned aversion in cancer patients. *The Behav. Therapist,* 1981, *4,* 3–4.

Redd, W. H., Andresen, G. V., & Minagawa, R. Y. Hypnotic control of anticipatory emesis in patients receiving cancer chemotherapy. *J. Consult. Clin. Psychol.,* 1982, *50,* 14–19.

Redd, W. H., & Andrykowski, M. A. Behavioral intervention in cancer treatment: Controlling aversion reactions to chemotherapy. *J. Consult. Clin. Psychol.,* 1982, *50,* 1018–1029.

Redd, W. H., Rosenberger, P. H., & Hendler, C. S. Controlling chemotherapy side effects. *Am. J. Hypn.,* 1982–1983, *25,* 161–172.

Rosencweig, M., Von Hoff, D. D., Slavik, M., & Muggia, F. M. Cis-diamine dichloro platinum (II): A new anticancer drug. *Ann. Intern. Med.,* 1977, *86,* 803–812.

Rosenthal, T. *How could I not be among you?* New York: Avon Books, 1973.

Scogna, D. M., & Smalley, R. V. Chemotherapy induced nausea and vomiting. *Am. J. Nurs.,* 1979, *79,* 1562–1564.

Seligman, M. E. P. Phobias and preparednes. *Behav. Ther.,* 1971, *2,* 307–320.

Siegel, L. J., & Longo, D. L. The control of chemotherapy-induced emesis. *Ann. Intern. Med.,* 1981, *95,* 352–359.

Swanson, D. W., Swenson, W. M., Huizenga, K. A., & Melson, S. J. Persistent nausea without organic cause. *Mayo Clin. Proc.,* 1976, *51,* 257–262.

Turkat, I. D. An investigation of parental modeling in the etiology of diabetic illness behavior. *Behav. Res. Ther.,* 1982, *20,* 547–552.

Wallston, K. A., Wallston, B. S., & DeVellis, R. Development of the Multidimensional Health Locus of Control (MHLC) Scales. *Health Educ. Monog.,* 1978, *6,* 161–170.

Whitehead, V. M. Cancer treatment needs better antiemetics. *N. Engl. J. Med.,* 1975, *293,* 199–200.

Wilcox, P. M., Fetting, J. H., Nettesheim, K. M., & Abeloff, M. D. Anticipatory vomiting in women receiving cyclophosphamide, methotrexate, and 5-FU (CMF) adjuvant chemotherapy for breast carcinoma. *Cancer Treatment Rep.,* 1982, *66,* 1601–1604.

Glucocorticoid Hormones and the Humoral Immune Response

E. K. Shkhinek and E. A. Korneva

Investigations of the past few years have shown that the response of an organism to antigens comprises an intricate complex of processes consisting not only of the specific reactions of the immune system but also of nonspecific changes in the functions of other systems, including the neuroendocrine system. The concrete mechanisms of interaction between specific and nonspecific factors involved in the expression of reactions to an antigen are as yet imperfectly understood. In particular, there are many vague and conflicting elements in the evaluation of the role of hormones of the hypothalamo-hypophysio-adrenocortical system (HHACS) in the development of the immune response in the whole organism. It is generally known that the administration to an organism of large pharmacological doses of glucocorticoid hormones produces an immunosuppressive effect. Numerous experiments have proved that this effect is due to the influence of the hormones upon the metabolism of the principal cellular populations involved in the immune reaction: T- and B-lymphocytes, and macrophages. Joining the cytoplasmic receptors and penetrating into the nucleus, the hormones change the metabolism of the cell, the production of enzymes and other proteins (see surveys by Uteshev & Babichev, 1974; Ahlqvist, 1976). It has been proved experimentally that the development of lymphoid tissue in the course of ontogenesis proceeds under the control of the endocrine system with the participation of the HHACS as well (e.g., Pierpaoli & Sorkin, 1967, 1969; Sorkin & Pierpaoli, 1970). Failure of the endocrine system results in immunological insufficiency: in hypophyseal animals, in particular, a grave immunodeficient condition develops. At the same time, inactivation of the pituitary body or the adrenal glands in maturity brings about widely differing results: no effect of those operations on the course of immune reactions and higher or lower immune responses were recorded (e.g., Lundin, 1960; Koputovskaya,

1970; Thrasher, Bernardis, & Cohen, 1971; Van Dijk, Testerink, & Noordegraaf, 1976; Eliseeva, 1977; Besedovsky, Del Rey, & Sorkin, 1979).

Many authors conclude that adrenalectomy produces stimulation of humoral and especially, cellular, immune response (Chebotarev, 1979). Adrenalectomy results in higher sensitivity of lymphoid cells to the stimulating effect of thymosin (Chebotarev, 1979) and in greater migration ability of immune system cells (Petrov et al., 1975, 1979).

On the basis of those facts a viewpoint is evolving about the "limiting", restraining role of glucocorticoids which normally restrict the reaction of the immune system cells to antigen effects, the lymphocyte being regarded as a target cell for the hormones of oppositely directed effect–glucocorticoids and thymosin (Chebotarev, 1979). At the same time, in animals which have no extra adrenal gland tissue, adrenalectomy results in lower humoral immune response (e.g., Antonenko et al., 1972; Chebotarev & Valueva, 1972).

According to the evidence obtained in lymphocyte tissue culture (Ambrose, 1970; Besedovsky & Sorkin, 1977; and others) physiological doses of glucocorticoids, far from inhibiting humoral immune response, are essential for its normal course. In the complete absence of hormones in the culture medium the immune reaction does not take place. It is well known that the development of normal immune response to antigens is attended by a higher level of glucocorticoids in the blood (Belovolova, 1975; Shkhinek, Tsvetkova, & Marat, 1973; Besedovsky et al., 1975; Korneva, Klimenko, & Shkhinek, 1978). Certain kinds of stress do not in any way affect the response of humoral antibodies in the whole organism (Yamada, Jensen, & Rasmussen, 1964; Solomon, 1969; Locke & Heisel, 1977; Bartrop et al., 1977; Escola et al., 1978), and sometimes a stress brings about not an inhibition but rather a stimulation of humoral immune response (Kinnaert, Mahieu, & Van Geertruyden, 1978, 1979).

The migration abilities of thymocytes and splenic cells increase under the effect of stress, the cells apparently migrating to the bone marrow (Zimin, 1979).

According to other evidence, even a single stress effect may substantially suppress the immune abilities of the cells for humoral response, especially if they are evaluated experimentally *in vitro* or in the event of the transmission of the cells to the organism of an irradiated recipient (Gisler & Schenkel-Hulliger, 1971; Joasoo & McKenzie, 1976; Lindemann, Wirth, & Müller, 1978). Administration of small doses of ACTH may intensify cellular immune reactions and only large doses of that hormone result in immunosuppression (Comsa, 1977; Comsa, Leonhart, & Schwartz, 1975). In some experiments ACTH produced no effect on the formation of IgG-antibodies (Szabo et al., 1975). Only the dose of ACTH which increases the level of corticosteroids in the blood fivefold inhibits the migration of immunocompetent cells, a twofold increase in the hormone concentration not affecting the process (Bezin et al., 1977).

The conflicting evidence obtained by different authors does not make it possible, at present, to characterize adequately the role of glucocorticoid hormones in the development of the immune response in an organism, although this is important both for a better knowledge of the involvement of the hormonal system in the regulation of immune reactions and for elaborating adequate schemes of hormonal correction of the disturbances of the immune process.

One efficient method for studying the involvement and role of hormonal factors in the development of specific reactions consists in investigating correlations between immunological and hormonal characteristics in the course of immune response development under different physiological and pathological conditions. Studies of this kind were conducted by us under conditions of normal immune response as well as with directed changes in the intensity of immune reactions or hormonal shifts.

In experiments carried out on rabbits, rats and mice it has been found that administration of antigen may be attended by a rise in the level of glucocorticoids in the blood, developing during the first hours after the immunization. The intensity and duration of the hormonal reaction depends upon the character and dose of the antigen (Figures 1, 2, 3). A higher dose of the antigen intensifies the hormonal reaction. However, the hormonal shift to the same antigen may be altogether different in different kinds of animals; specifically, the reaction to a single administration of a corpuscular antigen–sheep erythrocytes–is clearly marked in mice and rats but is nonexistent in rabbits, despite the fact that in all cases use was made of antigen doses which provoke a distinct immune reaction (Figures 4, 5). In a more detailed investigation conducted jointly by K. Abavary & Z. Acs (JEM, HAS, Hungary) it was found that not only the total 11-OCS content, but also the level of chromatographically separate (Underwood & Williams, 1972) glucocorticoids quantitatively measured by the radioreceptor method (Murphy, 1967), remained unchanged, i. e., the absence of the effect was not associated with a relative shift in individual hormone contents (Table 1). However, the same animals responded to a repeated administration of the same dose of sheep erythrocytes 28 days after the initial immunization (the secondary immune response model) by a pronounced increase in the 11-OCS concentration (Figure 5).

The rise in the glucocorticoid level during the period of the immune response's inductive phase apparently occurs at the expense of free glu-

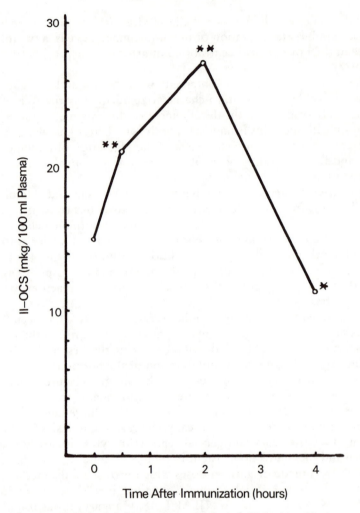

Fig. 1: Plasma 11-OCS level following immunization of CBA mice with sheep erythro-cytes (5×10^8 cells). *$p < 0.05$, **$p < 0.02$ difference from initial level.

cocorticoids not bound to protein. A study of the binding capacity of transcortin (Shkhinek, Acs, & Abavary, 1978) in rabbits immunized with the Vi-antigen of the typhoid bacillus has shown that the fixing ability of the protein drops substantially during the first two to 24 hours after immunization (Figure 6). In response to the administration of the antigen to rabbits, free 11-OCS content shows a reliable rise, whereas the concentration of the hormones bound to the proteins remains unchanged (Table II).

Table I. Variations of hydrocortisone concentration (mkg/100 ml) in rabbit blood plasma during the first hours after immunization.

Groups of animals	Number of animals	Hours after immunization			
		0	1	2	24
Immunization with Vi-antigen in a dose of 16 mkg/kg	6	0.3 ±0.07	0.5* ±0.1	0.45* ±0.09	0.5 ±0.1
Immunization with sheep erythrocytes in a dose of 6×10^9 cells	6	0.4 ±0.07	0.3 ±0.03	0.3 ±0.05	0.3* ±0.04

* Values reliably differing from the initial level at $p < 0.05$.

Table II. Protein-bound and free 11-OCS content in the blood plasma of rabbits immunized with Vi-antigen of typhoid bacillus in a dose of 16 mkg/kg with and without one hour of immobilization.

Animal's identification number	11-OCS content, mkg/100ml			
	Hours after immunization 0		Hours after immunization 2	
	protein-bound	free	protein-bound	free
Control				
1	10.3	3.0	7.5	4.4
2	14.3	6.2	12.9	10.3
3	16.8	5.6	10.3	10.0
4	8.8	7.0	14.0	8.5
Mean	12.2	5.45	11.2	8.8
%	100	100	91.8	152.3
Experimental				
1	16.3	7.8	13.5	9.6
2	17.6	5.5	12.3	8.2
3	18.9	7.7	16.8	17.1
4	16.6	6.5	18.5	9.5
Mean	17.3	6.9	15.3	11.1
%	100	100	88.4	160.8

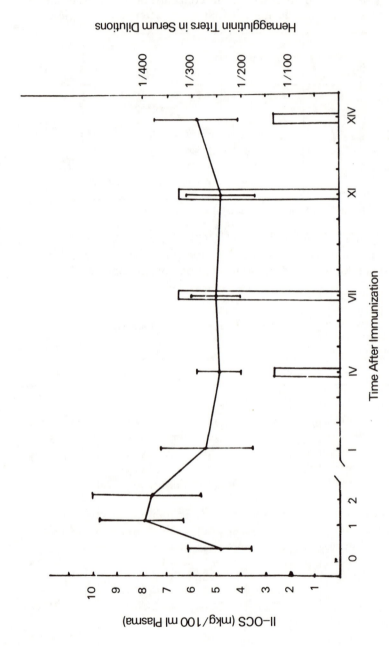

Fig. 2: Plasma OCS and antibody titers in rabbit blood serum at different periods after immunization with the Vi-antigen of typhoid bacilli in a dose of 8 mkg/kg. Arabic numerals on the abscissa denote hours, Roman numerals indicate days. Vertical lines at points are confidence intervals. Bars are antibody titers.

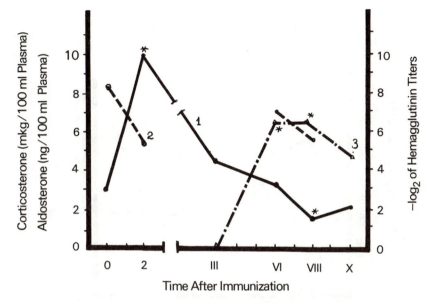

Fig. 3: Corticosterone (1) and aldosterone (2) plasma levels and hemagglutinin serum levels (3) in rats at different periods after immunization with sheep erythrocytes (5 × 10⁹ cells). Arabic numerals on the abscissa denote hours; Roman numerals, days. *p < 0.05 difference from initial level.

The mineralocorticoid function of the hypothalamo-hypophysio-adrenal system may also change in the course of the inductive phase of immune response development. Radioimmunological studies of the aldosterone level in rabbits and rats immunized with Vi-antigen or sheep erythrocytes (carried out jointly with Szalay (JEM, HAS, Hungary) have shown that the concentration of that hormone drops substantially one to two hours after the administration of allogeneic erythrocytes (Figure 3, 4). In the case of Vi-antigen immunization the same trend was noted (Figure 4).

In later periods, in the productive phase of immune reaction development, during the period of intensive antibody formation, no regular shifts in the hormone contents were found in our investigations; it was only in the case of application of horse serum that wave-like variations of the 11-OCS level were revealed which were not of regular character and which manifested themselves only in some of the animals (Shkhinek & Biryukov, 1977). It should be pointed out that in the experiments of some other authors certain (sometimes clearly marked) changes in the 11-OCS content were noted in the productive phase period. Specifically, Belovolova (1973) found phase changes in the 11-OCS concen-

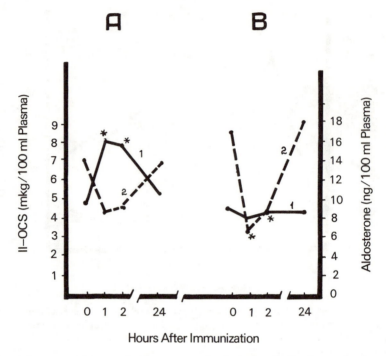

Fig. 4: Plasma 11-OCS (1) and aldosterone (2) levels during the first hours after immunization of rabbits with Vi-antigen of typhoid bacilli at a dose of 8 mkg/kg (A), and sheep erythrocytes in a dose of 6×10^9 cells (B). *$p < 0.05$ difference from initial level.

tration in rabbits after the administration of fraction 1 of the plague germ, repeated rises in the glucocorticoid level being noted within the first few hours as well as on the third and tenth days after immunization. Besedovsky et al. (1975) found two- and three-fold increases in the corticosterone level in blood serum after immunization of female rats with sheep erythrocytes, i. e., during the period of intensive increase in antibody-forming cells in the spleen. However, in our experiments the same antigen administered at the same dose to male rats produced no changes in the level of antibodies in the serum on the fifth to sixth day (Figure 3). It appears, therefore, that this fact does not reflect any general regularities, and it may be attributed to sex differences in the animals used.

Changes in the glucocorticoid level during the first hours after immunization are mediated through the nervous system. Hormonal shifts in response to antigenic stimuli (as with stimuli of a nonantigenic nature) increase reliably with electrolytic lesioning of the posterior hypo-

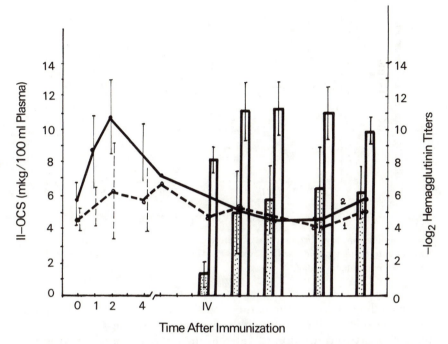

Fig. 5: Plasma 11-OCS level and serum antibody titers at different periods after primary and secondary immunization of rabbits with sheep erythrocytes (17.5×10^9 cells). Dashed curve 11-OCS following primary immunization; solid curve, after repeated immunization. Stippled bars, $-\log_2$ of antibody titers after primary immunization; blank bars, after repeated immunization. Arabic numerals on the abscissa denote hours; Roman numerals, days.

thalamus. The basal level of the hormones under such conditions is lowered (Shkhinek, 1975; Korneva et al., 1978).

The foregoing evidence justifies a conclusion that the HHACS is involved in the organism's reaction to an antigen, manifested by a more or less pronounced stimulation of 11-OCS production, in a lower binding capacity of transcortin, and a lower aldosterone level during the first few hours after antigen administration. However, under certain conditions there may be no stimulation of 11-OCS production in response to an antigen (no reaction to sheep erythrocytes in rabbits) despite a normally developing humoral immune reaction. Changes in the glucocorticoid function of the HHACS during the period of the productive phase of immune response are of a less regular character, being noted on the administration of only certain antigens. The manifestation of hormonal reaction in that period apparently depends upon many fac-

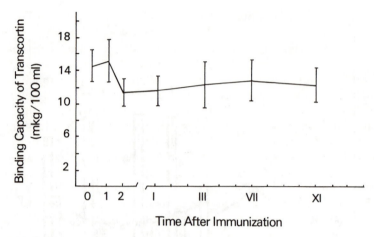

Fig. 6: Binding capacity of transcortin at different periods after immunization of rabbits with Vi-antigen of typhoid bacilli (8 mkg/kg). Arabic numerals on the abscissa denote hours; Roman numerals, days.

tors including, possibly, the nature and the dose of the antigen and the sex of the animal. In considering the mechanisms of the development of the glucocorticoid reaction to antigens, it is perhaps possible, as in the case of other stress factors, to allow for several possible avenues of development, including a direct or mediated reflex effect on the central part of the HHACS or some peripheral parts of the system. It has been shown by work in the laboratory of E. Stark in Hungary that the concrete effects of a stressful stimulus depend on the nature of the stimulus. Specifically, a direct affect upon the pituitary body and the adrenal glands has been proved for certain endotoxins (Stark et al., 1968; Makara et al., 1969). It is worthwhile to note that the observed changes in the mineralocorticoid function of the HHACS in response to certain antigens, as distinct from that of glucocorticoids, do not conform to the usual stress reaction scheme: the level of those hormones in response to sheep erythrocytes and Vi-antigen not only failed to rise but even showed a downward trend. It is not yet clear whether that is a characteristic property of the reaction to antigens or whether it reflects the distinguishing features of the method for the administration of the preparations (intravenous immunization).

Altogether open is the question as to what extent the hormonal reactions to the antigen are due to the effect of the stimulus itself or to that of the mediators released as a result of the contact of the antigen with immune system cells. It may be expected that practically all the elements involved in the specific response are capable of transmitting to the CNS information about the antigen. Moreover, serving as such a source may be those cells which are nonspecifically involved in the reaction to antigen as a result of the nonspecific action of the stimulus itself, or of the mediators released by specifically activated cells.

The physiological role of changes in the glucocorticoid function of the HHACS in the development of immune response was studied by a variety of methods. First of all, the correlation between the intensity of humoral immune response and the extent to which 11-OCS concentration rises due to an antigen was investigated. For this purpose hormonal and immune shifts were analyzed in normal immunized animals with high and low antibody titers, as well as in animals with directed suppression of immune response caused by the lysis of the posterior hypothalamic field. In either case no direct relationship was found to exist between the intensity of humoral response and the magnitude of hormonal shift due to antigen. The course of hormonal reaction was almost identical in animals with high and low antibody titers (Shkhinek et al., 1973; Korneva et al., 1978). Investigation into the same relationship in another model under conditions of competition between two antigens successively administered to mice has shown that the administration of rat erythrocytes three days after previous immunization of the animals with sheep erythrocytes results in about a four-fifths reduction in the humoral response to rat erythrocytes. In the meantime, the intensity of hormonal reaction to rat erythrocytes, i.e., the magnitude of the deviation of the hormone concentration in relation to the initial level, was greater in the controls, i.e., those animals with a higher immune response (Figure 7). The initial level of 11-OCS in the experimental group three days after the administration of sheep erythrocytes did not differ reliably from the hormonal concentration of the control group mice, while the rise in response to the administration of rat erythrocytes in absolute concentration units in the experimental group was the same as in the controls (Korneva et al., 1978).

At the same time, in experiments performed on female rats (Besedovsky et al., 1979) on a similar model (competition between horse and sheep erythrocytes successively administered after a period of six days), a lowering of the suppressive competition phenomenon (as measured by the plaque-formation level of splenic cells) after adrenalectomy was found. The authors are inclined to regard it as a result of eliminating the influence of glucocorticoids. However, in the same paper the phenomenon of competitive suppression was shown to manifest itself in tissue culture in the presence of the same glucocorticoid concentration at which the response to one antigen is sharply stimulated.

It appears that, in addition to glucocorticoids, other factors are involved in the concrete action of two antigens, the more so, as in our ex-

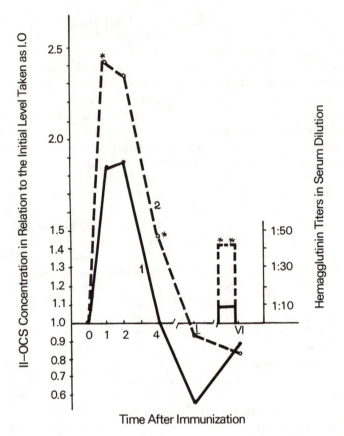

Fig. 7: Plasma 11-OCS levels in mice immunized with rat erythrocytes (2×10^7 cells) after previous injection of 2×10^9 sheep erythrocytes (1) and without previous injection of sheep erythrocytes (2). Solid bar, titers of antibody in group 1; broken bar, group 2. *$p < 0.05$, **$p < 0.01$ levels of significance in comparison to corresponding values of the experimental group.

periments the suppression of antibody synthesis in response to the second antigen also manifested itself whenever the latter was administered against the background of a normal, not higher, level of 11-OCS in the blood.

In order to elucidate the role played by a hormonal shift developing in the first few hours after immunization, use was made of a model with a centrogenous block of the HHACS function, produced by a single intraventricular administration of dexamethasone (0.4 mg) in rabbits. It had been previously established that dexamethasone itself, with its systemic administration in a dose ten times greater than that

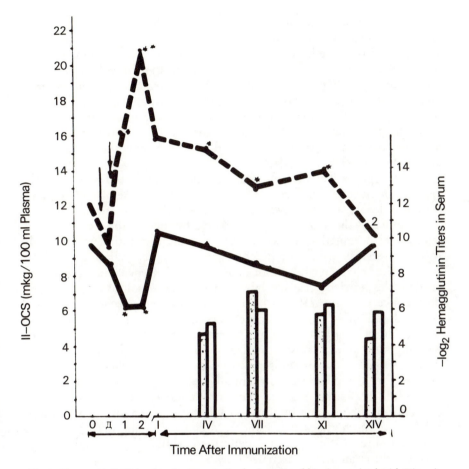

Fig. 8: Plasma 11-OCS level and serum antibody titers in rabbits immunized with Vi-antigen of typhoid bacilli (16 mkg/kg) following intraventricular injection of dexamethasone (1) or physiological solution (2). Arabic numerals on the abscissa denote hours; Roman numerals, days: Д, 3.5-hour period after injection of dexamethasone or physiological solution into the lateral ventricle of the brain. Blank bars, -log₂ hemagglutinin titers in group 1; stippled bars, in group 2. Single arrow, injection on dexamethasone or physiological solution; double arrow, injection of antigen. *p<0.05; **p<0.01 in comparison to corresponding values of the experimental group.

used for intraventricular injection, produced no substantial changes in the course of antibody production (Korneva et al., 1978). The preparation was administered 3–3¹/₂ hours before immunization. The level of 11-OCS in the blood had dropped by that time, and the administration of the Vi-antigen of the typhoid bacillus not only failed to stimulate

11-OCS secretion, which was characteristic for the control animals, but actually lowered the hormone level (Figure 8). However, there was no significant difference in the intensity of antibody production (as shown by the hemagglutinin content in the serum) in the control and experimental animals (Figure 8). Similar findings were obtained in experiments using sheep erythrocytes as antigen. Although during the first few hours after immunization the 11-OCS level among animals of the experimental group was reliably lower than in the controls (0.05), the antibody titers in the experimental and control groups showed no reliable difference (Figure 9).

The foregoing data testify once again to the fact that moderate changes in glucocorticoid content in the inductive phase of the immune response do not appreciably affect the level of antibody production.

Inasmuch as the drop in 11-OCS caused by the centrogenous administration of dexamethasone was of relatively short duration, it appeared to be of interest to investigate correlations between humoral and immunological characteristics under conditions of deeper and longer glucocorticoid deficiency caused by adrenalectomy. Analysis of published data concerning the effect of adrenalectomy upon response has revealed that in most studies no check was kept on the level of hormones in the blood even though this is very important, particularly when working with animals possessing extra adrenal gland tissue.

Exogenous glucocorticoids are known to change the functions of certain T-cell populations substantially (e.g., Anderson & Blomgren, 1970; Zak, 1977; and others). Therefore it was expedient to study the character of the immune response to a T-dependent antigen, evaluating the level of antibodies of IgG and IgM classes, an approach which allows an indirect estimation of T-cell function. In experiments on rats it was found that bilateral adrenalectomy brought about a drop in the level of 11-OCS one to two days after the operation, the hormone level lowering most appreciably in the first two to four days following the operation. The 11-OCS level in the plasma of adrenalectomized animals two days after the operation was 2.56 ± 0.4 mkg/100 ml when measured by the fluorometric method (Pankov & Usvatova, 1965) and 1.2 ± 0.4 mkg/100 ml as determined by the radioreceptor technique (Murphy, 1967), i. e., there was no absolute glucocorticoid deficiency. By the 10th–12th day after the operation the level of glucocorticoids in the blood had risen somewhat, a finding which is in line with those of some other authors (Desser-Wiest, 1976), and which appears to testify to the intensive functioning of the extra adrenal gland tissue. Antigen administration on the second day after the operation produced no hormonal shift in the control animals (Figure 10). Reliable differences in the 11-OCS level between the control and experimental immunized ani-

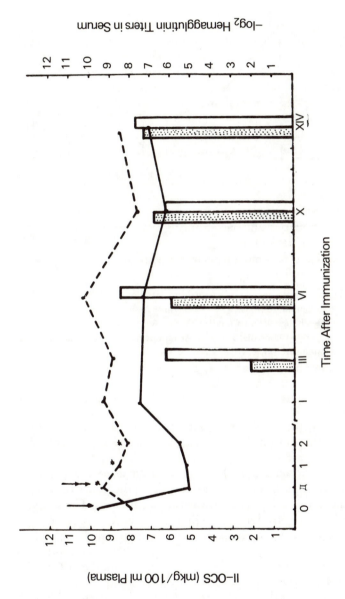

Fig 9: Plasma 11-OCS level and serum antibody titers in rabbits immunized with sheep erythrocytes (18×10^9 cells) following intraventricular injection of dexamethasone (solid curve) or physiological solution (broken curve). Arabic numerals on the abscissa denote hours; Roman numerals, days: II, 3.5-hour period after injection of dexamethasone or physiological solution into the lateral ventricle of the brain. Blank bars, $-\log_2$ hemagglutinin titers in dexamethasone group; stippled bars, in control group. Single arrow, injection of dexamethasone; double arrow, injection of antigen. *$p < 0.05$; **$p < 0.01$.

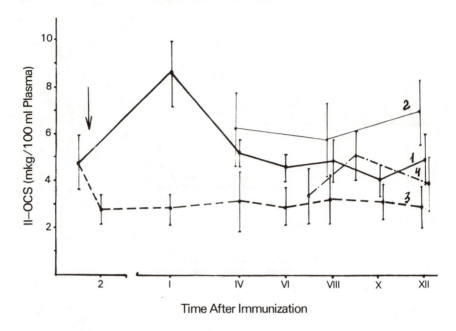

Time After Immunization

Fig 10: Plasma 11-OCS level of control and adrenalectomized rats at different periods in the development of the immune response to sheep erythrocytes (5×10^9 cells). Arabic numeral on abscissa denotes hours; Roman numerals, days. Arrow indicates time of immunization. Curve 1, unoperated controls; curve 2, pseudooperated; curve 3, adrenalectomized 2 days before immunization; curve 4, adrenalectomized 5 days before immunization.

mals remained up to the eighth day. Adrenalectomy performed on the fifth day after immunization did not bring about any significant drop in the 11-OCS concentration (Figure 10).

The general titers of hemagglutinins in the adrenalectomized animals did not differ reliably from those characteristic of the controls (Figure 11), although there was some trend towards their increase. The titers of IgG antibodies were considerably higher than in the control rats, whereas the titers of IgM antibodies showed no material changes (Figure 12). In rats adrenalectomized on the fifth day after immunization both the general antibody titers and the level of antibodies of classes IgG and IgM did not differ from those of the controls.

Thus, it appears that in the whole organism only intensive and lingering hormonal balance disturbances are capable of producing substantial shifts in humoral immune response. In rats, adrenalectomy, although

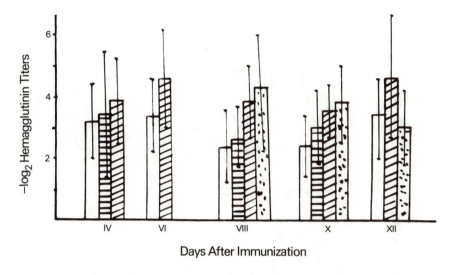

Fig 11: Total hemagglutinin titers in blood serum of control and adrenalectomized rats of different periods of immune response development. Clear bars, control animals; horizontal hatching, pseudooperated; oblique hatching, adrenalectomized 2 days before immunization; stippling, adrenalectomized 5 days before immunization.

causing a fairly long but rather slight glucocorticoid deficiency, probably leads to functional disturbances of those cellular populations which are most sensitive to hormones. Since the synthesis of IgG class antibodies has been shown to be a T-dependent function, proceeding with the indispensable participation of T-helpers (Miller, 1975), there is reason to believe that adrenalectomy disturbs the functions of those cells or alters the processes of cooperative interaction between the cells. Taking into account the data of Van Dijk et al. (1976) indicating a pronounced effect of adrenalectomy upon cellular elements of the monocytic series, it is possible that these cells, too, are involved in the effect.

The suggestion that transitory changes in the level of corticosteroids in blood cannot significantly change the intensity of antibody production in an intact organism is supported by the evidence obtained in studying the humoral immune response in rabbits exposed to the action of episodic stress during the preinductive and inductive phases of immune reaction. Stress was produced by the daily immobilization of the animals for one hour during two days prior to and two days after immunization with sheep erythrocytes or Vi-antigen of typhoid bacilli.

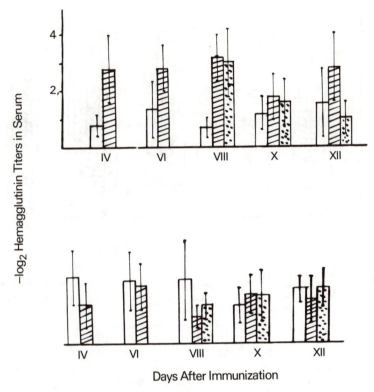

Fig 12: IgG (upper panel) and IgM (lower panel) titers in control and adrenalectomized animals at different periods of immune response development. Clear bars, control animals; hatching, adrenalectomized 2 days before immunization; stippling, adrenalectomized 5 days before immunization.

The stress induced a regular rise of the 11-OCS level in blood plasma by 100–200% relative to the initial level. The reaction's maximum was noted one hour after the beginning of immobilization, and one hour after its termination the hormone level was normal in most of the animals. Immunization was performed during the period of maximum 11-OCS rise. Neither the controls nor the stressed group had a hormonal response to sheep erythrocytes (Figure 13), whereas the reaction to Vi-antigen administration was approximately of the same intensity as in the controls (Figure 14). The level of humoral antibodies following immunization with sheep erythrocytes and with Vi-antigen showed no significant differences between control and experimental groups (Figures 13, 14). These findings are in agreement with the results obtained by some other authors who found no effect of episodic stress on hu-

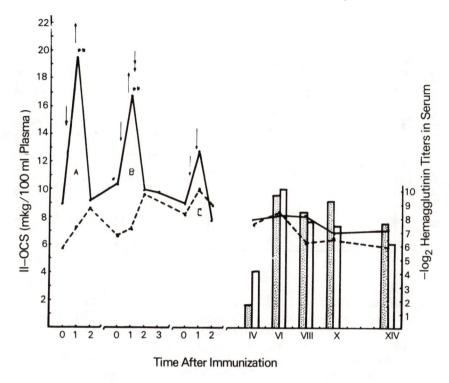

Fig. 13: Plasma 11-OCS level and serum antibody titers in rabbits immunized with sheep erythrocytes (7.5×10^9 cells) following immobilization and without it. Arabic numerals on the abscissa denote hours, Roman numerals, days. Dashed curve, 11-OCS concentration in the control group; solid curve, that in the stress group. Blank bars, antibody titers in the experimental group; stippled bars, those in the controls. Downward arrows, the beginning and upward arrows the end of immobilization. Double arrow, the time of immunization. A, hormonal reaction to the stress 2 days prior to immunization; B, on the day of immunization; C, on the day following immunization. *$p < 0.05$, **$p < 0.01$ in comparison to the corresponding values of the control group.

moral immune reactions (Solomon, 1969). The foregoing facts indicate that transitory stress also does not appreciably affect the level of antibody production when the antigen enters the organism at the time of maximum rise of the 11-OCS level due to a stressor.

The results outlined above show that pronounced and relatively brief changes in glucocorticoid concentration toward higher or lower values

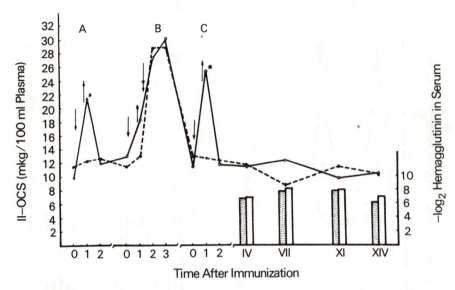

Fig 14: Plasma 11-OCS levels and serum antibody titers in rabbits immunized with Vi-an-tigen of typhoid bacilli following immobilization and without it. Arabic numerals on the abscissa denote hours, Roman numerals, days. Dashed curve, 11-OCS concentration in the control group; solid curve, that in the stress group. Blank bars, antibody titers in the experimental group; stippled bars, those in controls. Downward arrows the beginning and upward arrows the end of immobilization. Double arrow, the time of immunization. A, hormonal reaction to stress 2 days prior to immunization; B, on the day of immuniza-tion; C, on the day following immunization. *p < 0.05, **p < 0.01 in comparison to the corresponding values of the control group.

do not lead to any significant shifts of humoral immune response meas-ured by the level of antibodies in blood plasma. At the same time it has been found that in certain experimental situations a rise in the level of antibody production may correlate with a marked intensification of glucocorticoid shifts in the first few hours after the administration of antigen (secondary immune response to sheep erythrocytes in rabbits) and conversely, a drop in the immunological reactivity is attended by a lowering of hormonal reaction to antigen (model of antigen competi-tion in mice).

This evidence suggests that glucocorticoid hormones in a complex with other neurohumoral factors responding to antigen administration may contribute to the activation of cells of the immune system. The possibility of the activating effect of physiological concentrations of glucocorticoids on immunocompetent cells has been adequately proved in experiments with tissue cultures (Ambrose, 1970; Fauci et al., 1977).

However, our experiments have shown that hormonal shifts caused by antigens themselves (as well as slight episodic shifts due to other external stimuli in the inductive phase period) do not play a decisive role in the end result of the immune system's operation as measured by the level of antibodies in blood serum. This is so because the elimination of the shifts (centrogenous block of the HHACS) or their absence in certain immune models (primary immune response to sheep erythrocytes in rabbits) do not produce any appreciable changes in the intensity of humoral immune response. As pointed out above, no correlations were found in some of the immune models between hormonal and immunological indices (e.g., with immune response suppression following electrolysis of the posterior hypothalamus).

At the same time a protracted glucocorticoid deficiency due to adrenalectomy, brought about higher IgG antibody titers and a trend toward greater general hemagglutinin titers, attesting to the possibility of an inhibiting or a so-called limiting effect of physiological concentrations of glucocorticoids upon certain populations of immunocompetent cells—first of all, apparently, upon the subpopulations of T-lymphocytes (Chebotarev, 1979) and the cells of the monocytic series (Van Dijk et al., 1976). As for humoral immune response, that action of the hormones manifested itself in our experiments only under conditions of adrenalectomy, i.e., with a relatively protracted deficiency of the hormones and a complicated hormonal balance disturbance produced by the operation. Hormonal deficiency of short duration due to a centrogenous block of the HHACS did not affect immune response. It appears that either the potentialities for the limiting effect do not vary significantly within certain ranges of glucocorticoid concentrations, or the elimination of the limiting effect following adrenalectomy is not due solely to the influence of glucocorticoids, but has a more complex mechanism.

It should be emphasized that in our experiments we were concerned only with the integrative result of the operation of the entire immune system, immune response being estimated by the level of antibodies in blood serum. Taking into consideration present-day concepts relating to the morphofunctional peculiarities of different populations of lymphoid cells, their marked differences in sensitivity to glucocorticoid hormones—from complete resistance to high sensitivity (e.g., Levine & Claman, 1970; Anderson & Blomgren, 1970; Cohen, 1971; Claman, 1975)—due, apparently, to specific features of the receptor system of cells (Duval et al., 1976, 1977), the diversity of the effects induced by physiological shifts in hormone contents can be credited to the nonuniform sensitivity to hormones of lymphoid cells. Zak and colleagues (Zak, 1977; Zak et al., 1975) found that morphological changes in lymphocytes of different populations due to the effect of glucocorticoids testify to the suppression of functions of some cell populations and the stimulation of others, appreciable differences being noted between the effects of single and protracted administration of hormones.

There is a difference of opinion as to which particular cell populations are the most sensitive to glucocorticoids. Thus, Levine and Claman (1970) have found that bone marrow cells are hormone-resistant, T-dependent elements being the most sensitive. The authors attribute lower immunological reactivity of splenic cells in cortisone-treated mice to the diminution of the T-cell function. Similar results were obtained by some other authors (Mishell, Lucas, & Mishell, 1977). It has been found that following the administration of large doses of dexamethasone the number of plaque-forming cells in the bone marrow increases with their simultaneous decrease in the spleen (Benner & van Oudenaren, 1979). According to other findings there are sensitive cells in the bone marrow, as well as in the spleen and in the thymus, the largest number being in the thymus, where resistant cells account for only 5 to 6 percent, and the smallest number being in the bone marrow, where the resistant-cell population comprises about 80 percent. The number of resistant cells depends upon the dose of hormones: small doses of hydrocortisone diminish the total number of cells in the thymus but do not alter it in the spleen (Cohen, Fischbach, & Claman, 1970). The cortisone-resistant population of thymic cells is immunologically competent, and fully retains its ability to participate in humoral and cellular immune response. According to those data, thymus-dependent cell helpers as well as cell initiators of cellular response are cortisone-resistant (Cohen, 1971). It has been established that under certain conditions the immunological potencies of those cells (the capability for cellular response, in particular) can increase (Cohen et al., 1970). The lower capability of splenic cells for humoral immune response under the effect of glucocorticoids is attributed by the authors to damage of B- rather than T-cell elements, that ability, in their experiments, being restored by bone-marrow cells.

However, in certain cellular systems, e. g., when human lymphocytes are cultivated with sheep erythrocytes and mitogens, hydrocortisone induced stimulation of B-cell functions (Fauci, Pratt, & Whalen, 1977). It is important to note that the resistance of cells to glucocorticoids may vary under the influence of a number of factors. It has been found that after contact with antigen a sensitive cell acquires resistance, which, in particular, has been demonstrated for B-cells (Cohen, 1971) and T-cell helpers interacting with antigen carriers (Segal & Cohen, 1972).

According to some evidence thymic suppressor cells are cortisone-sensitive (Cohen & Gershon, 1975). Physiological concentrations of glucocorticoids in culture may weaken the suppressor effect of the cells on the immune response to sheep erythrocytes (Haynes & Fauci, 1979). Some authors believe that glucocorticoids influence the balance of positive and negative action of T-cells which regulate humoral immune response, this phenomenon manifesting itself only within 24 hours after the introduction of the antigen in the culture (Fauci et al., 1977).

Investigations in recent years have shown that glucocorticoid hormones are also capable of altering the functions of cells of the monocytic series, which are also known to participate in immune reactions, the character of that influence depending upon the dose of hormones: physiological concentrations of hormones can activate macrophages (Olivo & Shands, 1977), while large doses would suppress their functions (e. g., Slonecker & Lim, 1972; Gaumer et al., 1974).

The above findings appear to suggest that the "physiological" shifts in the level of glucocorticoid hormones, as well as their pharmacological influence, may induce dissimilar alterations in the functions of cells of different populations, the decisive role in the character of the ultimate effect of the hormonal influence on the level of antibodies being played by the intensity and duration of the hormonal shift. In the whole organism, there may also exist extra mechanisms providing protection against the effect of higher hormone concentrations.

The testing of immunological abilities of lymphoid cells in *in vitro* cultures and *in vivo* reveals a specific result of the hormonal influence, whereas a humoral response measured by the amount of antibody in the blood serum reflects the general level of operation of the system. This is probably what accounts for the fact that studies of the immunological capabilities of the cells of lymphoid organs, carried out by a number of authors, indicate sharp changes in immunological reactivity even after transitory and moderately intensive hormonal shifts, whereas humoral immune response, measured by titers of antibodies in the serum, is more resistant to such influences. Transitory variations of the glucocorticoid level may lead to significant alterations of the functions of certain cellular clones, which are noted if the immune response is tested, for instance, by means of the *in vitro* system, and the cellular material is taken at a certain period of time in relation to the hormonal effect. In the meantime, the antigen introduced into the cellular system being tested may affect only those isolated cells and, therefore, it is easier to detect changes in the immunological capabilities of the cell pool being investigated. In the entire organism, temporary changes in HHACS activity may induce the same functional disturbances in certain cell pools, but since the antigen stimulates a much wider circle of different cells, many of which are resistant to hormones, this may fail to affect the end result of the immune system activity, i. e., the intensity of antibody production measured by the titers of antibodies in the blood serum. Inasmuch as antigen-stimulated cells are not easily subjected to hormonal influence (Cohen, 1971), and polypotent bone marrow cells are resistant to hormones (e.g., Levine & Claman, 1970; Mishell et al., 1977), relatively brief hormonal influences in the whole organism do not materially alter the general synthesis of antibodies. In this connection an important role is probably played by the fact that antigens are present in the organism for a fairly long period of time, measured by days, whereas glucocorticoids induce irreversible changes in the cellular functions; therefore a prolonged and intensive hormonal effect is required for the marked suppression of antibody production in the whole organism.

From the viewpoint of the limiting influence of physiological concentrations of glucocorticoids upon the lymphoid cells in the whole organism, the role of those hormones may consist in inhibiting the activity of the cortisone-sensitive cells which are not directly involved in the immune process, but are nonspecifically activated as a result of the antigen entering the organism. Then the higher ratio of glucocorticoids to antigens in response to the introduction of an antigen may be regarded as suppressing the activation of lymphoid cells with a low affinity for antigens or with none at all (Besedovsky & Sorkin, 1977). In that case there may be no direct correlation between the system's immune response and the intensity of hormonal shift induced by the antigens, but the higher glucocorticoid concentration may play the role of the factor which limits the influence of the antigen upon those cells nonspecifically involved in the process, i.e., cells possessing no specific receptors to the antigen, but involved in the process indirectly – as a result, for example, of being affected by mediators released by specifically activated cells.

It is also possible that a hormonal shift induced by antigens under certain conditions (e.g. in the case of secondary immune response) limits the excessive activation of the cells which are directly concerned with the immune response. In that case its elimination should enhance the intensity of antibody production, which may be experimentally demonstrated on a model of secondary immune response under conditions of a functional block of the HHACS.

In evaluating the role of glucocorticoid hormones in the expression of the immune response in the whole organism it is probably important to take into account those neurohumoral shifts which accompany changes in the level of glucocorticoids under certain conditions. This concerns both the neurohumoral reactions induced by the antigens themselves which, apparently, may have their own distinctive features, depending upon the character of the antigen, and also reactions to other external stimuli against the background of which the immune response takes place.

Specifically, it is well known that stress induces complex disturbances of hormonal balance, and individual components of the neurohumoral shift induced by stress may affect the lymphoid cell functions in opposite directions. Considering the fact that glucocorticoids possess potentiating or permissive properties in relation to many biologically active substances (e.g., Lee, Charles, & Reed, 1977; Ambrose, 1970), the end result of a complex neurohumoral shift will depend upon its character.

Thus, in evaluating the role of physiological concentrations of glucocorticoids in the manifestation of the immune response in the whole organism, it is necessary to take into account not only the foregoing data on the nonuniformity of sensitivity to hormones of different cell populations of the immune system, but also the character of the general neurohumoral shift attending the development of the immune response.

The foregoing proves that in evaluating the physiological influence of HHACS hormones on immune reactions it is necessary to take into account the concrete conditions under which that influence takes place, as well as the level of immune system function at which that function is evaluated.

References

Ahlqvist, J. Endocrine influences on lymphatic organs, immune responses, inflammation and autoimmunity. *Acta Endocrinol.*, 1976, *83*, Suppl. 206, 136 pp.

Ambrose, C. T. The essential role of corticosteroids in the induction of the immune response *in vitro*. In G. E. W. Wolstenholme & J. Knight (Eds.), *Hormones and the immune response*. London: Churchill, 1970.

Anderson, B., & Blomgren, H. Evidence for a small pool of immunocompetent cells in the mouse thymus. Its role in the humoral antibody response against sheep erythrocytes, bovine serum albumin, ovalbumin and NIP determinant. *Cell. Immunol.*, 1970, *1*, 362–371.

Antonenko, A. V., Valueva, T. K., Starikova, O. N., & Chebotarev, V. F. Dynamics of development of slow-type hypersensitivity and antibody formation in adrenalectomized guinea-pigs. (In Russian). In: Aktualnye problemy fiziologii, biokhimii i patologii endokrinoi sistemy. Moscow: Meditsin, 1972.

Bartrop, R. W., Luckhurst, E., Lazarus, L., Kiloh, L. G., & Penny, R. Depressed lymphocyte function after bereavement. *Lancet*, 1977, *1*, 834–836.

Belovolova, R. A. Some aspects of neurohumoral regulation of immunogenesis. (In Russian). Author's abstract of candidate dissertation. Rostov on the Don: 1973, 19pp.

Benner, R., & van Oudenaren, A. Corticosteroids and the humoral immune response of mice. II. Enhancement of marrow antibody formation to lipopolysaccharide by high doses of corticosteroids. *Cell. Immunol.*, 1979, *48*, 267–275.

Besedovsky, H. O., Del Rey, A., & Sorkin, E. Antigenic competition between horse and sheep red blood cells as a hormone-dependent phenomenon. *Clin. Exp. Immunol.,* 1979. *37,* 106–113.

Besedovsky, H., & Sorkin, E. Network of immune-neuroendocrine interactions. *Clin. Exp. Immunol.,* 1977, *27,* 1–12.

Besedovsky, H., Sorkin, E., Keller, M., & Müller, J. Changes in blood hormone levels during the immune response. *Proc. Soc. Exp. Biol. Med.,* 1975, *150,* 466–470.

Bezin, G. J., Moroz, B. B., Petrov, R. V., Khaitov, R. M., Romashko, O. O., & Gavrilov, V. A. Migration and differentiation of hematopoietic truncal cells depending on the level of endogenous corticoids in the organism. (In Russian). In: Problemy gematologii i perelivaniya krovi. Moscow: 1977, *12,* 21–27.

Chebotarev, V. F. Endocrine regulation of immunogenesis. (In Russian). Kiev: Zdorovie, 1979.

Chebotarev, V. F., & Valueva, T. K. Effect of adrenalectomy on the development of antibody-forming cells in animals with delayed hypersensitivity. (In Russian). *J. Microbiol. Epidemiol. Immunol.,* 1972, *42,* 128–131.

Claman, H. N. How corticosteroids work. *J. Allergy Clin. Immunol.,* 1975, *55,* 145–151.

Cohen, J. J. The effect of hydrocortisone on the immune response. *Ann. Allergy,* 1971, *29,* 358–361.

Cohen, J. J., Fischbach, M., & Claman, H. N. Hydrocortisone resistance of graft vs. host activity in mouse thymus, spleen, and bone marrow, *J. Immunol.,* 1970, *105,* 1146–1150.

Cohen, P., & Gershon, R. K. The role of cortisone-sensitive thymocytes in DNA synthetic responses to antigen. *Ann. N. Y. Acad. Sci.,* 1975, *249,* 451–461.

Comsa, J. Influences hormonales sur les fonctions immunitaires. *Pediatrie,* 1977, *32,* 439–446.

Comsa, J., Leonhardt, H., & Schwartz, J. A. Influences of the thymus-corticotropin-growth hormone interaction on the rejection of skin allografts on the rat. *Ann. N. Y. Acad. Sci.,* 1975, *249,* 387–401.

Desser-Wiest, L. Corticosterone in serum of adrenalectomized male rats. *Osterr. Z. Onkol.,* 1976, *3,* 70–73.

Duval, D., Dardenne, M., Dausse, J. P., & Homo, F. Glucocorticoid receptors in corticosensitive and corticoresistant thymocyte subpopulations. II. Studies with hydrocortisone-treated mice. *Biochim. Biophys. Acta.,* 1977, *496,* 312–320.

Duval, D., Dausse, J. P., & Dardenne, M. Glucocorticoid receptors in corticosensitive and corticoresistant thymocyte subpopulations. I. Characterization of glucocorticoid receptors and isolation of a corticoresistant subpopulation. *Biochim. Biophys. Acta.,* 1976, *451,* 82–91.

Eliseeva, L. S. Connection of the adrenal glands with the regulatory function of the serotoninergic system in immunogenesis. (In Russian). Fiziologiya immunogo gomeostaza. Tezisy dokladov II vsesoyuznogo simpoziuma. Rostov on the Don: 1977, 61–62.

Escola, J., Ruuskanen, O., Soppi, E., Viljanen, M. K., Järvinen, M., Toivonen, H., & Kouvalainen, K. Effect of sport stress on lymphocyte transformation and antibody formation. *Clin. Exp. Immunol.,* 1978, *32,* 339–345.

Fauci, A. S., Pratt, K. R., & Whalen, G. Activation of human B lymphocytes. IV. Regulatory effects of corticosteroids on the triggering signal in the plaque-forming cell response of human peripheral blood B lymphocytes to polyclonal activation. *J. Immunol.,* 1977, *119,* 598–603.

Gaumer, H. R., Salvaggio, J. E., Weston, W. L., & Claman, H. N. Cortisol inhibition in immunologic activity in guinea pig alveolar cells. *Int. Arch. Allergy Appl. Immunol.,* 1974, *47,* 797–809.

Gisler, R. H., & Schenkel-Hulliger, L. Hormonal regulation of the immune response. II. Influence of pituitary and adrenal activity on immune responsiveness *in vitro. Cell. Immunol.,* 1971, *2,* 646–657.

Haynes, B. F., & Fauci, A. S. Mechanisms of corticosteroid action on lymphocyte subpopulations. IV. Effects of *in vitro* hydrocortisone on naturally occurring and mitogen-induced suppressor cells in man. *Cell. Immunol.,* 1979, *44,* 157–168.

Joasoo, A., & McKenzie, J. M. Stress and the immune response in rats. *Int. Arch. Allergy Appl. Immunol.,* 1976, *50,* 659–663.

Kinnaert, P., Mahieu, A., & Van Geertruyden, N. Stimulation of antibody synthesis induced by surgical trauma in rats. *Clin. Exp. Immunol.,* 1978, *32,* 243–252.

Kinnaert, P., Mahieu, A., & Van Geertruyden, N. Stimulation of antibody synthesis induced by surgical trauma in rats. Revised statistical analysis. *Clin. Exp. Immunol.,* 1979, *37,* 174–175.

Koputovskaya, L. P. The influence of the hypophyseal-adrenal system on immunogenesis in white mice. (In Russian). In: Sovremennye problemy immunologii i immunopatologii. Leningrad: 1970, 59–75.

Korneva, E. A., Klimenko, V. M., & Shkhinek, E. K. Neurohumoral maintenance of immune homeostasis. (In Russian). Leningrad: Nauka, 1978.

Lee, T. P., Charles, P., & Reed, E. Effects of steroids on the regulation of the levels of cyclic AMP in human lymphocytes. *Biochem. Biophys. Res. Commun.,* 1977, *78,* 998–1004.

Levine, M. A., & Claman, H. N. Bone marrow and spleen: Dissociation of immunologic properties by cortisone. *Science,* 1970, *167,* 1515–1517.

Lindemann, L., Wirth, W., & Müller, U. S. Altersabhängige Veränderungen streßbedingter Immunsuppression. *Z. Rheumatol.,* 1978, *31,* 23–32.

Locke, S. E., & Heisel, J. S. The influence of stress and emotions on the human immune response. *Biofeedback Self-regul.,* 1977, *2,* 320. (Abstract)

Lundin, P. M. Effect of hypophysectomy on antibody formation in the rat. *Acta. Pathol. Microbiol. Scand.,* 1960, *48,* 351–357.

Makara, G. B., Stark, E., Palkovits, M., Revesz, T., & Michaly, K. Afferent pathways of stressful stimuli: Corticotropin release after partial deafferentation of the medial basal hypothalamus. *J. Endocrinol.,* 1969, *44,* 187–193.

Miller, J. F. A. P. T-cell regulation of immune responsiveness. *Ann. N. Y. Acad. Sci.,* 1975, *249,* 9–26.

Mishell, R. I., Lucas, R., & Mishell, B. B. The role of activated accessory cells in preventing immunosuppression by hydrocortisone. *J. Immunol.,* 1977, *119,* 118–122.

Murphy, B. E. P. Some studies of the protein-binding of steroids and their application to the routine micro and ultramicro measurement of various steroids in body fluids by competitive protein-binding radioassay. *J. Clin. Endocrinol. Metab.,* 1967, *27,* 973–990.

Olivo, P., & Shands, J. W. Glucocorticoid modulation of LPS activation of murine peritoneal macrophages. *J. Reticuloendothel. Soc.,* 1977, *22,* Suppl., No. 561, A 18. (Abstract)

Pankov, Y. A., & Usvatova, I. Y. Fluorometric method for determining 11-OCS in peripheral blood plasma. (In Russian). In: Metody issledovaniya nekotorykh gormonov i mediatorov. No. 3, Moscow: 1965, 137–145.

Petrov, R. V., Khaitov, R. M., Bezin, G. I., & Rachkov, S. M. Regulatory influence of the hypophyseal-adrenal system on migration of truncal cells, T- and B-lymphocytes: The effect of adrenalectomy, ACTH and hydrocortisone. (In Russian). Neirogumoralnaya i farmakologicheskaya korrektsiya immunologicheskikh reaktsiy v eksperimente i klinike. Tezisy dokladov I vsesoyuznogo simpoziuma. Leningrad: 1978, 52–53.

Petrov, R. V., Maniko, V. M., Moroz, B. B., & Khaitov, R. M. Control of migration and differentiation of truncal cells. (In Russian). In: Kriokonservirovanie immunokompetentnoy tkani. Kiev: Naukova Dumka, 1979.

Pierpaoli, W., & Sorkin, E. Relationship between thymus and hypophysis. Nature, 1967, 215, 834–837.

Pierpaoli, W., & Sorkin, E. A study on antipituitary serum. Immunology, 1969, 16, 311–318.

Segal, S., & Cohen, J. Thymus-derived lymphocytes: Humoral and cellular reactions distinguished by hydrocortisone. Science, 1972, 175, 1126–1128.

Shkhinek, E. K. On the functional role of the posterior hypothalamic field in the expression of reactions of the hypothalamo-hypophysio-adrenal system in rabbits. (In Russian). Probl. Endocrinol., 1975, 21, 59–65.

Shkhinek, E. K., Acs, Z., & Abavary, K. Transcortin's binding capacity in the dynamics of immune process development. (In Russian). Probl. Endocrinol., 1978, 24, 94–99.

Shkhinek, E. K., & Biryukov, V. D. Concerning the role of endocrine factors in the development of the immune response. (In Russian). Patolog. Fiziol. i Exper. Terap.,1977,4,52–55.

Shkhinek, E.K., Tsvetkova, I. P., & Marat, B. A. Analysis of neuroendocrine influences of the posterior hypothalamus on the dynamics of specific defense reactions in rabbits. (In Russian). Fiziol. J. SSSR, 1973, 59, 228–236.

Slonecker, G., & Lim, W. C. Effects of hydrocortisone on the cells in an acute inflammatory exudate. Lab. Invest., 1972, 27, 123–128.

Solomon, G. F. Stress and antibody response in rats. Int. Arch. Allergy Appl. Immunol., 1969, 35, 97–104.

Sorkin, E., & Pierpaoli, W. Hormones and the capability of immunological response. In: Sovremenye problemy immunologii i immunopatologii. Leningrad, 1970.

Stark, E., Fachet, J., Makara, G. B., & Michaly, K. An attempt to explain differences in the hypophyseal-adrenocortical response to repeated stressful stimuli by their dependence on differences in pathways. Acta Med. Acad. Sci. Hung., 1968, 25, 251–260.

Szabo, T., Matus, F., Babiszky, L., Osire, I., Siman, J., & Janko, L. Az ACTH hatasa az IgG-tipusúellenanyagok termelésére kiséleti körülmények között. Tuberk. Estudobeteg., 1975, 28, 377–379.

Thrasher, S. G., Bernardis, L. L., & Cohen, S. The immune response in hypothalamic-lesioned and hypophysectomized rats. Int. Arch. Allergy Appl. Immunol., 1971, 41, 813–820.

Underwood, R. H., & Williams, G. H. The simultaneous measurement of aldosterone, cortisole and corticosterone in human peripheral plasma by displacement analysis. J. Lab. Clin. Med., 1972, 79, 849–862.

Uteshev, B. S., & Babichev, V. A. Inhibitors of antibody synthesis. (In Russian). M., 1974, 320 pp.

Van Dijk, H., Testerink, J., & Noordegraaf, E. Stimulation of the immune response against SRBC by reduction of corticosterone plasma levels: Mediation by mononuclear phagocytes. Cell. Immunol., 1976, 25, 8–14.

Yamada, A., Jensen, M. M., & Rasmussen, A. F., Jr. Stress and susceptibility to viral infection. III. Antibody response and viral retention during avoidance learning stress. *Proc. Soc. Exp. Biol. Med.,* 1964, *116,* 677–680.

Zak, K. P. New conceptions of the mechanism of glucocorticoid lymphocytopenia. (In Russian). In: Novoe o gormonakh i mekhanizme ikh deistviya. Kiev: Naukova Dumka, 1977.

Zak, K. P., Tsarenko, V. I., Filatova, R. S., Naumenko, N. J., Khomenko, B. M., Vinnitskaya, M. L., Liktsina, V. V., & Shlyakhovenko, B. S. Effect of hydrocortisone on the ultra-structure and intracellular metabolism of leukocytes of blood and leukopoietic organs in immunized rabbits. (In Russian). Neirogumoralnaya i farmakologicheskaya korrektsiya immunologicheskikh reaktsiy v eksperimente i klinike. Tezisy dokladov I vsesoyuznogo simpoziuma. Leningrad: 1975, 23–24.

Zimin, Y. I. Immunity and stress. (In Russian). Itogi nauki i tekniki. VINITI *Immunologiia,* 1979, *8,* 173–198.

Changes in Immune Response
and
Tumor Growth in Mice Depend
on the Duration of Stress

H. Teshima and C. Kubo[1]

Introduction

The influence of emotional stress on the prognosis of malignant diseases has been observed clinically and experimentally, and multidimensional analysis made. Psychosomatic studies have revealed personality characteristics and particular life styles of cancer patients (Bahnson & Bahnson, 1969; Booth, 1973; Greene, 1966; LeShan, 1978; Thomas & Duszynski, 1974), while basic experiments have clarified the relationship between emotional stress and cancer growth in laboratory animals with spontaneous, induced, or transplanted cancer (Andervont, 1944; Balitsky, Kapshuk, & Tsapenko, 1969; Kavetsky, Turkevich, & Balitsky, 1966; Levine & Cohen, 1959; Mühlbock, 1951; Rashkis, 1952). Although evidence was obtained for the influence of stress on the prognosis of cancer growth, these results did not elucidate the pathways by which emotional stress influences the growing cancer cells. The importance of functions related to self-defense mechanisms in the host has been given increasing attention and there are numerous clinical reports that immune reactions are closely linked to emotional stress (Rasmussen, Spencer, & Marsh, 1959; Solomon, 1969; Teshima et al., 1974; Wittkower, 1953). This would suggest that the immune system is an intermediate pathway through which emotional stress influences the prognosis of immunological diseases, and perhaps even malignancy.

From the standpoint of immunology, we have performed several types of experiments. C3H strain mice were used as recipients of heterogeneic and leukemia cells, and stress was given to the recipients before

[1] We are grateful to M. Ohara for assistance in preparation of the manuscript.
This research was supported by a grant from the Ministry of Health and Welfare, Japan.

and after the transplantation of the cells. The interval for rejection of the cells and the cytotoxic activity of killer T-cells in the recipients were compared for stressed and control mice. We found that rejection of the transplanted cancer cells was delayed due to suppression of the killer T-cells' cytotoxicity in the stressed mice.

Other studies in our laboratory have revealed the influence of stress on the function of macrophages, which play important roles in the immune system. When a carbon clearance test was carried out to measure the phagocytic activity of the macrophages at different points in the stress-reaction sequence, the elements of the phagocytic process were observed to change, depending on the duration of stress. Enhancement and suppression of phagocytosis were induced by different durations of stress. The same phenomenon was also observed in a starvation experiment in mice. Functions of the immune system were enhanced by short-term starvation and depressed with long-term starvation. Thus, there is a countershock phase against stress in the immune system. Analyzing the countershock phase, we have found that certain amounts of stress enhance the immune system and suppress cancer growth through acceleration of the anti-tumor immune response. We now present immunological and related data on the countershock phase.

Stress and T-cell Function

T-cells (thymus-derived lymphocytes), were separated into several subgroups. Included were killer T-cells or cytotoxic T-cells (Tc), amplifier T-cells, suppressor T-cells, helper T-cells, and effector cells of delayed-type hypersensitivity (Td cells). Among the functions of these cells, we evaluated the cytotoxicity of killer T-cells to clarify the pathway of influence of stress on T-cell functions. Killer T-cells play an important role in rejection of transplanted cells, removal of virus-infected cells and cytotoxicity to cancer cells.

The relationship between cytotoxic functions of killer T-cells induced by chicken red blood cells (CRBC) and stress was studied and the cytotoxicity of killer T-cells induced by cancer cells was then given attention.

CRBC (1.0×10^8 cells) or EL-4 leukemia cells (1.0×10^7 cells) were transplanted subcutaneously into inbred mice of the C3H/H strain (8 week old males). The EL-4 cells were originally thymic leukemia cells of C57BL/6 strain mice which had been maintained in a state of ascites.

Stress was given by buzzer and electricity before and after injection of the cells. The mice were left in the stress box, where stimulation with a 100 db buzzer and a 10 mA electric current was given every 15 seconds over a period of 15 minutes twice daily–morning and afternoon. After the stress, the behavior of the mice became aggressive; they bit each other and were hyperreactive to stimuli.

The mice were separated into four groups, according to the different times of induced stress. In group A, stress was given for three days before and three days after the transplantation of cells; in group B, it was given before the transplantation; in group C, it was given for three days after the transplantation; and in group D no stress was given (controls).

The level of function of killer T-cells was measured by the 51-Cr cytotoxicity test (Lavrin et al., 1973). 51-Cr-traced cells (target cells) and killer T-cells (effector cells) collected from spleen cells of the recipient mice on the 11th day after the transplantation of leukemia cells were mixed in a ratio of 1:50 and the preparation incubated for four hours. Those target cells damaged by effector cells released 51-Cr into the supernatant and counts per minute (cpm) were used as a measure of cytotoxic activity of the effector cells (Figure 1).

The body weight of the mice did not change with this stress. The thymus and the spleen weighed the same in the control and stressed groups. In experiments using CRBC, cytotoxicity was 3.3% in group A,

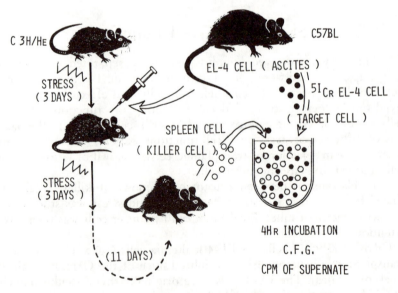

Fig. 1: Cytotoxicity of killer T-cells and stress. Stress was given using the stress box before and after transplantation of EL-4 leukemia cells. Killer T-cells (effector cells) from the spleens of recipient mice were incubated with 51-Cr labelled leukemia cells (target cells). 51-Cr released from damaged target cells into the supernatant was measured.

6.5% in group B, 6.5% in group C, and 14.6% in group D (controls). In the study on transplantation of leukemia cells, rejection of cancer cells was tested by palpation of the tumor. In stressed groups, tumors remained in eight out of nine of the stressed mice on the 11th day after transplantation of the cancer cells. In all three mice in the control group, the tumor was rejected. In the 51-Cr cytotoxicity test, cytotoxicity was 4.4% in group A, 2.3% in group B, 0% in group C and 10.6% in the control group. (Figures 2, 3).

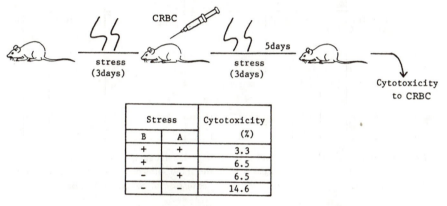

Stress		Cytotoxicity
B	A	(%)
+	+	3.3
+	-	6.5
-	+	6.5
-	-	14.6

Fig. 2: Cytotoxicity of killer T-cells against chicken red blood cells (CRBC). These killer T-cells were induced by heterogeneic antigens of CRBC and inhibition of their cytotoxicity was evident in the stressed group.

Thus the presence of stress led to a suppression of cytotoxicity of the killer cells when induced by CRBC (heterogeneic cells) and by allogeneic cancer cells. Rejection of the cancer cells by killer T-cells was delayed. The killer T-cells recognized heterogeneic antigens of CRBC and a specific tumor antigen on the cancer cells as nonself, and a cytotoxicity reaction occurred. In another experiment, the killer T-cells stimulated to activity by EL-4 cells were used to detect the specific function of killer T-cells in respect to tumor cells.

Although the weights of the thymus and spleen remained unchanged after the mice had been in the stress box, we could not rule out an effective impact on these organs, since the stress which induced no major damage of these organs did, nevertheless, suppress certain functions. The changed behavior of the stressed mice also clearly showed the impact of the stress procedure.

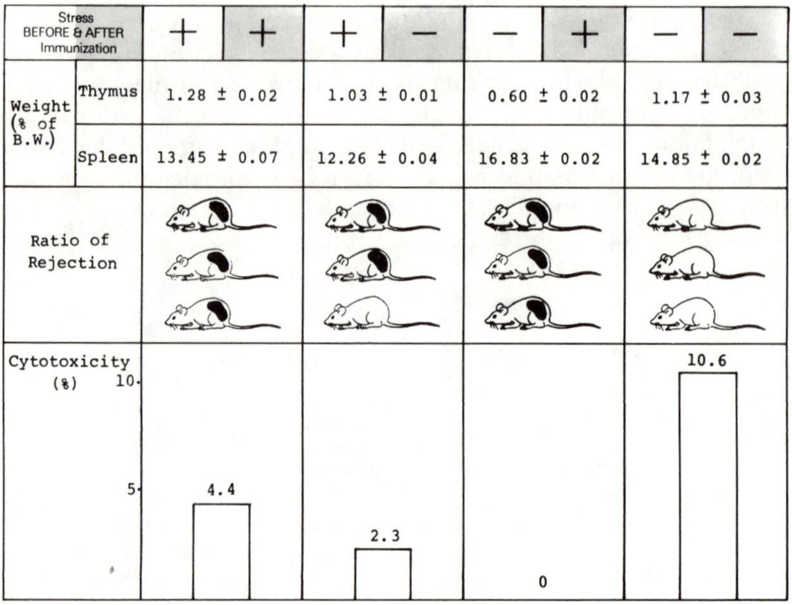

Stress BEFORE & AFTER Immunization		+	+	+	−	−	+	−	−
Weight (% of B.W.)	Thymus	1.28 ± 0.02		1.03 ± 0.01		0.60 ± 0.02		1.17 ± 0.03	
	Spleen	13.45 ± 0.07		12.26 ± 0.04		16.83 ± 0.02		14.85 ± 0.02	
Ratio of Rejection									
Cytotoxicity (%)		4.4		2.3		0		10.6	

Reproduced from Teshima, H., Kubo, C., Kihara, H., Nagata, S., Imada, Y., & Ago, Y. Psychosomatic aspects of skin diseases from the standpoint of immunology. *Psychother. Psychosom.,* 1982, *37,* 165–175, with the kind permission of S. Karger AG, Basel.

Fig. 3: Comparison between stressed and control groups as to weights of the spleen and the thymus, and cytotoxic activity. Changes in cytotoxic activity were statistically significant (Teshima, H. et al., 1982).

Stress and Macrophages

Macrophages play important roles such as particulate phagocytosis, recognition of antigen, and phagocytosis against nonself cells, in particular tumor cells. Using stressed AKR mice, the carbon clearance test was employed to assess changes in the phagocytic activity of macrophages, under conditions of different periods of stress.

Mice (8-week old females, AKR strain) were separated into five groups of four, each being subjected to a different period of stress. AKR strain mice have defects in serum complement component C5, one of the opsonic and chemotaxic factors. Stress was given using the stress box as explained above, and also by immobilization or restraint. Stress was given for 0, 2, 4, 5, and 6 days using the stress box, and for 0, 4, 8, 12, and 24 hours of immobilization.

A carbon clearance test was done, following the procedure of Biozzi, Benacerraf, and Halpern (1953). Carbon (C 11/1431 Gunther Wagner, Hanover, West Germany) was dissolved in 30 mg per ml saline with 1% gelatin. Three hundred mg of carbon per kg of mouse body weight was given intravenously. Every three minutes after the injection of carbon, a 0.02ml blood sample was hemolyzed by 0.1% NaCO$_3$ and measured by spectrophotometer at OD 660 mµ. Calculation of the carbon clearance rates is shown in Figure 4.

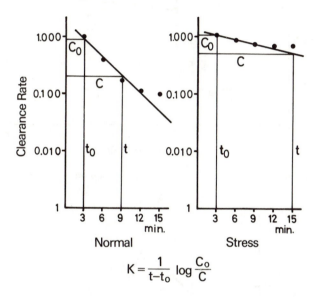

$$K = \frac{1}{t-t_0} \log \frac{C_0}{C}$$

Fig. 4: Calculation of carbon clearance rates of AKR mice in stressed and control groups. The clearance rate (K) was calculated using the formula shown.

In the case of stress induced using the stress box, the carbon clearance rate was 0.083 in the controls, 0.059 on the second day, 0.062 on the fourth day, 0.066 on the fifth day, and 0.058 on the sixth day. On the fourth and fifth days, the clearance rate decreased significantly and on the second and sixth days, the clearance rate was also suppressed (Figure 5).

In the case of immobilization, the carbon clearance rates were 0.077 in the controls and 0.095, 0.120, 0.068 and 0.025 after 4, 8, 12, and 24 hours of restraint, respectively. Following up to eight hours of restraint, the clearance rate was increased by stress. After that a rapid decrease in the clearance rate occurred (Figure 6).

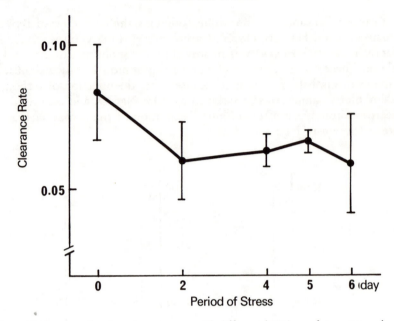

Fig. 5: Fluctuation of carbon clearance rate with different durations of stress (stress box).

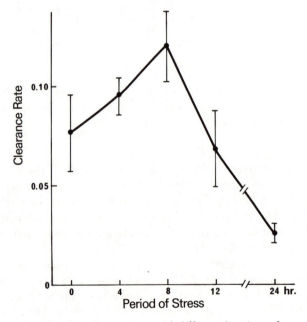

Fig. 6: Fluctuation of carbon clearance rate with different durations of stress (restraint).

In the next experiment, the supplementation of control mouse serum produced no recovery. Normal mouse serum (0.3 ml) was given to the stressed mice after 24 hours of restraint, and 30 minutes later the clearance rates were measured. There was no improvement of the depressed function of macrophages in the stressed mice, as seen in Figure 7. This means that the decreased function of macrophages could not be restored, even by supplementation of humoral factors from normal mice.

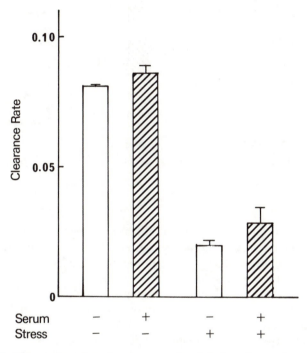

Fig. 7: Changes in carbon clearance rate after infusion of normal serum.

Next, before restraint, *Corynebacterium parvum*, which increases the immune response nonspecifically, was injected to activate phagocytosis by macrophages. Following activation of macrophages, the stress experiment was carried out using restraint as the stressor. When one mg of *Corynebacterium* was administered intraperitoneally seven days before restraint, there was an enhancement of clearance rate in the normal mice from 0.075 to 0.097 (Figure 8). Activation of macrophages by *Corynebacterium* reduced the suppression of clearance rate, changing it from 0.016 to 0.047.

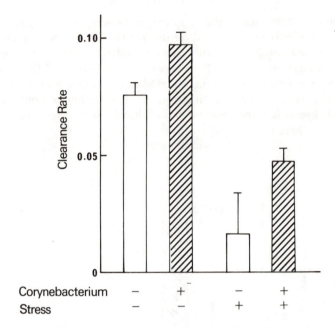

Fig. 8: Changes in carbon clearance rate after enhancement by *Corynebacterium*.

In the experiment using immobilization stress, activity of macrophages, which was determined for intervals of restriction up to eight hours, presumably reflected the countershock phase of the organism's response to the stress, as reported by Selye (1936). This phenomenon was not found in experiments involving the stress box. Thus stress induced by the stress box and by immobilization produced different responses in mice.

The decrease of macrophage phagocytosis by stress did not occur secondary to a decrease of humoral factors, for example an opsonic factor, in the serum. Saba (1970) showed that suppression of macrophage phagocytosis by surgical stress recovered after infusion of normal serum into rats, and it was concluded that supplementation of complement overcame the decrease in opsonic activity induced by the stress. Phagocytosis by macrophages was recovered in our experiment, and supplementation of serum enhanced phagocytosis in the control mice, but not in the mice stressed by immobilization. These differences in findings were probably caused by the different forms of stress, different both qualitatively and quantitatively, which were used. AKR strain mice have fewer humoral factors, since the serum is deficient in complement component C5, one of the opsonic and chemotaxic factors. Thus our study, in which AKR mice were used, suggests the existence of a pathway through which stress acts on macrophages directly.

Stress influences the autonomic nervous system (ANS). The next experiment was carried out to detect participation of the ANS in phagocytosis by macrophages, using ANS-reacting drugs. Epinephrine (10 mg per kg), propranolol (10 mg per kg) and diazepam (10 mg per kg) were administered subcutaneously after 24-hour restraint stress and one hour before the carbon clearance test (Figure 9). Propranolol enhanced phagocytosis in control and stressed mice, and epinephrine suppressed phagocytosis in control mice and produced no amelioration of the decreased macrophage function in the stressed mice. Macrophages seem to be particularly sensitive to drugs acting on the ANS.

After release from 24-hour restraint the carbon clearance rate recovered gradually to 70% after 24-hours (Teshima et al., 1982). This re-

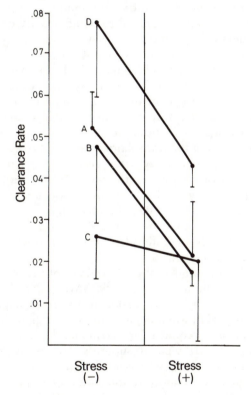

Fig. 9: Autonomic nervous system-related drugs and phagocytosis by macrophages. The mice were restrained for 24 hours and given drugs subcutaneously one hour before the carbon clearance test. A: control; B: diazepam; C: epinephrine; D: propranolol.

covery of phagocytosis in the absence of stress suggests that, while the restraint stress suppressed the functions of the macrophages, the cells were not destroyed.

Time Course of the Tumor Growth of Mice Exposed to Different Periods of Stress

In experiments on the cytotoxicity of T-cells, we found that stress suppressed anti-tumor reactions by suppressing function of killer T-cells. In other experiments, stress generally suppressed phagocytosis by macrophages, but a certain amount of stress did induce an enhancement of macrophage activity. This phenomenon was attributed to the countershock phase described by Selye (1936). We confirmed that stress does lead to a suppression of the immune system but that a certain amount of stress will enhance the coping activity of the organism. We then considered that some stress may enhance anti-tumor activity by activating the immune system. For clarification, the following experiment was done. Eight-week old female AKR strain mice were given transplanted EL-4 leukemia cells and these mice were separated into three groups: group A, the controls, were given no stress; group B animals were exposed to stress by restraint for eight hours; and group C animals were exposed for 24 hours to restraint stress. The sizes of the tumors developing from the transplanted cancer cells were measured on the fifth, eighth and tenth day after grafting the leukemic cells. In group B, inhibition of tumor growth was noted on the fifth, eight and tenth day. In group C, growth of the tumor was not suppressed, especially on the eighth and tenth day (Figure 10).

These results suggest that the immune system's capability of coping with the tumor growth was intensified at the phase when phagocytosis by macrophages was enhanced.

To analyze the mechanism of enhancement of the immune system in more detail, we measured levels of cyclic AMP and cyclic GMP in plasma under various durations of exposure to stress (Figure 11). After eight hours of restraint, when coping with tumor growth and phagocytosis by macrophages were at their maximum, the levels of cyclic AMP also peaked. Cyclic AMP tends to suppress cell-mediated immunity and leukocyte functions (Smith, Steiner, & Parker, 1971). The functions of cyclic AMP depend on concentration, stage of reaction, etc. A slight elevation enhances mitosis of T cells, while large elevations lead to inhibition. Cyclic AMP augments the functions of helper T-cells early in the stages of response, and inhibition then follows (Schied et al., 1975).

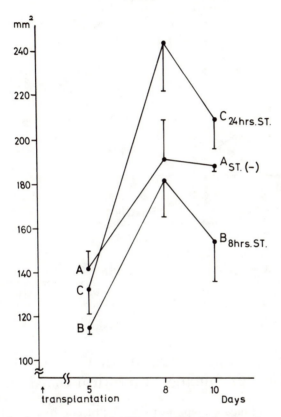

Fig. 10: Growth of tumor in stressed AKR mice. EL-4 leukemic cells were transplanted into stressed mice. Group A, the controls, were given no stress, group B were given eight hours of restraint before the transplantation, and group C were given 24 hours of restraint.

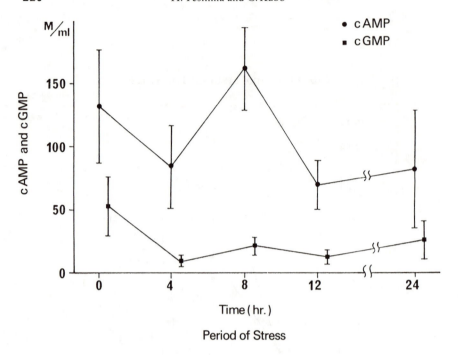

Fig. 11: Changes in plasma levels of cyclic AMP and cyclic GMP in mice given different periods of restraint stress. Cyclic AMP and cyclic GMP were measured by radioimmunoassay.

Changes in Functions of the Immune System During Starvation of Mice

Starvation and acute hyponutrition represent one form of stress which alters several functions of the organism. Starvation has been prescribed as a medical treatment in the Orient since ancient times; however, the mechanisms involved have not been clarified.

We used starvation stress in mice and found evidence for the countershock phase when examining immune function. AKR mice (8 week-old females) were deprived of food for up to six days, but water was given *ad libitum*. A pronounced effect was a decrease in the weight of various organs such as thymus, spleen and liver, as well as that of the whole body (Figure 12). On the second day of starvation the weight of the whole body and of various organs decreased rapidly and thereafter the weight loss was gradual. The carbon clearance rates were enhanced

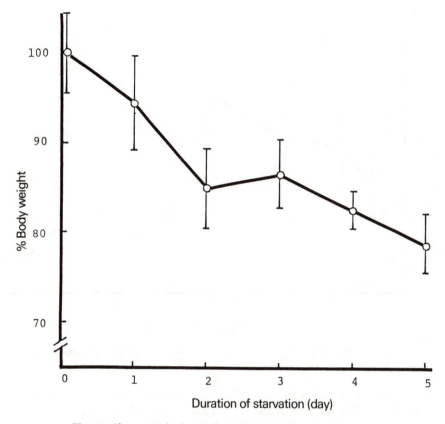

Fig. 12: Changes in body weight during starvation in AKR mice.

on the second and third day of starvation but declined substantially after the fourth day of starvation (Figure 13).

In the starvation study, we investigated the effect on functions of lymphocytes in the spleen (T-cell transformation by the mitogen concanavalin A and B-cell transformation by the mitogen *E. coli* lipopolysaccharide), delayed hypersensitivity, cytotoxicity and antibody production. The T-cell mitogen response was enhanced on the second day of starvation and was suppressed strongly after the third day. B-cell mitogen response was enhanced up to the fifth day and was then suppressed.

Injection of CRBC induced three types of reactions in mice: delayed hypersensitivity, cytotoxicity and antibody production (Kubo et al., 1977). These immune reactions were all enhanced on the second day of starvation and were suppressed after the fourth day (unpublished ob-

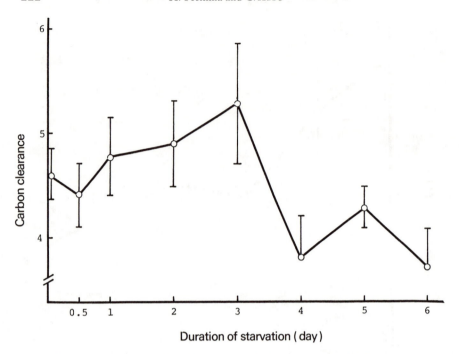

Fig. 13: Changes in carbon clearance rate during starvation in AKR mice.

servation). Recovery to the levels of the controls did not occur until seven days after the end of starvation, except for delayed hypersensitivity, which seems to be more strongly influenced by starvation. These results indicate that short-term starvation enhances immune function while long-term starvation suppresses this system's activity.

Conclusion

Andervont (1944) reported that isolation stress advanced the growth of breast cancer in C3H strain mice. Mühlbock (1951) reported similar results. He found as well that the incidence of tumors was decreased, and the stress presumably diminished, when mice were given access to activity wheels. Rashkis (1952) reported that forced swimming inhibited chemically induced sarcoma in Swiss mice. Levine and Cohen (1959) reported that stress by handling was associated with a decreased survival rate in DBA/2 mice with leukemia. Kavetsky found that C3H mice with experimentally induced neurosis seemed more apt to contract breast cancer (see Kavetsky, Turkevich, & Balitsky, 1966). All of these observations show relationships between stress and cancer growth *in vivo*.

We estimated cellular immunity, the cytotoxicity of killer T-cells and phagocytosis by macrophages in stressed mice. Suppression of cytotoxicity of T-cells with stress was clearly evident. Killer T-cells of the host seemed to recognize the tumor-specific antigen on the surface of cancer cells and reacted cytotoxically, and the stress inhibited these functions of the killer T-cells.

Selye (1936) described the countershock phase of response, in which stress enhances reactivity in the organism. In the macrophage experiment, we noted such a phase in the immune system function of immobilized mice. Enhancement of macrophage phagocytosis was also found in the early stage of starvation in AKR mice.

The prognosis of cancer patients often seems dependent on their life style and suggests the existence of a countershock phase in the human anti-tumor defense mechanism. If such a phase does indeed exist, its prolongation may be relevant.

The cell surfaces of killer T-cells and macrophages have various receptors which respond to peripheral stimuli. The receptors for hormones and drugs related to the ANS probably play some role in this picture. The presence of β-adrenergic and prostaglandin receptors on mast cells has been demonstrated (Lichtenstein & Henney, 1974). The concentrations of cyclic AMP and cyclic GMP also have a definite influence.

References

Andervont, H. B. Influence of environment on mammary cancer in mice. *J. Natl. Cancer Inst.,* 1944, *4,* 579–581.

Bahnson, M. B., & Bahnson, C. B. Ego defenses in cancer patients. *Ann. NY Acad. Sci.,* 1969, *164,* 546–559.

Balitsky, K. P., Kapshuk, A. P., & Tsapenko, V. F. Some electrophysiological peculiarities of the nervous system in malignant growth. *Ann. NY Acad. Sci.,* 1969, *164,* 520–525.

Biozzi, G., Benacerraf, B., & Halpern, B. N. Quantitative study of the granulopectic activity of the reticuloendothelial system. II. A study of the kinetics of the granulopectic activity of R. E. S. in relation to the dose of carbon injected: Relationship between the weight of the organs and their activity. *Br. J. Exp. Pathol.,* 1953, *34,* 441–457.

Booth, G. Psychobiological aspects of "spontaneous" regressions of cancer. *J. Am. Acad. Psychoanal.,* 1973, *1,* 303–317.

Greene, W. A. The psychosocial setting of the development of leukemia and lymphoma. *Ann. NY Acad. Sci.,* 1966, *125,* 794–801.

Kavetsky, R. E., Turkevich, N. M., & Balitsky, K. P. On the psychophysiological mechanism of the organism's resistance to tumor growth. *Ann. NY Acad. Sci.,* 1966, *125,* 933–945.

Kubo, C., Nomoto, K., Sato, M., & Takeya, K. Direct cytotoxicity against chicken eryth-
    rocytes in mice. I. Fundamental nature of T cell-mediated cytotoxicity. *Immunology,*
    1977, *33,* 895–905.
Lavrin, D. H., Herberman, R. B., Nunn, M., & Soares, N. *In vitro* cytotoxicity studies of
    murine sarcoma virus-induced immunity in mice. *J. Natl. Cancer Inst.,* 1973, *51,*
    1497–1508.
LeShan, L. *You can fight for your life.* New York: M. Evans and Co., 1978.
Levine, S., & Cohen, C. Differential survival to leukemia as a function of infantile stimu-
    lation in DBA/2 mice. *Proc. Soc. Exp. Biol. Med.,* 1959, *102,* 53–54.
Lichtenstein, L. M., & Henney, C. S. Adenylate cyclase-linked hormone receptors: An im-
    portant mechanism for the immunoregulation of leukocytes. In L. Brent & J. Holborow
    (Eds.), *Progress in immunology II* (Vol. 2). New York: American Elsevier, 1974.
Mühlbock, O. Influence of environment on the incidence of mammary tumors in mice.
    Acta Union Int. Contra Cancrum, 1951, *7,* 351–353.
Rashkis, H. A. Systemic stress as an inhibitor of experimental tumors in Swiss mice.
    Science, 1952, *116,* 169–171.
Rasmussen, A. F., Jr., Spencer, E. S., & Marsh, J. T. Decrease in susceptibility of mice to
    passive anaphylaxis following avoidance-learning stress. *Proc. Soc. Exp. Biol. Med.,*
    1959, *100,* 878–879.
Saba, T. M. Mechanism mediating reticuloendothelial system depression after surgery.
    Proc. Soc. Exp. Biol. Med., 1970, *133,* 1132–1136.
Scheid, M. P., Goldstein, G., Hammerling, U., & Boyse, E. A. Lymphocyte differentiation
    from precursor cells *in vitro. Ann. NY Acad. Sci.,* 1975, *249,* 531–540.
Selye, H. A syndrome produced by diverse nocuous agents. *Nature,* 1936, *138,* 32.
Smith, J. W., Steiner, A. L., & Parker, C. W. Human lymphocyte metabolism: Effects of
    cyclic and non-cyclic nucleotides on stimulation by phytohemagglutinin. *J. Clin. In-
    vest.,* 1971, *50,* 442–448.
Solomon, G. F. Stress and antibody response in rats. *Int. Arch. Allergy Appl. Immunol.,*
    1969, *35,* 97–104.
Teshima, H., Inoue, S., Ago, Y., & Ikemi, Y. Plasminic activity and emotional stress. *Psy-
    chother. Psychosom.,* 1974, *23,* 218–228.
Teshima, H., Kubo, C., Kihara, H., Nagata, S., Imada, Y., & Ago, Y. Psychosomatic
    aspects of skin diseases from the standpoint of immunology. *Psychother. Psychosom.,*
    1982, *37,* 165–175.
Thomas, C. B., & Duszynski, K. R. Closeness to parents and the family constellation in a
    prospective study of five disease states: suicide, mental illness, malignant tumor, hyper-
    tension, and coronary heart disease. *Johns Hopkins Med. J.,* 1974, *134,* 251–270.
Wittkower, E. D. Studies of the personality of patients suffering from urticaria. *Psycho-
    som. Med.,* 1953, *15,* 116–126.

Opponent Processes, Neurohormones and Natural Resistance

A. H. Greenberg, D. G. Dyck and L. S. Sandler[1]

Introduction

Over the past thirty years researchers have expended considerable effort in an attempt to describe the relationship between parameters of aversive stimulation and host resistance to tumors. Experimentation has involved a wide variety of aversive stimuli, species and strains of animals, tumor induction methods and types of transplantable tumors. The upshot of this activity is a rapidly growing, but sometimes confusing literature which implicates the central nervous system in host resistance. As researchers in this area are well aware, the confusion stems from the fact that different aversive stimulation procedures produce very different effects on host resistance. Aversive stimulation has been found just as frequently to increase host resistance as to decrease it. However, in their excellent review of this literature, Sklar and Anisman (1981) noted that many of the apparently inconsistent effects were systematically related to two factors: namely the chronicity of the regimen and the availability of "coping" responses. More specifically, they suggested that tumor growth was enhanced when aversive stimulation was acute and inescapable but unaffected or inhibited under chronic or repeated stimulation conditions.

The variables identified by Sklar and Anisman as affecting host resistance have also been found to affect neurochemical and neurohormonal functioning in predictable ways. For example, the characteristic

[1] We wish to thank Mr. Peter Gregor and Ms. Lenka Joralim for their technical assistance, and Michael Dresel and Bill Pohajdak for their enthusiastic contributions. We are also grateful to Ms. Susan Diamond for typing this manuscript in record time. This work was supported by grants from the Children's Hospital Research Foundation, Manitoba Mental Health Research Foundation, National Cancer Institute of Canada and the National Science and Engineering Research Council of Canada.

neurochemical response to acute inescapable aversive stimulation is an increase in catecholamine usage and synthesis, specifically that of nor-epinephrine and dopamine, resulting in a depletion of available amines. However, this is not typically observed with acute escapable shock or with chronic inescapable shock (see Anisman, 1978). Similar adaptive changes have been found with neurohormonal responses to aversive stimulation. For example, acute inescapable stress enhances secretion of adrenocorticotropic hormone (ACTH) from the pituitary and increases synthesis and release of corticosteroids (Stein, Keller, & Schleifer, 1979). Escapable shock on the other hand increases plasma corticoster-one levels to a lesser extent than inescapable shock (see Anisman, 1978; Weiss, Glazer, & Pohorecky, 1976), and chronic exposure to various forms of aversive stimulation results in a decrease in those changes in-duced by acute stimulation.

It seems, then, that adaptation to aversive stimulation is heightened both by chronic exposure and by the availability of behavioral coping responses under conditions of acute exposure. Further, adaptation to aversive stimuli appears to be a general phenomenon which is seen at virtually all levels of biobehavioral functioning. Two implications fol-low from these generalizations. First, adaptive phenomena have multi-ple bases. During initial exposure to aversive stimulation, behavioral control processes are principally involved in the modulation of adaptive adjustments. However, following repeated exposure to aversive stimuli which cannot be ameliorated through behavioral adjustments, the burden of physiological adaptation falls primarily on the shoulders of endogenous processes. In some sense the data we shall present here re-flect our current attempts at the identification and conceptualization of endogenous neurohormonal processes and their relation to host resist-ance to tumors. The second implication derives from the generality of adaptive phenomena at various levels of functioning. That similar neu-rochemical, neurohormonal, and perhaps immunological adjustments occur in response to aversive stimulation indicates that adaptation in-volves the whole organism. It is nontrivial that changes in neurochemi-cal function are likely to be paralleled by changes at other levels. It means that in order to elevate our understanding of host-tumor inter-actions it will be necessary to describe the interactions between various levels of functioning.

In the present research we were interested in cataloguing the possible interactions between neurohormonal functioning and a specific form of host resistance to tumors called natural resistance. Our broad strategy was to examine first the neurohormonal responses to various parame-ters of aversive stimulation, and then to relate these neurohormonal changes to host resistance phenomena. In particular, our goal was to identify homeostatic relationships between various neurohormones, and to note their effects on peripheral mechanisms.

Previous research suggests that immunity is among the peripheral responses which neuroregulatory mechanisms may affect. For example, the observation that hormonally deficient hypopituitary Snell-Bagg (dw) mice are also immunologically deficient (Pierpaoli et al., 1969), and that hypophysectomy results in suppression of natural killer (NK) cell lysis of tumors (Saxena et al., 1982), suggest that the hypothalamic-pituitary axis has at least a permissive role in regulating immune activity. Endorphins also have the ability to augment or suppress immune responsiveness (Palacios & Sugawara, 1982; McCain et al., 1982; Gilman et al., 1982), raising the further possibility that neuropeptides can actively regulate the ongoing immune response. One of the better known neurohormonal immunoregulatory pathways is the response to glucocorticoids occurring after pituitary ACTH activation of adrenocortical activity (Palacios & Sugawara, 1982; Gisler & Schenkel-Hulliger, 1971). Our subsequent studies of neurohormonal modulation of anti-tumor immunity were therefore directed at identifying a role for these two neurohormones, β-endorphin (βEND) and ACTH, in host resistance.

Natural Resistance

The dominant theory of immune surveillance of tumors until the mid-1970's, as postulated by Burnet (1970), held that lymphocytes of the T (thymus-dependent) lineage were the major mediators of anti-tumor immunity. Rigorous testing of this hypothesis, most notably in the congenitally athymic (nude) mouse (Rygaard & Povlssen, 1974), failed to confirm this traditional view and led to a rethinking of tumor immunology (Moller & Moller, 1976). Work in the last five years has led to the description of host defense mechanisms which act independently of T cell immunogenicity. These are referred to as "natural" resistance mechanisms. Cellular and humoral mediators of this host defense include natural killer (NK) cells and macrophages (see Herberman, 1982) and T-independent natural antibodies (Greenberg, Chow, & Wolosin, 1983).

Two main assay systems have been used to evaluate natural resistance in vivo: the frequency of tumors following the injection of subthreshold inocula (Greenberg & Greene, 1976) and the rate of elimination of ^{131}I- or ^{125}I-UdR labelled tumor cells (Carlson et al., 1980). The latter assay, and the one we have chosen for the subsequent experiments, is a rapid and convenient method of evaluating NK activity in vivo (Riccardi et al., 1980). To establish that resistance to a given tumor is NK mediated, and not dependent on other natural resistance mechanisms, several critical tests of NK dependence should be made in which ablation or augmentation of NK activity is correlated with the hosts' anti-tumor resistance.

Table I illustrates three experimental models in which the NK dependence of the intraperitoneal elimination of SL2–5 lymphoma cells was examined. 1) The bg/bg mutant which is deficient in NK cell activity is more susceptible to NK-sensitive (NK^S) tumors compared to its heterozygous littermates (Karre et al., 1980). Low NK levels in bg/bg mice were associated with increased whole body tumor retention of the SL2–5 lymphoma; 2) stimulation of DBA/2 mice with poly I:C, an interferon and NK inducer (Riccardi et al., 1980), produced a decrease in tumor load relative to untreated and poly I-treated controls; and 3) Asialo GMl is an NK membrane antigen, and intravenous inoculations of antiserum to this ganglioside reduces NK activity and increases susceptibility to transplanted tumors (Gorelik et al., 1982). Treatment of DBA/2 mice with the antiserum slowed the elimination of the lymphoma. These results, then, indicate that NK cells play a major role in the elimination of the SL2–5 tumor in this natural resistance assay.

Table I
Natural Resistance to SL2–5 is NK Dependent

Exp	Treatment	Strain	% ^{131}I Retained ± S.E. (20 hours)	% NK Lysis ± S.E.		
				150:1	*75:1*	*37:1*
1.	–	bg/bg	51.2±4.3	6±1	3±0.5	1±0.5
	–	bg/+	31.5±2.5*	23±2	13±3	7±2
2.	–	DBA/2	41.5±2.0	15±2	12±2	5±1
	Poly I:C	DBA/2	12.4±3.2**	58±3	41±4	30±3
	Poly I	DBA/2	39.4±3.7	14±2	11±2	6±1
3.	–	DBA/2	59.7±4.7	59.4	46.8	38.7
	Anti-Asialo GMl	DBA/2	79.0±3.4*	3.6	2.1	0
	NRS	DBA/2	–	62.1	45.1	37.5

Note. Poly I:C (or Poly I) 100 µg was given IP 20 hours before injection of 2 × 10⁶ ^{131}I-labelled SL2–5 or removal of splenocytes for the NK assay. Anti-Asialo GMl antiserum (20 µl) or normal rabbit serum (NRS) was injected IV 20 hours before natural resistance or NK assays. All natural resistance assays were conducted with 5 mice/group, and splenocytes from 3 mice were used in the NK assays.

Statistical Analysis: Students 't' test (*) p<.05, (**) p<.01

The Effects of Acute Inescapable Shock on Natural Resistance to Tumors

The model we have chosen to study the effects of neuroendocrine activation is the response to inescapable tail shock. Practically, inescapable shock provided us with an aversive procedure which was quantifiable, did not require extensive handling of individual animals, and gave us a way of testing simultaneously groups of 5 or more animals needed for reproducibility in the natural resistance assay. Further, manipulating the parameters of tail electroshock (TES) is a relatively straightforward matter. In addition to these practical considerations our selection of TES was influenced by the large amount of previous biobehavioral neuroendocrine research with this variable. This is desirable since it allows us to compare our results more readily with those obtained by other researchers in the field.

In our typical experimental design we compared inescapably shocked mice to those receiving restraint (Sham-TES) or no shock. Although we did not include an escapably shocked condition, we were satisfied on the basis of previous research that such a condition would not differ from restrained or unhandled controls. That inescapable shock produces a wide variety of behavioral and physiological deficits not seen in animals exposed to equivalent amounts of escapable shock and no shock is well established (cf. Maier & Seligman, 1976). For example, inescapable shock retards the subsequent acquisition of escape from shock (Overmier & Seligman, 1967) and frustration cues (Rosellini & Seligman, 1975), and interferes with both aversive (Maier & Jackson, 1979) and appetitive choice behavior (Rosellini, DeCola, & Shapiro, 1982). In addition, pain inhibition which is reversible by opiate antagonists (Maier & Jackson, 1979; Maier et al., 1983) as well as decreased shock-elicited aggression (Maier, Anderson, & Lieberman, 1972) and social dominance (Rapaport & Maier, 1978) have also been reported with inescapable, but not escapable shock.

As noted previously in their review of the neurochemical, hormonal, and immunological changes associated with inescapable stressors generally, and inescapable shock specifically, Sklar and Anisman (1981) indicated that the chronicity of exposure was an important variable determining the effects. Thus a single session of shock is likely to produce neurochemical depletion (e.g., of norepinephrine), increased neuroendocrine activity, and immunosuppression, while multiple sessions of shock produce effects that are typically reduced and in some cases reversed. The most relevant result in this regard is Sklar and Anisman's (1979) finding that tumor growth is enhanced by one session of inescapable shock, relative to escapable shock or no shock. However, this effect was reduced following 5 sessions of shock and reversed after 10 sessions, relative to no shock controls.

Since we were interested in documenting the effects of inescapable shock on tumors known to be regulated by T-independent mechanisms, and tracing the activity of several neurohormones in relation to tumor elimination, we decided to use acute exposure in our initial experiments. Although we were ultimately interested in identifying the neurohormonal correlates of adaptation to aversive stimulation in this system, our first objective was to produce an effect (i. e., immunosuppression) which could be used as a benchmark for adaptation phenomena in our later studies.

Shock Intensity

In our first experiments we examined the intensity of TES that was necessary to produce an effect on tumor elimination. Four groups of five DBA/2 mice received either 150 µA, 275 µA, or 400 µA six-second tail shocks for a 15 minute period, while unhandled controls (no shock condition) were left untouched in their cages. Immediately (10–30 min.) following TES, ^{131}IdUR-labelled SL 2–5 was injected intraperitoneally and whole body retention of labelled tumor was assessed for three days. It may be seen in Figure 1 that as shock intensity increased, the tumor elimination rate was progressively suppressed; however, statistical significance was reached only at the 400 µA level.

Using this condition we then examined the reproducibility of the phenomenon (Table II). In 9 experiments, the elimination of the SL 2–5 tumor was consistently slower in TES mice than in unhandled controls. Statistical significance was reached in 7 out of the 9 individual experiments while analysis of all data by a paired 't' test was highly significant ($p < .001$) on each day of whole body counting.

Shock and Restraint

In five experiments the effects of sham TES were examined where all aspects of the handling procedure were identical except for the shock variable (Table II). Inhibition of tumor elimination was also observed in these mice compared to unhandled controls, and paired 't' tests showed that statistical significance was reached on day 1 ($p < .025$) and day 2 ($p < .03$), but not day 3 of the experiments. In four experiments

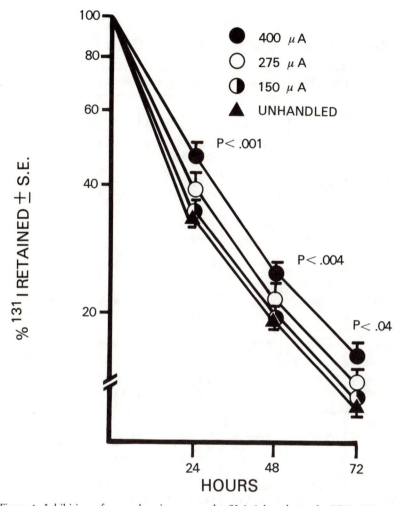

Figure 1: Inhibition of natural resistance to the SL 2–5 lymphoma by TES. Mice were placed in plexiglass restrainers designed so that the mouse's tail rested on two stainless steel plates. The tails were abraded with a nail file, coated with electrode jelly at that point of contact, and then taped to the electrodes. Resistance of each mouse was measured and in no case did it exceed 5 Kohms. TES was delivered by a Model E 13–35 Coulborn Instruments programmable, feedback-regulated shocker. Groups of 5 DBA/2 mice were connected in series and placed in sound-attenuated Model E 10–20 Coulborn isolation cubicles. The inside of each cubicle was illuminated by a house light, and a 70 db white noise was presented throughout the session. The mice received fifteen random 6-second TES (1/min) and were then immediately injected IP with 2×10^6 ^{131}IUdR-labelled tumor cells. Progressively greater slowing of tumor elimination was observed with increasing shock amperage. Significant inhibition of anti-tumor resistance was noted only at the 400 µA level.

Table II

Suppression of Natural Resistance after TES and Sham TES

Exp	Tumor	Inoculum	Treatment	% [131] IUdR Retained ± S. E.[1]		
				Day 1	Day 2	Day 3
1.	SL 2–5	2×10^6	Control	21.0 ± 3.8	9.8 ± 1.3	7.5 ± 0.9
			TES	43.4 ± 5.5[+]	17.6 ± 1.8*	13.4 ± 1.3**
2.	SL 2–5	2×10^6	Control	54.8 ± 5.0	20.1 ± 1.5	12.7 ± 1.2
			TES	55.2 ± 4.1	34.7 ± 3.3**	23.0 ± 2.5**
3.	SL 2–5	2×10^6	Control	41.7 ± 0.9	22.7 ± 0.7	14.4 ± 0.2
			TES	56.0 ± 3.4**	28.4 ± 3.2	16.5 ± 1.9
4.	SL 2–5	2×10^6	Control	36.8 ± 2.9	18.2 ± 1.6	11.8 ± 0.9
			TES	44.3 ± 1.0	20.9 ± 1.1	13.8 ± 0.6
5.	SL 2–5	2×10^6	Control	41.9 ± 0.9	21.5 ± 1.6	14.7 ± 0.9
			TES	48.8 ± 1.7[+]	26.9 ± 1.7	18.0 ± 1.3
6.	SL 2–5	2×10^6	Control	35.2 ± 2.2	18.8 ± 1.4	12.2 ± 0.6
			Sham TES	39.5 ± 2.9	20.1 ± 1.3	13.3 ± 0.8
7.	SL 2–5	2×10^6	Control	26.1 ± 1.1	12.4 ± 0.7	9.6 ± 0.5
			Sham TES	30.7 ± 3.6	13.4 ± 2.2	9.3 ± 1.2
			TES	39.1 ± 4.2[+]	18.5 ± 1.8*	12.4 ± 2.1[+]
8.	SL 2–5	2×10^6	Control	30.5 ± 2.2	16.1 ± 1.2	11.7 ± 0.4
			Sham TES	31.2 ± 2.8	18.1 ± 1.2	12.4 ± 0.7
			TES	40.0 ± 3.3	21.8 ± 2.2	14.8 ± 1.6
9.	SL 2–5	2×10^6	Control	36.4 ± 1.8	21.1 ± 0.8	14.7 ± 0.7
			Sham TES	45.3 ± 2.2*	25.8 ± 1.3[+]	16.7 ± 1.2
			TES	48.1 ± 2.2**	26.2 ± 0.8*	16.7 ± 0.9
10.	SL 2–5	2×10^6	Control	26.6 ± 4.0	14.4 ± 0.9	9.6 ± 1.1
			Sham TES	31.1 ± 2.3	16.4 ± 1.1	10.4 ± 0.6
			TES	41.8 ± 5.1[+]	19.9 ± 1.1	12.7 ± 0.8

[1] Students 't' test analysis comparing TES or sham TES to unhandled controls ([+]) p < .05, (*) p < .02, (**) p < .01

Statistical analysis by a paired 't' test: TES vs control (df = 8), day 1, t = 5.67, p < .005; day 2, t = 5.91, p < .004; day 3, t = 4.27, p < .03.

where TES and sham TES conditions were compared, tumor elimination was always slower in the TES group and this difference was significant on day 2 (p < .05) of the assay.

NK^S and NK^R Tumors

If the inhibitory effects described above resulted from NK suppression we would predict that host resistance to another NK^S tumor (YAC-1.3) should also be retarded while an NK-resistant (NK^R) line (P815–16) would not be affected. Accordingly the YAC-1.3 and P815–16 were injected into DBA/2 mice after TES (Table III). Significant inhibition of elimination was noted with the YAC-1.3 and SL2, while the NK^R P815–16 was unaffected.

Table III
Suppression of Natural Resistance to NK^S and NK^R Tumors

Exp	Tumor[1]	Inoculum	Treatment	% ^{131}I Retained ± S.E.[2]		
				Day 1	*Day 2*	*Day 3*
1.	YAC-1.3	2×10^6	Control	66.9±2.7	48.0±2.5	39.2±2.5
			TES	81.0±1.6**	64.7±0.8^{++}	52.2±1.3^{++}
2.	SL2–5	2×10^6	Control	26.6±4.0	14.4±0.9	9.6±1.1
			TES	41.8±5.1$^+$	19.9±1.1$^+$	12.7±0.8
3.	P815–16	2×10^6	Control	62.9±1.9	53.9±2.4	46.0±2.6
			TES	61.1±4.6	53.7±9.3	44.9±4.1

[1] The YAC-1.3 and SL2–5 are NK^S lymphomas and the P815–16 is an NK^R mastocytoma.
[2] Students 't' test analysis comparing TES and unhandled controls (+) p<.05, (**) p<.01, (++) p<.001.

Tumor Load

To appreciate the quantitative effect of our manipulation on the handling of the tumor, we related tumor inoculum size to IdUR retention at 20 hours (Figure 2). We estimated that the rate of elimination slowed by 7% between 10^4 and 10^5 tumor cell inocula, 10% between 10^5 and 10^6, and approximately 12% between 10^6 and 10^7 cells (estimated from extrapolation). Since the mean 20-hour retention in the control group was 36% and the mean difference (Δ) between control and TES groups was 12.4%, we estimated that the slower tumor elimination was equivalent to the inoculation of at least tenfold more tumor into control mice. Fourfold and twofold differences were calculated in this manner when comparing sham TES and TES, or control and sham TES experiments, respectively.

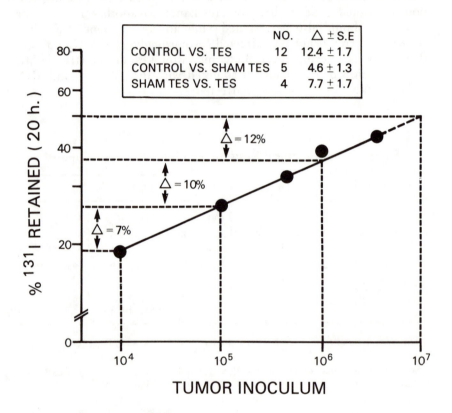

Figure 2: Quantitative relationship between the tumor inoculum size and the retention of radiolabel. Five groups of DBA/2 mice were injected IP with 10^4, 10^5, 10^6 and 4×10^6 [131]IUdR-labelled SL2-5, and whole-body isotope retention was assessed 20 hours later. The mean differences (Δ) ± S.E. between control, TES, and sham TES treatments in Table II are given in the box insert. Comparison with the regression line calculated from the control dose-response curve reveals that the Δ of control versus TES groups represents a tumor retention equivalent to more than a ten-fold increase in inoculum size. Sham TES versus TES and control versus sham TES differences represent four-fold and two-fold increases, respectively.

The Suppression of Natural Resistance: Neurohormonal Mediators

Inescapable Shock, Restraint and Corticosteroids

Reports of suppressive effects of corticosteroids on NK activity (Hochman & Cudkowicz, 1979; Lotzova, 1980) led us to examine both the production of corticosterone in groups of mice exposed to the TES and restraint conditions and the effects of hydrocortisone on natural resistance to the SL2–5 lymphoma. Corticosterone levels in mice receiving either TES or restraint for 15 or 60 minutes were highly elevated (p < .001) compared to unhandled controls. However, no differences in levels were detected between the handled groups (Table IV).

Table IV

Serum Corticosterone Levels in TES and Sham TES-Treated Mice

Group	Time (min)	No. of Mice	Serum Corticosterone (nM/L)
Control	–	9	63 ± 13
TES	15	9	698 ± 74*
Sham TES	15	9	642 ± 106*
TES	60	9	742 ± 75*
Sham TES	60	9	589 ± 61*

Note. All groups were significantly greater than unhandled controls (* = p < .001). No difference was detected between TES or sham TES at either 15 or 60 minutes.

In Table V a provocative test of the hypothesis that corticosteroids are suppressive was made by injecting DBA/2 mice with hydrocortisone sodium succinate (Upjohn Co., Don Mills) 30 minutes before tumor inoculation. A significant slowing of tumor elimination was noted, showing maximal effects at 1.0 mg of hydrocortisone, while higher doses (10 mg) were less effective.

The experiments reported to this point demonstrated that a transient suppression of natural resistance to an NK sensitive tumor occurs following inescapable tail electroshock and restraint, and this is associated with a rapid increase in serum corticosterone levels. In addition, the administration of corticosteroids to these mice can suppress host anti-tumor resistance. It would, however, be incorrect to conclude that the suppression of natural resistance was due entirely to enhanced corticosterone production. For example, mice exposed to sham TES conditions were significantly less affected than TES treatment mice (Table II), yet corticosterone levels were equivalent (Table IV). The inability to correlate quantitative serum corticosterone responses, and presumably ACTH, to suppression of natural resistance led us to examine the role of other hypophyseal hormones.

Table V
The Effect of Hydrocortisone on Natural Resistance

Treatment	No. Mice	% ^{131}I Retained ± S. E.		
		Day 1	Day 2	Day 3
Control	5	19.2 ± 2.8	9.2 ± 1.3	6.5 ± 0.8
0.5 mg HC	5	22.7 ± 2.8	11.9 ± 3.1	7.9 ± 1.0
1.0 mg HC	5	33.2 ± 2.6*	17.2 ± 1.2**	10.9 ± 0.9+
10.0 mg HC	5	24.9 ± 2.8	7.4 ± 1.1	4.9 ± 0.7

Note. Hydrocortisone (HC) sodium succinate in HBSS (0.1 ml) was injected IP 30 minutes before 2×10^6 SL2-5 lymphoma.

Statistical analysis by students 't' test ($^+$) $p < .02$; (*) $p < .01$; (**) $p < .001$ comparing means of experimental to control groups.

Naltrexone Reversible Suppression

The endogenous opiate βEND is derived from a large precursor molecule, pro-opiomelanocortin, that also bears the ACTH sequence (Imura & Nakai, 1981). Release of both ACTH and βEND into serum following the initiation of electroshock occurs simultaneously, and within minutes (Guillemin et al., 1977; Rossier et al., 1977). Since βEND binds to cells through μ opiate receptors, one test of the *in vivo* activity of this hormone is to administer the long acting opiate receptor antagonists naloxone or naltrexone (Endo Laboratories, Montreal) (Lord et al., 1977). These drugs bind to the receptor with high affinity but are inactive, and therefore effectively block receptor activation by endogenous βEND. In Table VI we report two experiments in which naltrexone (7 mg/kg) or vehicle were administered IP to mice just before being placed in restrainers and given 15 or 60 TES. Naltrexone treatment significantly augmented tumor elimination at both time points compared to the vehicle control. The increased tumor elimination was equivalent to a tenfold decrease in the size of the tumor inoculum ($\Delta = 10.6\% \pm 2.2$) (see Figure 2). Administration of μ receptor antagonists naloxone or naltrexone to unhandled animals produced a slight but not significant slowing of tumor elimination, indicating that the effect of the drugs was limited to TES groups only. These observations implicate the stimulation of μ opiate receptors in the suppression of natural resistance noted after TES. The phenomenon, then, could be a result of the combined effect of both corticosteroids and stimulation of the μ opiate receptor by βEND. This might also explain the differences between tumor elimination in TES and sham TES groups. Endorphins mediating analgesia are released during electroshock stimulation (Maier et al., 1980), and our observations may reflect a quantitative difference in the endorphin response to simple handling (sham TES) versus the administration of the shock stimulus (TES). The conclusion that this immunosuppression is a βEND-mediated effect, however, must be tempered by the need for confirmatory experiments using μ receptor agonists or morphine-cross tolerance (Sawynok et al., 1979).

Repeated Neurohormonal Stimulation Augments Natural Resistance

Intrasession Adaptation

In the next group of experiments, examining the TES conditions on tumor elimination, we studied the effect of the number of shocks on resistance to the SL2–5 tumor in DBA/2 mice (Figure 3). The shock delivery procedures were identical to those described for the experiments in Table II with the exception that one group received 15 and the other 60 TES. It may be seen that in each case, mice in the 15 TES condition group eliminated the tumor more slowly than the controls. The effect of the 60 TES manipulation on the elimination of the tumor was lower than that of the 15 TES group in all of the experiments. In two out of three comparisons, (A) and (C), 15 TES produced significantly slower elimination of the tumor than 60 TES. Relative to unhandled controls the 60 TES condition did not differ (A), slowed (B), or accelerated (C) the elimination of the tumor.

The final experiment in this series (shown in panel D) makes the simple but important point that the elimination of heat-killed tumor is rapid and is unaffected by these experimental conditions. This indicates that the differences observed are the result of modulated resistance to live tumors and do not reflect nonspecific clearance of tumor debris.

An examination of the corticosterone levels in mice receiving 15 and 60 TES trials revealed that both were highly elevated compared to unhandled controls, but interestingly, did not differ significantly from each other (Table IV). The reversal of the TES-induced suppression noted after increasing the number of treatments (Figure 3) was therefore not accompanied by any decrease in corticosterone production.

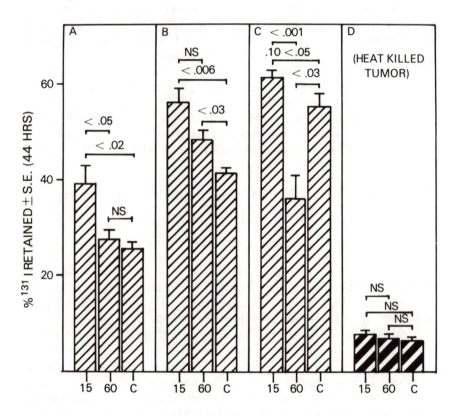

Figure 3: Reversal of inhibitory effects of TES during prolonged TES trials. Mice were handled as described in Table 2 with the addition of a 60 TES trial group in each of the four experiments. Results are given for [131]IUdR retention at 20 hours, but the identical relationship was observed on all three days of the experiment. Note the consistent and significant drop in tumor retention after 60 trials compared to the 15 trial groups in experiments A, B and C (in the correspondingly lettered panels). *P* values are given for Student's 't' test analysis in each exeriment. C refers to the unhandled control group. In experiment D, no difference was detected in the elimination of heat-killed tumor among the 15 or 60 TES groups and controls.

Table VI
The Effect of μ Opiate Receptor Antagonists on Natural Resistance in TES-Treated Mice

Exp	Treatment	TES	%[131]IUdR Retained ±S.E.		
			Day 1	Day 2	Day 3
1.	Vehicle	15 min.	61.4±2.5	33.9±2.1	20.0±2.2
	Naltrexone		49.6±3.5	29.5±3.5	18.8±2.2
	Vehicle	60 min.	44.3±1.0	20.9±1.1	13.8±0.6
	Naltrexone		31.5±2.9	16.4±1.5	11.3±0.9
2.	Vehicle	15 min.	44.4±3.7	21.1±1.0	13.6±0.6
	Naltrexone		30.8±4.9	16.3±2.4	11.1±1.5
	Vehicle	60 min.	36.1±5.1	21.1±2.5	13.8±0.9
	Naltrexone		23.0±4.0	18.1±1.2	13.2±1.5
3.	Vehicle	Nil	30.9±5.3	15.1±2.8	10.7±1.9
	Naloxone		38.1±6.1	20.7±2.6	13.1±1.4
4.	Vehicle	Nil	46.3±2.4	24.5±1.6	15.5±1.1
	Naltrexone		48.5±4.5	23.8±2.1	15.8±1.5
5.	Vehicle	Nil	25.8±1.2	15.0±0.9	9.4±0.7
	Naloxone		33.4±2.7	15.1±2.8	12.1±0.5

Note. In experiments 1 and 2, groups of 5 DBA/2 mice were injected with Naltrexone (7 mg/kg) or HBSS vehicle just prior to placing them in restrainers for the 15 or 60 min TES treatment groups. All mice received 2×10^6 SL2–5 IP immediately following TES. Statistical analysis of the four groups indicated a significant enhancement of tumor elimination in the Naltrexone-treated mice by a paired 't' test on day 1 (p<.02), day 2 (p<.002) and day 3 (p<.04) of the experiment.

In experiments 3, 4 and 5 unhandled mice were given either Naloxone (7 mg/kg) or Naltrexone (7 mg/kg) just before tumor injection. No significant effect was noted, although a slight slowing in tumor elimination rate was detected in naloxone and naltrexone-treated mice.

This set of experiments, then, showed that although relatively intense, acute tailshock reliably suppresses the elimination of NK sensitive tumors, there is some intrasession adaptation. Although intersession adaptation effects using other tumor systems have been reported (e.g., Sklar & Anisman, 1979), we were somewhat surprised to find such effects occurring within a single session. It is interesting that both Visintainer et al. (1982) and Sklar and Anisman (1979), found 60 inescapable footshocks to inhibit host resistance to tumors. While there are a number of procedural differences which may account for the seemingly more rapid adaptation seen in our experiments, we think that the restraint variable in our work may be the most significant. The mice which received inescapable shock were restrained while in the aforementioned studies animals could move around freely. It is possible that endogenous processes designed to modulate the impact of pain are more quickly engaged when the opportunities for making gross behavioral responses are minimized. Another possibility for rapid adaptation in our work is that the T-independent responses we were observing may adapt more rapidly than the T-dependent responses detected in other assays.

Intersession Adaptation and Enhanced Natural Resistance

In the following experiment we examined the effect of repeatedly stimulating mice by sham TES (restraint) treatment prior to the inoculation of the SL 2–5 tumor cells. In these experiments the mice were treated daily for three days by placing them in restrainers for 60 min., then on the day of tumor injection they were given either TES, sham TES, or left unhandled prior to tumor injection. A parallel group of mice was bled for serum corticosterone determinations. In three experiments, tumor elimination in all treatment conditions was significantly greater than in unhandled controls (Figure 4). Corticosterone levels, on the other hand, were significantly elevated only in groups handled on the day of tumor injection (Table VII). This indicated that while stimu-

Table VII

Serum Corticosterone Levels in Prestimulated Mice

Treatment		No. Mice	Corticosterone nM/L $\pm$ S. E.
Day 1–3	*Day 4*		
(a) Sham TES	Sham TES	5	923 ± 92*
(b) Sham TES	TES	5	1040 ± 27*
(c) Sham TES	Nil	5	200 ± 42
(d) Nil	Nil	5	88 ± 60

Note. Mice were placed in restrainers (Sham TES) for 60 min/day on day 1–3 of the experiment and on day 4 either (a) TES, (b) Sham TES treated or (c) left unhandled prior to bleeding. A control group (d) was unhandled throughout the experiment.

Statistical analysis by 't' test, comparing group (d) with (a) and (b); (*) $p < .001$. Groups (d) and (c) were not significantly different.

lation of the mice prior to tumor injection resulted in an enhancement of host resistance, high levels of serum corticosterone on the day of tumor injection were not associated with a suppression of host resistance mechanisms under these experimental conditions.

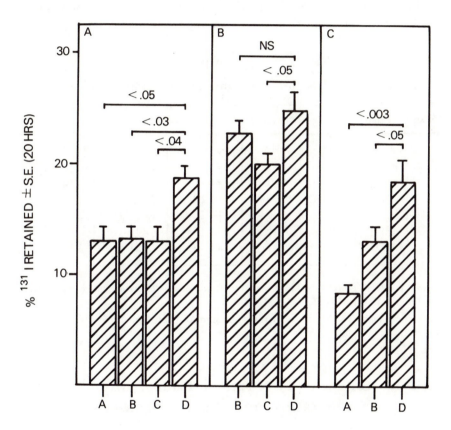

Figure 4: Augmentation of natural resistance following repeated aversive stimulation. Elimination of radiolabelled SL 2–5 in control (unhandled) DBA/2 mice (D) was compared to groups that had been sham-TES treated daily for 60 min. for three days (Day 1–3). On the day of the experiment (Day 4), just prior to tumor injection, these mice were given either TES (A) or sham TES (B), or left unhandled (C). Significant enhancement of natural resistance was observed in all treatment conditions. The same results were obtained on other days of whole-body counting.

ACTH Enhances Natural Resistance

A further experiment, in which four inoculations of ACTH were given prior to the injection of the tumor, tested the hypothesis that repeated stimulation of the pituitary-adrenal axis via the release of ACTH was responsible for the phenomenon of enhanced tumor elimination following repeated sham TES treatments. In the two experiments outlined in Table VIII, ACTH-treated mice were indeed more resistant to the tumor than control or vehicle-treated animals.

Table VIII
Enhancement of Natural Resistance by Pretreatment with ACTH

Exp	Treatment	No. Mice	% ^{131}I Retained ±S.E.		
			Day 1	Day 2	Day 3
1.	Control	5	51.0±3.7	31.1±3.5	14.9±0.9
	Vehicle SC (×4)	5	46.2±3.5	24.4±0.7	20.0±1.0
	ACTH 25 µg SC (×4)	5	31.5±2.2*	17.2±1.0+	13.3±0.8
2.	Control	5	34.1±3.1	15.0±1.3	8.7±0.4
	ACTH 25 µg SC (×4)	5	13.2±0.9**	6.9±0.6**	4.8±0.4**
	ACTH 25 µg IP (×4)	5	17.8±0.8*	8.8±0.6**	6.3±0.2*

Note. Four injections of ACTH (Cosyntropin) or vehicle were given at 12 hour intervals before the IP injection of 2×10^6 SL 2–5 tumor.

Statistical analysis by 't' test, comparing control to ACTH treated groups; (+) p < .02, (*) p. < .01, (**) p < .001.

Discussion and Theoretical Issues: Biobehavioral Adaptation and Neurohormones

A general issue raised by the present results concerns the biobehavioral basis of adaptation to repeated neurohormonal stimulation. Our results indicate that although natural resistance to tumors is initially suppressed by inescapable shock, repeated stimulation of the pituitary axis actually increases natural resistance. Other investigators have reported similar results with different methods of stimulation and tumor systems. Thus the phenomena we have observed with the natural resistance assay are quite general. Although the mechanisms underlying the adaptation of organisms to aversive stimulation are not well understood we think there is sufficient evidence to merit a distinction between two broad sets of adaptive phenomena with somewhat different underlying mechanisms. The first, and most frequently emphasized in the behavioral literature, identifies the importance of operant contingencies of control in biobehavioral adaptations. The mechanisms here are identified with operant conditioning and behavioral coping. It is proposed that operant control processes are most critically involved in adaptations to acute aversive stimulation. However, when organisms are subjected to repeated aversive stimulation from which they cannot escape (e. g., chronic exposure to inescapable shock or restraint) adaptation involves the recruitment of endogenous compensatory processes which are designed to modulate the impact of intense hedonic stimuli. This long-term habituation process involves endogenous responses which may be conditioned to environmental cues associated with repeated system stimulation. In contrast to the short-term process with its emphasis on behavioral control, the long-term process emphasizes the influence of Pavlovian conditioning.

Behavioral Control and Short-Term Adaptation

The effect of variations in operant control on behavioral and physiological adaptations has been widely studied by behavioral researchers. This emphasis has particularly characterized research involving the effects of aversive stimulation. In this context operant control is usually operationalized as the presence versus absence of controllability over the offset of the aversive stimulus. As we have noted previously, the effect of behavioral control in such work is well documented and wide-ranging (cf. Maier & Seligman, 1976, for a review). In short, there is evidence for both associative and motivational deficits as a result of exposure to inescapable, but not escapable shock (cf. Maier & Jackson, 1979).

The physiological effects of inescapable shock appear to depend on the chronicity of exposure to the environmental contingency. Thus, in examinations of the effect of the controllability variable on tumorigenicity both Sklar and Anisman (1979) and Visintainer et al. (1982) found that host resistance to tumor was decreased by a single session of inescapable shock. However, Sklar and Anisman showed that these effects were reduced following 5 sessions of shock, and reversed following 10 sessions. The behavioral control variable then seems to affect tumorigenicity under acute, but not chronic exposure conditions. As previously noted in the introduction, this effect is consistent with other research which has shown similar effects on neurochemical and neurohormonal changes (cf. Sklar & Anisman, 1981). On the basis of these results it may be argued that behavioral control factors are principally involved in short-term adaptations to stressful stimuli. However, the impressive adaptations to long-term inescapable stressors necessarily involve other factors. Quite generally, it appears that when animals are repeatedly unable to extricate themselves from aversive settings, physiological mechanisms are activated which allow for habituation to such environmental events. Although the idea that nervous system(s) are designed with the capacity to oppose disturbances of physiological and neural equilibrium is an old one (Cannon 1932/1963), the evidence for conditioning in such regulation is a relatively recent development. This issue is dealt with in the next section and in the summary.

Conditioning Opponent States and Long-Term Adaptation

Recent evidence suggests that many conditioned responses (CRs) to pharmacological agents (UCSs) are opposite to the initial responses (UCRs) to such agents (cf. Bower & Hilgard, 1981). For example, if antisialosis is repeatedly induced in dogs by atropine administration, a placebo manipulation produces hypersalivation (e. g., Korol, Sletten, & Brown, 1966). When animals with a history of epinephrine administration (with its resulting decreased gastric secretion, tachycardia, and hyperglycemia) are given a placebo injection they show increased gastric secretion (Guha, Dutta, & Pradhan, 1974), bradycardia, and hypoglycemia (Russek & Pina, 1962). In response to a placebo, rats that have repeatedly had their glucose levels decreased by injections of insulin show a hyperglycemic response (Siegel, 1972; Woods & Shogren, 1972). These and other compensatory conditioned reactions have been summarized elsewhere (e. g., Siegel, 1978; Wikler, 1973).

The most extensively analyzed form of systemic stimulation is that of morphine. Siegel (1975, 1976, 1977, 1978) as well as Mitchell and colleagues (Adams, Yeh, Woods, & Mitchell, 1969; Ferguson, Adams, & Mitchell, 1969; Kayan & Mitchell, 1969) have furnished evidence that tolerance to the pyretic and analgesic effects of morphine is consistent with a Pavlovian conditioning model (see also Tiffany & Baker, 1981). On this model, tolerance derives in part from the learning of an association between the systemic reactions to a drug and those environmental stimuli that reliably precede and hence come to signal the systemic reactions. The development of an association between the two events is most frequently assessed by presenting the cues associated with the drug administration ritual (CS) without the actual systemic stimulation which defines the UCS, i.e., by sham injection. Siegel and others have shown that with repeated systemic stimulation the effects of the drug are increasingly cancelled by the development of compensatory responses which have been conditioned to environmental cues. Thus the response to a sham injection in rats previously exposed to repeated morphine injections is hyperalgesia and hypothermia. That these latter responses are CRs is indicated by the observation that they are situation-specific, extinguish, and show latent inhibition effects.

Experiments on morphine tolerance and other compensatory CRs are readily interpreted within the framework of opponent-process theory (Solomon & Corbitt, 1974; Schull, 1979). According to the theory, adaptation to repeated stimulation is determined by the net product of two underlying processes: the primary process and the opponent process. The primary process which is elicited by the onset of a stimulus is assumed to be maximal and not to change as a function of repeated stimulation. The opponent process is a slave process, more sluggish than the primary process but dependent on it. The opponent is hypothesized to become stronger over repeated stimulation, and to become more resistant to decay. The net effect of these two underlying processes is to decrease the amplitude of the manifest response with repeated stimulation. Further, if the cues but not the systemic stimuli are presented, the manifest response reflects only the opponent, thereby producing rebound phenomena, compensatory CRs, and the like. Schull (1979) in particular has interpreted the compensatory CRs as manifestations of conditioned opponent states.

Although much of our description of compensatory CRs has thus far focused on experimental manipulations involving pharmacological agents, there is a substantial literature involving the behavioral and physiological effects of shock which may also be interpreted within this framework. For example, a number of experiments have shown that the response to painful and other aversive stimuli is inhibited by endogenous analgesic mechanisms involving the endorphins (e.g., Cannon, Liebeskind, & Frenk, 1978; Sherman & Liebeskind, 1980). Thus, the endogenous opiates may be viewed as an expression of an opponent process which functions to inhibit the impact of painful stimuli. This interpretation is favored by the finding that rats prefer signaled shock to unsignaled shock. According to the theory, the preference may indicate that signaled shocks hurt less because they are more effectively opposed than unsignaled shocks (see Schull, 1979). Consistent with the idea that endogenous opiates are differentially released during signaled and unsignaled shock, Fanselow and Bolles (1979) found that the preference for signaled shocks is cancelled by pre-experimental administration of naloxone.

The conditioned-opponent theory places conditioning phenomena in an adaptive context. In short, it allows us to view responses to systemic stimulation within a total homeostatic system in which the compensatory CRs reflect the action of a corrective feedback loop which is responsive to the systemic disturbance caused by the UCS. These notions provide us with a language for describing the effects of repeated aversive stimulation on behavioral and physiological systems in chronic situations where the organism has no visible behavioral control over the UCS. While touting the heuristic and integrative functions of this type of analysis, it is important to recognize that this, or any other behavioral model, does not specify the mechanisms at the physiological level. Thus we may search for compensatory CRs using the theory as a guide; however, the theory does not name the mechanisms. Below we consider the relative merits of postulating compensatory CRs at the central neurohormonal level versus the peripheral effects of neurohormones.

Opponent Processes, Neurohormones, and Natural Resistance

In the experiments reported earlier we demonstrated that a transient suppression of natural resistance to an NK-sensitive tumor occurs following tail electroshock, and that this was associated with a rapid increase in serum corticosterone levels. In addition, the administration of corticosterone to these mice was found to suppress host anti-tumor resistance. Since we had also found that a major effector for host natural resistance to this tumor was the NK cell, these observations are consistent with earlier reports that glucocorticoids suppress NK activity in both *in vitro* and *in vivo* assays (Hochman & Cudkowicz, 1979; Lotzova, 1980). In exploring a similar phenomenon, Riley (1981) found that corticosterone production induced following rotational disorientation of mice was associated with suppression of host responses to transplanted histoincompatible lymphosarcoma in C3H/He mice, and to Murine Sarcoma Virus (MSV)-induced tumors following MSV injection into BALB/c mice. In both of these tumor "regressor" models, rejection was also reversed by the administration of corticosterone. Further support for a corticosteroid-based immunosuppressive mechanisms comes from earlier reports by Rettura et al. (1973), using the MSV model, in which it was demonstrated that tumor formation could be inhibited by feeding mice metyrapone, an inhibitor of 11-β-hydroxylase and corticosterone production. Although the syngeneic natural resistance model we have described depends on a T-independent (NK) immune mechanism in contrast to the T-dependency of the rejection of histoincompatible and MSV-induced tumors, the similarities in the responses to corticosterone and corticosterone-inducing manipulations are evident. Although it could be argued that corticosterone acts as a suppressive signal, the effects of this hormone did not discriminate between restraint and acute shock (although these variables produced differential effects on natural resistance.) Further, in the multiple stimulation experiment which produced enhanced natural resistance, corticosterone levels differed among groups receiving shock, restraint, and unhandled controls on the fourth day, yet natural resistance did not. While these findings do not deny the possible interaction of corticosterone with other hormones in natural resistance, the empirical inconsistencies noted above indicate that factors other than corticosterone play an important role in immunoregulation.

Our observations that naltrexone partly reverses the TES effects suggests that endogenous opiates may be involved in the initial immunosuppression. Although it is difficult to imagine an account of adaptation to painful stimulation that does not accord the endogenous opiates a principal role, it must be noted that reports of endorphin immunomodulation are conflicting. Both βEND enhancement (Gilman et al., 1982) and suppression (McCain et al., 1982) of mitogen-induced T cell proliferative responses have been observed, and in both cases were not reversed by μ receptor antagonists. Naloxone-insensitive opiate receptors on lymphocytes have also been described (Hazum et al., 1979). Potent naloxone-reversible suppression of T-dependent and T-independent antibody responses by α-endorphin, as well as lesser effects by (Leu) and (Met)enkephalin, as well as β- and γ-endorphin were reported by Johnson et al. (1982). Structural and functional similarities between interferon, a major NK regulator, and endorphins are intriguing (Blalock & Smith, 1980; Jornvall et al., 1982), although not all investigators agree with these latter investigators' conclusions (Wetzel et al., 1982; Epstein et al., 1982). Very recently Mathews et al. (1983) reported that βEND and (Met)enkephalin, but not (Leu)enkephalin, α-endorphin or morphine, could amplify human NK cell activity *in vitro*. This enhancement was dose-dependent and naloxone-reversible, and increased the number of tumor-killer cell conjugates, suggesting that the drug was able to increase the number of active killer cells. These effects appear to be similar to interferon in their ability to increase NK activity, but unlike interferon, βEND augments tumor-killer cell conjugate formation. Considering these data on NK modulation by βEND as well as our own observations on the role of μ opiate receptor stimulation in the suppression of NK-mediated natural resistance, βEND may be able to both amplify and suppress NK activity, not unlike its effect on T cell responsiveness.

With the activation of immunosuppressive hormonal mechanisms (βEND and corticosteroids) following acute unsignaled shock, it follows that a compensatory hormonal and/or immunological response must also be available to the organism to maintain its biological homeostasis. In the absence of this kind of homeostatic response, immunosuppression resulting from, for example, painful tissue injuries would leave the organism at a life-threatening disadvantage when confronted with pathogens. If βEND can also amplify NK activity (Mathews et al., 1983), it may be able to reverse the initial suppressive effects and eventually amplify host resistance. Just how this hormone can be both immunosuppressive and immunostimulatory is problematic and necessitates postulating the existence of a regulatory system for NK cells which includes at least two cell types of opposing activity, each bearing endorphin receptors. Immunoregulatory mechanisms involving amplifier and suppressor cells are well known in the T-dependent immune response, and have also been implicated in natural resistance (see Saksela, 1981). For example, suppression of NK cells by hydrocortisone appears to be the result of the activation of carbonyl iron-adherent suppressor cells (Hochman & Cudkowicz, 1979). Corticosterone and βEND may, then, rapidly generate suppressor signals with activation of this type of cell. Subsequent stimulatory effects of βEND on NK precursors and/or activation of NK activity would overcome this initial immunosuppression and eventually lead to amplification of host resistance. ACTH may also participate in immunoenhancement, since repeated ACTH administration augmented natural resistance (Table VIII). This effect may, however, not be directly on NK cells. Interferon and interleukin-2 are both NK amplifiers and originate in several cell types including the macrophage and T cell as well as the NK cell itself (Djeu et al., 1979; Timonen et al., 1980; Suzuki et al., 1983).

Other neuropeptides that could potentially be involved in the activation of NK cells include growth hormone and prolactin. Growth hormone can apparently restore NK activity in hypophysectomized mice (Saxena at al., 1982). Although growth hormone production drops quickly with increasing corticosteroid production during aversive handling (Lennox et al., 1980), later recovery of growth hormone levels could be associated with the amplification in host resistance seen over longer stimulation periods. Prolactin, on the other hand, increases sharply in serum with aversive stimulation (Lennox et al., 1980), but in our hands had no effect when injected into unstimulated mice (unpublished observations). If this latter hormone has a role to play, it would have to be similar to that proposed for growth hormone since it does not appear to have a direct effect on anti-tumor responses.

Neurohormones then could act as either amplifiers or suppressors of natural resistance depending on a number of interdependent phenom-

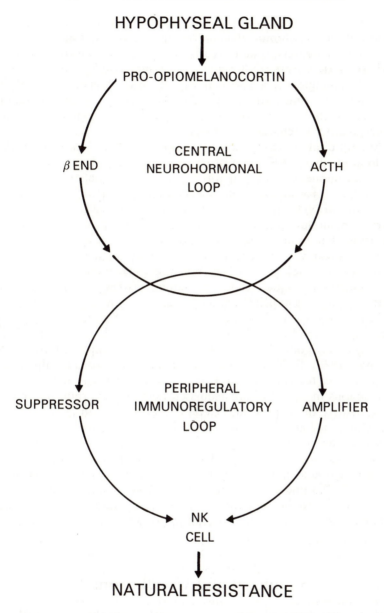

Figure 5: Postulated opponent processes for immunological homeostasis in natural resistance. Interacting homeostatic mechanisms occur at two levels: (A) a central neurohormonal loop in which pro-opiomelanocortin-derived hormones, βEND and ACTH, interact as opponent processes, and (B) a peripheral immunoregulatory loop in which NK activity is determined by amplifier and suppressor signals generated in response to the central neurohormonal stimulation.

ena. For example, ACTH and βEND are derived from a single precursor molecule, pro-opiomelanocortin; ACTH activates natural resistance, yet its daughter hormone, corticosterone, is immunosuppressive; βEND similarly activates NK activity, yet it may also be capable of acting via an immunosuppressive pathway. If these observations hold up to further experimentation, this ACTH-βEND immunoregulation would fulfill the criteria for the predicted bidirectional homeostatic neuroregulatory mechanism (Figure 5).

While we think it is necessary to invoke a peripheral immunoregulatory loop involving NK suppressors and amplifiers, the central effects of neurohormones cannot be ignored. The two hormones which are the best candidates for involvement in a central homeostatic loop are again ACTH and βEND (Figure 5). This notion is favored by a number of observations in addition to their opposite effects in the natural resistance assay. For example, these hormones share a common precursor (Imura & Nakai, 1981), yet they seem to produce opposite neurochemical and neurophysiological effects. When pharmacological doses are injected into the periaqueductal gray matter, rats become analgesic and sedated in response to βEND, and hyperalgesic, agitated, and hypermobile in response to ACTH injections (Jacquet, 1978). Similarly, at the neurochemical level it has been reported that βEND and ACTH have opposing effects on adenyl cyclase in the hippocampus (Botticelli & Wurtman, 1980). βEND inhibited (Klee, 1978) and ACTH stimulated adenyl cyclase (Ide et al., 1972). Finally, it has been suggested that morphine actions in the CNS are regulated both by endorphin receptors, which mediate the depressant effects of morphine, and ACTH receptors, which mediate the excitatory actions of morphine. The coincidence that identical CNS cells are affected by these two hormones with such opposite actions suggests that they participate in a homeostatic loop which functions to maintain biobehavioral equilibrium (Jacquet, 1979, 1980). To understand homeostasis, then, it will be necessary to define two interacting opponent processes, a central neurohormonal loop and a peripheral immunoregulatory loop for natural resistance.

Summary and Conclusions

The present series of experiments clearly supports the hypothesis that neuroendocrine activation arising from exposure to inescapable aversive events alters natural resistance to NK-sensitive lymphomas. Further, the degree and direction of change in the organism's handling of the tumor is highly dependent on the chronicity of the stimulation.

That is, brief aversive stimulation suppressed elimination of the tumor while repeated stimulation enhanced anti-tumor resistance.

The present results also provide information on the relation between several well known neurohormones and natural resistance. In particular, the release of corticosterone into the serum accompanying aversive stimulation, and the ability of hydrocortisone to suppress natural resistance, implicates ACTH-activated adrenocorticosteroid production in the phenomenon. However, serum corticosterone levels did not quantitatively correspond to relative differences in tumor elimination among shocked and restrained groups, and more importantly, failed to affect the increased elimination of the tumor following repeated stimulation. The shock-induced suppression of natural resistance was reversed by the μ opiate receptor antagonist naltrexone, thereby suggesting that endogenous opiates–possibly βEND–released during aversive stimulation, were immunosuppressive. Although βEND and corticosterone could be implicated in the initial immunosuppressive events, the observation that repeated ACTH injections increased host resistance and that βEND can amplify NK activity (Mathews et al., 1983) suggests that these hormones may participate in a bidirectional immunoregulatory loop to maintain homeostasis after aversive stimulation.

Our discussion of homeostatic mechanisms has emphasized the role of conditioning factors. In particular, we find Schull's (1979) extension of opponent-process theory to provide a useful theoretical framework for understanding biobehavioral adaptations to chronic inescapable aversive events. To some readers it may seem odd that we have chosen to interpret our results within a conditioning framework since none of our experiments contained either formal manipulations or measures of such processes. Although the need to provide direct evidence of conditioning in our experiments is obvious, and something we have begun to do recently, we believe that the current emphasis is defensible for at least two reasons. First, the phenomenon of contextual conditioning is well established in the literature (see Bower & Hilgard, 1981). Although it is beyond the scope of the present discussion to detail the evidence, it can be safely stated that animals have been found to develop associations to handling and other routine background stimuli. Indeed, many conditioning phenomena such as blocking and latent inhibition are now interpreted as effects which reflect conditioning to contextual cues. In our repeated stimulation experiments there was ample opportunity for contextual stimuli (e.g., handling, white noise, etc.) to become associated with aversive stimulation. As a result, the modulation of pain and other aversively based response systems could very easily have come under the control of contextual stimuli. Second, the plausibility of the conditioning analysis of adaptation is furthered by evidence indicating the susceptibility of immune responses to such procedures (see Ader, 1981, for a historical overview of the conditioned immune response literature). For example, Ader and Cohen (1975) have reported conditioned immunosuppression using a taste-aversion paradigm (e.g. Garcia & Koelling, 1966), while Gorczynski, McRae, and Kennedy (1982) have shown complementary immunoenhancement effects with skin graft (CS) and alloantigen (UCS) pairings. Such demonstrations support the idea that conditioning processes are involved in immunological adaptations. Further, when such demonstrations are taken together with the evidence for contextual conditioning, it seems quite likely that the natural resistance phenomena reported here were affected by conditioning processes.

Our enthusiasm for a conditioning analysis of homeostatic immune responses must, however, be tempered by the recognition that there is to date no direct evidence of compensatory immune CRs. In Ader's work as well as that of Gorczynski and colleagues the CRs mimicked the UCRs. Although it is possible that different conditioning parameters would have produced different results in these studies it is nevertheless the case that our account of natural resistance adaptation in terms of central or peripheral conditioned opponents rests on indirect evidence at this time. It remains for future research to elucidate both the physiological mechanisms of homeostasis and their dependence on environmental cues. Since homeostasis involves the whole organism it is our view that a complete understanding of this complex process will emerge only through analysis at a number of different levels.

References

Adams, W. H., Yeh, S. Y., Woods, L. A., & Mitchell, C. L. Drug-test interaction as a factor in the development of tolerance to the analgesic effect of morphine. *J. Pharmacol. Exp. Ther.,* 1969, *168,* 251–257.

Ader, R., & Cohen, N. Behaviorally conditioned immunosuppression. *Psychosom. Med.,* 1975, *37,* 333–340.

Ader, R. An historical account of conditioned immunobiologic responses. In R. Ader (Ed.), *Psychoneuroimmunology.* New York: Academic Press, 1981.

Anisman, H. Neurochemical changes elicited by stress. In H. Anisman & G. Bignami (Eds.), *Psychopharmacology of aversively motivated behavior.* New York: Plenum Press, 1978.

Blalock, J. E., & Smith, E. M. Human leukocyte interferon: Structural and biological relatedness to adrenocorticotropic hormone and endorphins. *Proc. Nat. Acad. Sci. USA,* 1980, *77,* 5972–5974.

Blankstein, J., Fujeda, K., Reyes, F. I., Faiman, C., & Winter, J. S. D. Aldosterone and corticosterone in amniotic fluid during various stages of pregnancy. *Steroids,* 1980, *36,* 161–165.

Botticelli, L.J., & Wurtman, R.J. Endorphin and corticotrophin regulate the activity of septal-hippocampal colinergic neurons. In E.L. Way (Ed.), *Endogenous and exogenous opiate agonists and antagonists.* Oxford: Pergamon, 1980.

Bower, G.H., & Hilgard, E.R. *Theories of learning.* Englewood Cliffs, N.J.: Prentice Hall, Inc., 1981.

Burchfield, S.R., Woods, S.C., & Elich, S.E. Effects of cold stress on tumor growth. *Physiol. Behav.,* 1978, *21,* 537–540.

Burnet, F.M. *Immunological surveillance.* London: Pergamon, 1970.

Cannon, J.T., Liebeskind, J.C., & Frenk, H. Neural and neurochemical mechanisms of pain inhibition. In R.A. Sternbach (Ed.), *The psychology of pain.* New York: Raven Press, 1978.

Cannon, W.B. *The wisdom of the body.* (Originally published, 1932; revised, 1939). New York: Norton, 1963.

Carlson, C.A., Menychuk, D., & Meeker, M.J. H-2 associated resistance to leukemia transplantation antigens: Natural killing *in vivo. Int. J. Cancer,* 1980, *25,* 111–122.

Djeu, J.Y., Heinbaugh, J.A., Holden, H.T., & Herberman, R.B. Role of macrophages in the augmentation of mouse natural killer cell activity by poly I:C and interferon. *J. Immunol.,* 1979, *122,* 182–188.

Epstein, L.B., Rose, M.E., McManus, N.J., & Choi, H.L. Absence of functional and structural homology of natural and recombinant human leukocyte interferon (IFN-α) with human α-ACTH and β-endorphin. *Biochem. Biophys. Res. Commun.,* 1982, *104,* 341–346.

Fanselow, M.S., & Bolles, R.C. Triggering of the endorphin analgesic reaction by a cue previously associated with shock: Reversal by naloxone. *Bull. Psychonomic Soc.,* 1979, *14,* 88–90.

Ferguson, R.K., Adams, W.J., & Mitchell, C.L. Studies on tolerance development to morphine analgesics in rats tested on the hot plate. *Eur. J. Pharmacol.,* 1969, *8,* 83–92.

Garcia, J., & Koelling, R.A. Relation of cue to consequence in avoidance learning. *Psychonomic Sci.,* 1966, *4,* 123-124.

Gilman, S.C., Schwartz, J.M., Milner, R.J., Bloom, F.E., & Feldman, J.D. β-endorphin enhances lymphocyte proliferative responses. *Proc. Natl. Acad. Sci. USA,* 1982, *79,* 4226–4230.

Gisler, R.H., & Schenkel-Hulliger, L. Hormonal regulation of the immune reponse II. Influence of pituitary and adrenal activity on immune responsiveness *in vitro. Cell. Immunol.,* 1971, *2,* 646–657.

Gorelik, E., Wiltrout, R.H., Okumura, K., Habu, S., & Herberman, R.B. Role of NK cells in the control of metastatic spread and growth of tumor cells in mice. *Int. J. Cancer,* 1982, *30,* 107–112.

Gorczynski, R.M., MacRae, S., & Kennedy, M. Conditioned immune response associated with allogeneic skin grafts in mice. *J. Immunol.,* 1982, *129,* 704–709.

Greenberg, A.H., Chow, D.A., & Wolosin, L.B. Natural antibodies: Origins, genetics, specificity and role in host resistance to tumors. In R.B. Herberman (Ed.), *Natural mechanisms of immunity. Clinics in allergy and immunology.* Philadelphia and London: W.B. Saunders, 1983.

Greenberg, A.H., & Greene, M.I. Non-adaptive rejection of small tumor inocula as a model of immune surveillance. *Nature,* 1976, *264,* 356–359.

Guha, D., Dutta, S. N., & Pradhan, S. N. Conditioning of gastric secretion by epinephrine in rats. *Proc. Soc. Exp. Biol. Med.,* 1974, *147,* 817–819.

Guillemin, R., Vargo, T., Rossier, J., Minick, S., Long, N., Rivier, C., Vale, W., & Bloor, F. β-Endorphin and adrenocorticotropin are secreted concomitantly by the pituitary gland. *Science,* 1977, *197,* 1367–1369.

Hazum, E., Chang, K-J., & Cuatrecasas, P. Specific nonopiate receptors for β-endorphin. *Science,* 1979, *205,* 1033–1035.

Herberman, R. B. *NK cells and other natural effector cells.* New York: Academic Press, 1982.

Hochman, P. S., & Cudkowicz, G. Suppression of natural cytotoxicity by spleen cells of hydrocortisone-treated mice. *J. Immunol.,* 1979, *123,* 968–976.

Ide, M., Tanaka, A., Nakamura, M., & Okabayashi, T. Stimulation by ACTH analogs of rat adenyl cyclase activity: Correlation with steroidogenic activity. *Arch. Biochem. Biophys.,* 1972. *149,* 189–196.

Imura, H., & Nakai, Y. "Endorphins" in pituitary and other tissues. *Ann. Rev. Physiol.,* 1981, *41,* 265–278.

Jacquet, Y. F. Opiate effects after adrenocorticotropin or β-endorphin injection in the peri-aqueductal gray matter of rats. *Science,* 1978, *201,* 1032–1034.

Jacquet, Y. F. β-Endorphin and ACTH: Opiate peptides with coordinated roles in the regulation of behavior? *Trends in Neurosciences,* 1979, *2,* 140–143.

Jacquet, Y. F. β-Endorphin and ACTH: Inhibitory and excitatory neurohormones of pain and fear. Commentary on R. C. Bolles and M. S. Fanselow's model for fear and pain. *Behav. Brain Sci.,* 1980, *3,* 312–313.

Johnson, H. M., Smith, E. M., Torres, B. A., & Blalock, J. E. Regulation of the *in vitro* antibody response by neuroendocrine hormones. *Proc. Natl. Acad. Sci. USA,* 1982, *79,* 4171–4174.

Jornvall, H., Persson, M., & Ekman, R. Structural comparisons of leukocyte interferon and pro-opiomelanocortin correlated with immunological similarities. *FEBS Letters,* 1982, *137,* 153–156.

Karre, K., Klein, G. O., Kiessling, R., Klein, G., & Roder, J. C. *In vitro* NK activity and *in vivo* resistance to leukemia: Studies in beige, beige/nude and wild type hosts on C57 background. *Int. J. Cancer,* 1980, *26,* 789–797.

Kayan, S., Woods, L. A., & Mitchell, C. L. Experience as a factor in the development of tolerance to the analgesic effect of morphine. *Eur. J. Pharmacol.,* 1969, *6,* 333–339.

Klee, W. A. Dual regulation of adenylate cyclase: A biochemical model for opiate tolerance and dependence. In J. Fishman (Ed.), *The basis of addiction.* Berlin: Dahlem Konferenzen, 1978.

Korol, B., Sletten, I. W., & Brown, M. L. Conditioned physiological adaptation to anticholinergic drugs. *Am. J. Physiol.,* 1966, *211,* 911–914.

Lennox, R. H., Kant, G. J., Sessions, G. R., Pennington, L. L., Mangey, E. H., & Meyerhoff, J. L. Specific hormonal and neurochemical responses to different stressors. *Neuroendocrinology,* 1980, *30,* 300–308.

Lord, J. A. H., Waterfield, A. A., Hughes, J., & Kosterlitz, H. W. Endogenous opioid peptides: Multiple agonists and antagonists. *Nature,* 1977, *267,* 495–499.

Lotzova, E. Analogy between rejection of hemopoietic transplants and natural killing. In R. B. Herberman (Ed.), *Natural cell mediated immunity against tumors.* New York: Academic Press, 1980.

Maier, S. F., Anderson, C., & Lieberman, D. A. Influence of control of shock on subsequent shock-elicited aggression. *J. Comp. Physiol. Psychol.,* 1972, *81,* 94–100.

Maier, S. F., Dowies, S., Grau, J. W., Jackson, R. L., Morrison, D. H., Maye, T., Madden, J., & Barchas, J. D. Opiate antagonists and long term analgesic reaction induced by inescapable shock in rats. *J. Comp. Physiol. Psychol.,* 1980, *94,* 1172–1183.

Maier, S. F., & Jackson, R. L. Learned helplessness: All of us were right (and wrong): Inescapable shock has multiple effects. In G. H. Bower & J. T. Spence (Eds.), *The psychology of learning and motivation.* (Vol. 13). New York: Academic Press, 1979.

Maier, S. F., & Seligman, M. E. P. Learned helplessness: Theory and evidence. *J. Exp. Psychol. [Gen.],* 1976, *105,* 3–46.

Maier, S. F., Sherman, J. E., Lewis, J. W., Terman, G. W., & Liebeskind, J. C. The opioid/ nonopioid nature of stress-induced analgesia and learned helplessness. *J. Exp. Psychol. [Anim. Behav.],* 1983, *9,* 80–90.

Mathews, P. M., Froelich, C. J., Sibbitt, W. L., & Bankjurt, A. D. Enhancement of natural cytotoxicity by β-endorphin. *J. Immunol.,* 1983, *130,* 1658–1662.

McCain, H. W., Lamster, I. B., Bozzone, J. M., & Grbic, J. T. β-endorphin modulates human immune activity via non-opiate receptors. *Life Sci.,* 1982, *31,* 1619–1624.

Moller, G., & Moller E. The concept of immunological surveillance against neoplasia. *Transplant. Rev.,* 1976, *28,* 3–16.

Overmier, J. B., & Seligman, M. E. P. Effects of inescapable shock upon subsequent escape and avoidance learning. *J. Comp. Physiol. Psychol.,* 1967, *63,* 28–33.

Palacios, R., & Sugawara, I. Hydrocortisone abrogates proliferation of T cells in autologous mixed lymphocyte reaction by rendering the interleukin-2 producer T cells unresponsive to interleukin-1 and unable to synthesize the T-cell growth factor. *Scand. J. Immunol.,* 1982, *15,* 25–31.

Pierpaoli, W., Baroni, C., Fabris, N., & Sorkin, E. Hormones and immunological capacity II. Reconstitution of antibody production by somatotropic hormone, thyrotropic hormone and thyroxin. *Immunology,* 1969, *16,* 217–230.

Rapaport, P. M., & Maier, S. F. Inescapable shock and food competition in rats. *Anim. Learn. Behav.,* 1978, *6,* 160–165.

Rettura, G., Seifter, J., Zisblatt, M., Levenson, S. M., Levine, N., & Seifter, E. Metyrapone-inhibited oncogenesis in mice inoculated with Murine Sarcoma Virus. *J. Natl. Cancer Inst.,* 1973, *6,* 1983–1985.

Riccardi, C., Santoni, A., Barlozzari, T., Puccetti, P., & Herberman, R. B. In vivo natural reactivity of mice against tumor cells. *Int. J. Cancer,* 1980, *25,* 475–486.

Riley, V. Psychoneuroendocrine influences on immunocompetence and neoplasia. *Science,* 1981, *212,* 1100–1109.

Rosellini, R. A., De Cola, J. P., & Shapiro, N. R. Cross-motivational effects of inescapable shock are associative in nature. *J. Exp. Psychol. [Anim. Behav.],* 1982, *8,* 376–388.

Rosellini, R. A., & Seligman, M. E. P. Learned helplessness and escape from frustration. *J. Exp. Psychol. [Anim. Behav.],* 1975, *1,* 149–158.

Rossier, J., French, E. D., Rivier, C., Ling N., Guillemin, R., & Bloom, F. E. Foot shock induced stress increases β-endorphin levels in blood but not brain. *Nature,* 1977, *270,* 618–620.

Russek, M., & Pina, S. Conditioning of adrenalin anorexia. *Nature,* 1962, *193,* 1296–1297.

Rygaard J., & Povlssen, C. O. The nude mouse vs. the hypothesis of immunological surveillance. *Transplant. Rev.,* 1976. *28,* 46–60.

Saksela, E. Interferon and natural killer cells. In I. Gresser (Ed.), *Interferon.* London: Academic Press, 1981.

Sawynok, J., Pinsky, C., & LaBella, F. S. On the specificity of naloxone as an opiate antagonist. *Life Sci.,* 1979, *25,* 1621–1632.

Saxena, Q. B., Saxena, R. K., & Adler, W. H. Regulation of natural killer activity in vivo. III. Effect of hypophysectomy and growth hormone treatment on the natural killer activity of the mouse spleen cell population. *Int. Arch. Allergy Appl. Immunol.,* 1982, *67,* 169–174.

Schull, J. A conditioned opponent theory of Pavlovian conditioning and habituation. In G. H. Bower & J. T. Spence (Eds.), *The psychology of learning and motivation* (Vol. 13). New York: Academic Press, 1979.

Sherman, J. E., & Liebeskind, J. C. An endorphinergic, centrifugal substrate of pain modulation. Recent findings, current concepts and complexities. In J. J. Bonica (Ed.), *Pain.* New York: Raven Press, 1980.

Siegel, S. Conditioning of insulin induced glycemia. *J. Comp. Physiol. Psychol.,* 1972, *78,* 233–241.

Siegel, S. Evidence from rats that morphine tolerance is a learned response. *J. Comp. Physiol. Psychol.,* 1975, *89,* 498–506.

Siegel, S. Morphine analgesic tolerance: Its situation specificity supports a Pavlovian conditioning model. *Science,* 1976, *193,* 323–325.

Siegel, S. Morphine tolerance acquisition as an associative process. *J. Exp. Psychol. [Anim. Behav.],* 1977, *3,* 1–13.

Siegel, S. A Pavlovian conditioning analysis of morphine tolerance. In N. A. Krasnegor (Ed.), *Behavioral tolerance: Research and treatment applications.* (National Institute of Drug Abuse Research Monograph No. 18; U. S. Department of Health, Education, and Welfare Publication No. (ADM) 78–551). Washington, D. C.: U. S. Government Printing Office, 1978.

Sklar, L. S., & Anisman, H. Stress and coping factors influence tumor growth. *Science,* 1979, *205,* 513–515.

Sklar, L. S., & Anisman, H. Stress and cancer. *Psychol. Bull.,* 1981, *89,* 396–406.

Solomon, R. L., & Corbitt, J. D. An opponent-process theory of motivation. *Psychol. Rev.,* 1974, *81,* 119–145.

Stein, M., Keller, S., & Schleifer, S. Role of the hypothalamus in mediating stress effects on the immune system. In B. A. Stoll (Ed.), *Mind and cancer prognosis.* Chichester, England: John Wiley & Sons, Ltd., 1979.

Suzuki, R., Handa, K., Itoh, K., & Kumagai, K. Natural killer (NK) cells as a responder to interleukin 2 (IL 2). 1. Proliferative response and establishment of cloned cells. *J. Immunol.,* 1983, *130,* 981–992.

Tiffany, S. T., & Baker, T. B. Morphine tolerance in rats: Congruence with a Pavlovian paradigm. *J. Comp. Physiol. Psychol.,* 1981, *95,* 747–762.

Timonen, T., Saksela, E., Virtanen, I., & Cantell, K. Natural killer cells are responsible for the interferon production induced in human lymphocytes by tumor cell contact. *Eur. J. Immunol.,* 1980, *10,* 422–427.

Visintainer, M. A., Volpicelli, J. R., & Seligman, M. E. P. Tumor rejection in rats after inescapable or escapable shock. *Science,* 1982, *216,* 437–439.

Weiss, J. M., Glazer, H. I., & Pohorecky, L. A. Coping behavior and neurochemical changes: An alternative explanation for the original "learned helplessness" experiments. In G. Serban & A. Kling (Eds.), *Animal models in human psychobiology.* New York: Plenum Press, 1976.

Wetzel, R., Levine, H. L., Hagman, J., & Ramachandran, J. Human leukocyte interferon has no structural and biological relationship to corticotropin. *Biochem. Biophys. Res. Commun.,* 1982, *104,* 944–949.

Wikler, A. Conditioning of successive adaptive responses to the initial effects of drugs. *Cond. Refl.,* 1973, *8,* 193–210.

Woods, S. C., & Shogren, R. E., Jr. Glycemic responses following conditioning with different doses of insulin in rats. *J. Comp. Physiol. Psychol.,* 1972, *81,* 220–225.

Coping Styles and Other Psychosocial Factors Related to Medical Status and to Prognosis in Patients with Cutaneous Malignant Melanoma

Lydia Temoshok and Bernard H. Fox

Introduction

Recently, there has been increasing recognition of the need to expand the conventional biomedical model of health and illness to encompass a multifaceted *biopsychosocial* model (e.g., Engel, 1977) which incorporates individuals' personalities, bodily constitutions, lifestyles, attitudes, and environmental transactions. Such a biopsychosocial model becomes more relevant as the leading cause of death in Western countries has shifted from infectious to chronic diseases, most notably heart disease and cancer. Cancer, even more than heart disease, evokes emotional distress, and provokes numerous psychosocial problems that conceivably could affect the course of the disease.

"Repressive" Coping Styles and Cancer

Coping may be defined as cognitive and behavioral efforts to manage and control the stress of environmental and internal demands and conflicts (e.g., Lazarus, 1966). In the acute phase of coping with extreme stress, there may be a minimization of the threat, or a defensive distortion of the impact of the event. These coping efforts have often been labeled "denial" or "repression". In some persons, the terror of cancer may be of such proportion that they can only cope by minimizing or denying medical problems, by postponing or even avoiding treatment. Objective facts and amount of information alone do not facilitate adaptation (Averill, 1973).

A sample of psychosocial studies of cancer patients reveals some consistencies in emotional coping style. Stavraky et al. (1968) found that those with the most favorable outcome were strikingly characterized by "strong hostile drives without loss of emotional control," whereas stage-matched controls of average or of least favorable outcome lacked such drives. Bahnson & Bahnson (1969) reported that their cancer patients repressed and denied such unpleasant affects as anxiety, hostility, and guilt more than did matched controls. Similarly, Greer & Morris (1975) found that women with breast cancers suppressed anger and other emotions more than did matched controls with benign tumors. Further, they found (1981) that cancer patients with "fighting spirit" survived longer than those without.

Derogatis, Abeloff & Melisaratos (1979) found that women with metastatic breast cancer who died within one year from baseline had significantly lower levels of hostility and higher levels of positive mood (as measured by several instruments) than patients who lived longer than one year. The latter group demonstrated more psychiatric symptomatology, and higher levels of depression, anxiety, hostility, and negative attitudes toward their physicians.

Rogentine et al. (1979) found that malignant melanoma patients who indicated, on average, the need for a considerable amount of personal adjustment to cope with having melanoma and surgery for it were less likely to suffer relapse within one year than patients reporting that a low or average amount of adjustment was needed.

The studies discussed above, while similar in focusing on coping style as a psychosocial concept, operationally measured different dimensions of coping: emotional, cognitive, or behavioral. It is not clear whether such dimensions of coping play a role in cancer induction and/or progression; nor how such potential roles are enacted. For example, certain ways of coping cognitively, emotionally, or behaviorally with the stress of having or suspecting cancer could contribute to poor medical prognosis by facilitating patients' delay in seeking necessary medical attention, or noncompliance with medical recommendations. An alternative possibility is that certain types of coping responses may be associated with hormonal, neuroendocrine, and/or immune-system responses that may exacerbate tumor growth and metastasis, and/or weaken the body's resistance to the malignant process. For example, Pettingale, Greer & Tee (1977) reported that before breast tumor biopsy, serum IgA levels were significantly higher in patients who showed extreme suppression of anger than in those displaying extreme expression or "normal" emotional response. The same authors found that serum IgA levels were significantly correlated with advancing metastatic spread of breast cancer, which suggests a biologically mediated connection between emotional suppression and cancer progression. A third possibility (in retrospective studies) is that having cancer itself may alter behaviors, emotional states, and perhaps even personality traits. These changes occasioned by cancer and/or its treatment may be biochemical or psychosocial in origin, but in either case could result in a psychosocial configuration that when examined *post facto* may not resemble the *pre facto* condition.

A Focus on Malignant Melanoma: The Clinical Picture

Several cancer researchers have argued persuasively that types of cancer are so different from each other in terms of risk factors, etiologic complications, prognosis, and psychological consequences that it would be advantageous for studies to focus on one type and/or location of cancer, or at least to differentiate cancer types as separate variables in studies with a larger sample size (e.g., Fox, 1978).

The present chapter is concerned with cutaneous malignant melanoma, a tumor arising from the pigment-producing cells (melanocytes) in the skin. In contrast to the more frequent types of skin cancer such as basal cell and squamous cell carcinomas, which rarely metastasize, *untreated* malignant melanomas usually metastasize, sometimes early in their development. Details about the epidemiology of melanoma can be found elsewhere (e.g., Ackermann & Su, 1979; Greene & Fraumeni, 1979; Holman et al., 1980; MacKie & Aitchison, 1982), as well as about treatment (e.g., Gumport, Harris, Roses, & Kopf, 1980).

Prognosis for malignant melanoma is directly related to the size and invasiveness of the primary lesion. Research indicates that the five-year survival rate decreases progressively with either increasing level of tumor invasion in the skin–designated as Clark level (Clark, From, Bernardino, & Mihm, 1969) or with thickness of the primary lesion–Breslow's criterion (Breslow, 1970).

Malignant melanoma often strikes productive people in the prime of life. The diagnosis of melanoma is likely to come as a great shock, even with older persons. This reaction is sometimes exacerbated by family, friends, or acquaintances who, fearing the worst, or simply not knowing how to respond, may avoid the patient or discussion of melanoma with the patient. Their avoidance, and in many, their negative emotional reactions can impose major emotional stress on the patient.

One significant factor that impedes diagnosis of early melanotic lesions is patient delay in seeking medical care on observing a suspicious symptom. While a relatively small proportion of those knowing they have cancer persist in denial after diagnosis, both among those who know and those who only suspect or worry that they might have cancer, denial of a lesion's existence and its frequent sequela, delay, can be hypothesized to be considerably more prevalent. It is usually assumed that patients' delay will be associated with increased tumor invasion and a poorer diagnosis of such lesions, yet only a few studies have provided any quantitative assessment of the relationship between delay and the histopathologic stage of the melanotic tumor at the time of diagnosis. For example, Worden & Weisman (1975) have examined the possible effect of psychosocial considerations upon delay; however, their analysis was based on too small a sample of melanotics ($N = 17$) to permit confident conclusions.

Cassileth et al. (1982) found no relationship between delay and tumor thickness in 245 patients with superficial spreading melanoma (SSM). Although not specified in their paper, one might assume that all of their coincidentally diagnosed patients (lesion discovered during a doctor's examination being done for other reasons) were defined as having zero delay. If so, growth of their tumors probably ranged over a long time period, with associated high variability in tumor thickness. In that case a lower correlation would be forced by such a procedure. Further, 36 percent of their patients had "delays" of over two years (Cassileth, 1982), eight patients "delaying" more than a decade, one as long as 40 years (Cassileth et al., 1982), in sharp contrast to the present study, in which only one patient delayed more than two years. It is obvious that for many of the patients in the study by Cassileth et al., the delay was measured from the time when a mole was *noticed,* rather than when a lesion became suspicious, as was the case for the present study. A mole may be present for a long time without changes occurring that signify malignancy. For those patients, true tumor growth tended to be shorter than the interval labelled "delay," further attenuating any actual relationship of growth parameters and "true delay," defined as inaction after noticing a suspicious symptom or change.

Current Research Findings on Psychosocial Factors and Melanoma

We present here two sets of studies on psychosocial factors and malignant melanoma. The thrust of these studies is consistent with previous work in the field discussed above. For the sake of enhancing comprehension, our work will be presented separately: a series of studies completed at the University of California San Francisco Medical Center, and one study with continuing follow-up conducted at the National Cancer Institute in Bethesda, MD Following these presentations, we shall attempt to integrate the findings, discuss them in terms of the relevant issues, and arrive at a tentative position regarding research in this area.

Work at the University of California San Francisco Medical Center

Behavior Patterns and Somatic Disease: Hypotheses about Type A, Type B, and Type C

In 1979, one of us (L.T.) began interviewing patients in the UCSF Malignant Melanoma Clinic (MMC) at the invitation of the clinic's co-directors, Drs. Marsden S. Blois and Richard W. Sagebiel. They noted that their patients had reported severe life stresses within 5 years of developing melanoma and that they exhibited certain consistent behavioral patterns, which could be represented as being excessively nice or passive. They also wondered whether psychosocial interventions might alter patients' psychological reactions or perhaps the course of their disease.

After pilot interviews with more than 50 patients in the UCSF MMC, we (L.T. and Dr. Bruce Heller) confirmed the impressions of the clinic directors. Further, we were struck by the observation that these patients demonstrated characteristics that were the *polar opposite* of the Type A behavior pattern identified by Drs. Friedman and Rosenman (e.g., 1959), and found in several larger prospective studies (Rosenman et al., 1975; Brand, Rosenman, Sholtz et al., 1976) to be an important risk factor for coronary heart disease. Compared with the Type A descriptors of angry, fast, tense, aggressive, in control, and so forth, these melanoma patients could be described as extremely cooperative, patient, passive, lacking assertiveness, appeasing, and accepting – descriptions consistent with the literature on cancer patients. These adjectives do not describe the Type B pattern, which is usually seen simply as the absence of Type A characteristics. The Type B individual is more relaxed, confident, unhurried, and more concerned with personal satisfaction and enjoyment than with achievement and competition. This suggested the hypothesis that, in addition to Type A and Type B, there might exist a *Type C pattern.* Type A individuals strive to assert and maintain a sense of environmental mastery with control over their "weaker" emotional expressions, and a view of themselves as autonomous and competent. In sharp contrast, Type C individuals hypothetically work at maintaining a sense of pleasant interpersonal atmosphere with control over angry expressions, and a sense of themselves as well liked. The Type C individual may resemble a Type B, since both may appear easy going and pleasant, but the difference lies in the emotional expressivity associated with each type. While the Type B easily expresses anger, fear, sadness, and other emotions, the Type C individual, in our view, suppresses or represses "negative" emotions, particularly anger, while struggling to maintain a strong and happy facade. It would make sense to speculate that the Type C individual may be prone to suffer a poorer melanoma prognosis than other individuals who lack such a behavior pattern but who do have the same diagnosis and similar epidemiological and medical risk factors (Temoshok & Heller, 1981).

A series of three studies (Temoshok, DiClemente, Sweet, et al., 1983; Temoshok, Sweet, Sagebiel, et al., 1983a; Temoshok, Sweet, Sagebiel, et al., 1983b) was completed with 106 patients at the MMC at the University of California San Francisco and Children's Hospital, San Francisco.[1] Two features emerge clearly from the complex pattern of results relative to prognosis: delay in seeking medical attention and the hypothesized "Type C" behavior pattern. A component of the Type C pattern—non-expression of dysphoric emotion—was found significantly more strongly in melanoma patients who had died or relapsed during the 18-month follow-up than in nonrelapsers.

Patient Sample and Study Design

Patients seen at the two clinics mentioned above who had a biopsy-confirmed diagnosis of malignant melanoma were asked at their first visit to either clinic to participate in a psychosocial study. More than 90% of the patients agreed to be subjects. Nearly all patients were seen within a month of biopsy. Most knew at the time of the study that they had melanoma, but few had been told explicitly the severity of their lesions, or what this implied prognostically. Patients were referred to the two clinics for confirmatory diagnosis and treatment recommenda-

---

[1] This research was supported in part by a University of California San Francisco Academic Senate Research Grant, and by American Cancer Society, Inc., California Division, contract no. 529-5-E, both to Dr. Temoshok, and by National Cancer Institute grant no. 5301CA26655 to Dr. Marsden S. Blois. Dr. Martin Kamp, Director of the University of California San Francisco Computer Center, and the Environmental Epidemiology Branch of the National Cancer Institute, generously provided partial support for the data analyses. We wish to thank Dr. Lynn E. Spitler, Director of the Melanoma Clinic at Children's Hospital, San Francisco, Drs. Marsden S. Blois and Richard W. Sagebiel, Co-Directors of the UCSF Melanoma Clinic, for their consistent support and cooperation. The contributions of Dr. Bruce W. Heller, who conducted half the structured patient interviews, and who helped conceptualize and operationalize the "Type C" construct, are gratefully acknowledged. Appreciation is also due to Ms. Judy Curtiss and Mr. Marc L. Gold for the videotaped interviews, and to Mr. David M. Sweet and Mr. Ralph J. DiClemente, who conducted the data analyses. We are especially indebted to the patients who participated in our research.

tions; additionally, some patients seen at Children's Hospital were entered into a randomized transfer factor protocol. Patients ranged in age from 18 to 72 years; 48% fell within the age range 30–49. Sex distribution was 55% male and 45% female, which is comparable to other large-scale study samples.

The sample differs from that described in the National Cancer Institute Study (to follow) in the sex ratio and in that only 23 of this study's 106 patients were either in clinical Stage II (regional lymph node invasion) or in unfavorable prognostic categories of Stage I, using the same criteria as the NCI study.

Clinical Variables and Psychological Testing

Histopathology and Medical Status

Each patient was initially interviewed and examined by a physician and the case was reviewed by the clinic consultants. Two histopathologic indices were rated on the basis of this conference and the pathology report: Clark level (Clark et al., 1969) and Breslow's thickness criterion (Breslow, 1970). These two attributes were correlated .71 (p < .0001) in this sample. All biopsy specimens were reviewed by a single pathologist.

Medical follow-ups were obtained from patients' medical records, or in some cases, from contacting the patient's referring physician or surgeon. Stage at follow-up was rated on a 15-point scale elaborating degrees of Stage I (localized), Stage II (regional lymph-node involvement), Stage III (distant lymph-node metastases, distant cutaneous or subcutaneous lesions, or visceral spread), or death.

Physical Risk

Skin, eye and hair coloring were rated separately on 5-point scales of increasing pigmentation. A composite scale of "at risk" complexion included these three attributes plus a scale of relative number of freckles. Sun exposure and degree of tanning were rated on separate 5-point scales on the basis of inquiry in the psychological interview.

Psychological Measures

a. *The structured videotaped interview.* After the physical examination, patients were interviewed on videotape by a clinical psychologist. All 106 subjects were asked about possible delay in seeking medical attention after noticing a symptom or change in the lesion and related questions. Of these subjects, 59 were asked additional questions pertaining to thoughts about and emotional reactions to the diagnosis of melanoma, cancer, and general health/illness issues; behaviors used to cope with the current medical problem; stresses within the last 5 years and how these were dealt with; and characteristic responses to everyday stresses.

The interviews were later rated according to a precise coding manual by two masters-level psychologists who were uninformed as to the patients' medical status. Because the coding format was highly structured, interrater reliabilities were quite high across all attributes, generally ranging from 87%–99% agreement between observers (with one low 58% agreement). For delay-related variables, agreement between observers was 93% for amount of delay, 99% for reason for seeking medical attention, 93% for reason for delay, 87% for previous knowledge of melanoma, and 87% for patients' understanding of treatment.

The variables were aggregated into 15 indices on an *a priori* basis. Five of the indices (4, 6, 8, 10, 13) were intended to capture various dimensions of a "Type C" construct. The goal of including other indices was to describe the opposite, "Type A" (3, 6, 7, 9), or intermediate, "Type B" (11, 14), patterns. Strong expression of emotion, also thought to contrast with the "Type C" pattern, was reflected in indices 5, 12, and 15. The remaining indices reflected other hypotheses about psychosocial factors in cancer (1, 2).

(1) Familial alcoholism: Degree of alcoholism in family members, relatives, or close friends. (2) Prior stress: Total sum of stresses within five years of developing melanoma. This included the *number* of: (a) deaths of close friends or relatives from cancer or other occurrences; (b) serious illnesses/accidents/surgeries for self or significant other; (c) divorce/separation/breakup of significant relationship; (d) changes in occupation; (e) seriousness of drinking problem in significant other; (f) major change in personal life. (3) Type A: "Type A" Behavior Pattern responses to abbreviated structured interview questions about coping with everyday strains in work or other activities. (4) Type C: "Type C" responses to questions about coping with everyday interpersonal strains in work or other activities. (5) Discouraged: Visibly discouraged and/or depressed responses to questions about work, family, and mood. (6) Nonverbal type: Coder's rating of subjects' nonverbal expressiveness on 22 semantic differential scales, as either more "Type A" (low) or more "Type C" (high). (7) Internal attitudes: An internal locus of control, attitudinally, regarding cancer. (8) External attitudes: An external locus of control, attitudinally, regarding cancer. (9) Type A melanoma coping: Using "Type A" strategies to cope with having melanoma (i.e., taking control, attacking the problem). (10) Type C melanoma coping: Using "Type C" strategies to cope with having melanoma (i.e., accepting, persevering, keeping busy). (11) Type B coping: "Type B" emotional expressiveness (i.e., humor, sharing, communicating feelings) used to cope with having melanoma. (12) Dysphoric expressiveness: The

expression of dysphoric feelings (shock, anger, fear, anxiety, sadness, crying) about the diagnosis of melanoma, as this was reported and observed in the interview. (13) Denial: Denying, minimizing, or avoiding the facts about and/or the seriousness of malignant melanoma. (14) Optimism: Optimistic attitudes about melanoma and the subject's own condition. (15) Catastrophic reaction: An extremely distressed reaction to having melanoma, which is viewed as an overwhelming disruption of the subject's life.

b. *Self-report instruments.* After the interview, the 59 subjects who were coded on the complete psychosocial interview were given a packet of self-report instruments, and asked to complete them within a day and mail them back to the principal investigator. Return rate was 73%. These instruments were: the Marlowe-Crowne Social Desirability Scale (Crowne & Marlowe, 1960), Beck's Depression Inventory (Beck et al., 1961), the Psychological Distress Scale from the Minnesota Multiphasic Personality Inventory (MMPI) (McLachan, 1977), the Taylor Manifest Anxiety Scale (Bendig, 1956), McNair's Profile of Mood States (McNair et al., 1971) and Temoshok's Character Style Inventory, (Temoshok & Grand, 1983).

With the exception of the new Character Style Inventory, there is an extensive literature on reliability, validity, and standardization of these measures. However, the Beck Scale, having been standardized for clinical depression, may have yielded a distribution more skewed than the standardizing populations. These self-report measures were used partly to provide independent measures related to the constructs hypothesized to underlie the 15 indices derived from the Structured Interview. Ten out of the 15 correlations between the pairs of derived indices and standardized measures, all hypothesized to be positive, were above + 0.10, and six of these were statistically significant. Similarly, negative relationships of certain other measures to the Type C constellation were hypothesized. Sixteen out of the 24 correlations were above 0.10 in the predicted direction, 11 of these significantly. Other possible correlations were predicted to be weakly negative.

Similar relationships in respect to dysphoric emotional expression were determined. Positive relationships among those measures were strikingly related (18/21 correlations very significant). Of predicted negative correlations, 13/21 were significant. Details of the above relationships can be found elsewhere (Temoshok & Heller, 1983).

The same subject sample and methodology were used to derive results for two studies that have been previously reported (Temoshok, DiClemente et al., 1983; Temoshok et al., 1983b). These results, as well as those of another longitudinal study of the same subjects (Temoshok et al., 1983a), will be summarized below.

Factors Associated with Prognosis of Melanoma

This study (Temoshok et al., 1983b) was concerned with the relationship between the most reliable prognostic estimation, thickness of the primary malignant melanoma tumor, and a comprehensive set of psychosocial variables that were coded from the videotaped interviews of 59 of the total 106 subjects. Variable domains included: physical risk (skin/hair coloring, sun exposure), demographic (age, sex, occupational status), psychosocial (emotions, attitudes, coping style), behavioral (delay in seeking medical attention), and situational (prior life stresses and prior knowledge of melanoma).

Delay in seeking medical attention was correlated $r = 0.31$ ($p < .001$) with tumor thickness. Age was correlated $r = 0.26$ ($p < .01$). As a situational variable, less previous knowledge of melanoma (on the following scale: "knew nothing about it, knew a little, knew the definition and had read about it, and knew someone who had the disease") was associated with thicker lesions ($r = .25$, $p < .01$).

With respect to psychosocial variables, higher scores on Type C Melanoma Coping ($r = .27$, $p < .05$), Nonverbal Type C ($r = .23$, $p < .11$) and External Attitudes ($r = .28$, $p < .05$) were correlated with thicker lesions. "Type C" Melanoma Coping is characterized by patients' acceptance of having melanoma, having more concern for family members than for themselves, trying not to think about it, coping by perseverance and trying to keep busy, trying to think positively, keeping feelings inside, and being considered strong and capable at handling things. Nonverbal Type C is the rater's assessment of the videotaped interview on 22 semantic differential scales of relative "Type C" (e.g., passive, bland, cooperative, helpless) characteristics. "External attitudes" refers to believing that getting melanoma is something that just happens, that prayer can work miracles, that it is important to place one's faith in God and the doctors, and that what one doesn't know won't hurt one. Of the self-report measures, only Histrionic and Narcissistic character styles, from the Character Style Inventory (Temoshok and Grand, 1983), were significantly (negatively) correlated with tumor thickness ($r = -.31$, $p < .05$; $r = -.33$, $p < .05$, respectively). These Type C variables were all independent of delay behavior. Semi-partial correlations (Cohen & Cohen, 1975) showed that while age was positively correlated with the psychosocial variables, these variables, rather than age, explained the variance in tumor thickness.

Multiple regression was used to determine (a) how well the group of variables significantly correlated with thickness were able to estimate thickness as the dependent variable, and (b) which variables accounted for the most variance in thickness. A step-up regression was computed using the 9 variables that were individually significantly correlated with thickness. Type C Melanoma Coping Style accounted for the most variance in thickness as the dependent variable (21.9%) and was entered first by the step-wise procedure. Patient delay in seeking medical treatment was entered second and accounted for an additional 9.9% of the variance. Histrionic character style added 6.1% to the total variance. The remaining variables each contributed less than 3% to the total variance. The overall step-wise model accounted for 46.5% of the variance in tumor thickness.

While it is relatively easy to understand how delay leads to increasingly thicker and more invasive primary lesions, it is more difficult to explain the association of these psychosocial variables with less favorable histopathologic indicators. The Type C Coping Style may be construed as a "mature," other-oriented, outwardly strong, selfless style that is paralleled by attitudes that are also more "externally" or other oriented. The reverse of this picture may be generally construed as "immature": the emotionally labile, dramatic or *histrionic* style and the self-oriented, self-enhancing *narcissistic* style. Speculatively, there may be a conflict between what is considered psychosocially desirable (i.e., "maturity") and those psychosocial characteristics associated with medically unfavorable indicators.

Factors Associated with Delay in Seeking Medical Attention

This study (Temoshok, DiClemente et al., 1983) investigated the relationship between patient delay in seeking medical attention for suspicious lesions on the one hand, and on the other, tumor characteristics, and demographic and psychosocial factors for 106 patients with cutaneous malignant melanoma (although psychosocial factors were coded for only 59 of the 106 subjects).

Patients with less readily accessible lesions (i.e., on the back) delayed significantly longer (mean = 6 months) than those with lesions of the head or neck (mean = 2.9) or extremities (mean = 3.6) ($p < 0.02$ for back vs. all other sites combined). The prognostically unfavorable trunk lesions were found more frequently during visits to physicians for unrelated problems than detected by patients themselves (46.2% versus 30.3%).

As for psychosocial variables, patients with less knowledge of melanoma or its appropriate treatment than others had significantly longer delays ($p < .01$). Patients who minimized the seriousness of their condition were more likely to seek treatments sooner than those with no minimization ($p < .0001$). While the reasons for this remain an open question, it is possible that minimization of seriousness reduced fear and anxiety about the disease, and thus might have made seeking treatment less foreboding. Patients with *some* understanding of treatment minimized more than patients with either very little or with considerable understanding. This result suggests that *some* understanding of treatment may allay fear and promote seeking treatment sooner.

These findings are highly relevant to public health programs designed for early detection of melanoma. An important implication is that physician and patient alertness to suspicious lesions in less visually accessible places may reduce patient delay in getting medical attention. Further, public health education based on enhancing understanding of melanoma without making dire health warnings may have a positive impact on early detection of cutaneous malignant melanoma.

Factors Associated with Progression of Melanoma

Interpreting the findings that certain measures within the Type C constellation were associated with tumor thickness (Temoshok et al., 1983 b) poses a problem in that this association could be explained by the effects of having melanoma, knowledge of it, its biological sequelae, or its impact on individuals' coping styles. These problems have plagued much of the research in the literature on psychosocial factors and cancer. Therefore, a longitudinal study (Temoshok et al., 1983 a) was undertaken to investigate factors associated with melanoma *progression*. Medical status follow-ups were obtained on 100 of the 106 patients who were initially interviewed, on average, 18 months earlier. While the two groups did not differ significantly on thickness of the primary lesion or level of dermal invasion, they were significantly different on four scales from the Profile of Mood States (i.e., tension-anxiety, depression-dejection, anger-hostility, and confusion). These scales were administered at the time of the initial interview. Compared with patients in Group 1, patients who relapsed or died had initially reported significantly *less* dysphoric emotion on these scales. However, these patients were rated by coders of the videotaped interview (who were uninformed about patients' prognosis or actual follow-up status) as showing significantly *more* depression ($p < .02$) than patients who ended up in stable condition at follow-up. This difference between self-reported denial of dysphoric emotion and raters' assessments of significant depression in patients who at follow-up had died or relapsed may be interpreted as suppression or repression of dysphoric emotion in these patients.

Other initially assessed variables on which patients who were stable at follow-up (Group 1) were significantly different from those who relapsed or died (Group 2) included: (a) delay in seeking medical attention for the primary lesion (patients in Group 2 had delayed, on average, 3 weeks longer than those in Group 1); (b) minimizing the seriousness of melanoma in general, or of one's own condition (Group 1 > Group 2 for both variables); and (c) externalizing attitudes (Group 2 > Group 1).

A step-wise multiple regression was completed using nine variables that were not significantly intercorrelated but were separately correlated with change in medical status from initial presentation to the last follow-up. Clark level accounted for the most variance in the dependent variable, which was change in disease status (17.7%, $p < .03$), followed by initial stage of disease, which added 9.3% ($p < .02$) to the total variance. The psychosocial variable, "minimizing the seriousness of one's condition," entered third in the equation and added another 7% ($p < .02$). The tension-anxiety scale from the Profile of Mood States added 2% to the total variance ($p < .04$). The remaining five variables, including delay, each contributed 1% or less.

In order to provide a quasi-replication of the NCI melanoma study (Rogentine et al., 1979), discriminant analyses were conducted with a variable analogous to the melanoma adjustment score (MAS) used in that study. (The current variable was scored on a scale of 1–5 instead of 1–100.) Using only this one melanoma adjustment variable, 45/46 of Group 1 and $1/11$ of Group 2 were correctly classified as to follow-up status. This was the same percentage correctly classified when the three best medical prognostic indicators (level of invasion, initial stage, and tumor thickness) were used in a separate discriminant analysis.

Discussion: A "Type C" for Cancer?

Numerous authors (see review by Cox & Mackay, 1982) have provided descriptions that are consistent with our Type C notion of individuals who develop cancer (e.g., Bahnson & Bahnson, 1966; Huggan, 1968; Le Shan, 1969) or who have unpromising disease progression (e.g., Derogatis, Abeloff, & Melisaratos, 1979). Further, several authors have previously used the term "Type C" to refer to a cancer-prone personality as the opposite of the Type A personality (Levy, 1982; Ragland, Brand, Rosenman, Fox, & Moss, 1982), with low anxiety and little expression of anger (Morris & Greer, 1980), or a helpless-hopeless personality with depressive tendencies (Shiloh, 1982). None of these authors, however, actually *tested* the hypothesis of a "Type C" construct in a psychosocial study of cancer patients, as was done in the UCSF study.

Further, the UCSF study elaborated the Type C construct on the basis of the Type A behavior pattern that has been successfully linked in a number of prospective studies with the development of coronary heart disease (CHD).

In the UCSF study, the Type C construct was operationally defined as a constellation of (a) attitudes, (b) cognitive and emotional proclivities, (c) verbal and nonverbal expressive patterns, (d) specific coping strategies and tendencies, and (e) more general character styles. The notion of a constellation of different dimensions is different from the emphasis on behavior in the Type A literature.

It is likely that certain dimensions in such a Type C constellation will be differentially associated with various medical outcome criteria. The UCSF study did not look at incidence of melanoma; therefore, there is no test of Type C as a cancer-prone style. However, the study of factors associated with unfavorable prognostic indicators (thicker primary lesions) found that several Type C measures (of behavioral and cognitive coping strategies, nonverbal expression, and character style) were significantly correlated with these indicators. Delay behavior appears to be independently asssociated with unfavorable prognosis.

As for disease *progression,* another dimension of the Type C construct—lower self-report of dysphoric emotion—emerged as significant in differentiating patients who were disease free at follow-up from those who had recurrences or metastases.These results are consistent with other reports relating disease progression to lower self reports of depression, anxiety, and hostility in breast cancer patients (Derogatis, Abeloff, & Melisaratos, 1979) and with preliminary findings by Levy & Lippman (reported in Levy, in press) that in contrast to breast cancer patients who were disease free at one-year followups, patients who died or had progressing disease expressed *less* psychiatric distress at baseline. The UCSF findings are also consistent with previous observations of cancer patients as emotionally constrained (Kissen, 1963; Magarey, Todd, & Blizard, 1977); repressive and denying of unpleasant affect (Bahnson & Bahnson, 1969); and characteristically suppressive of anger (Greer & Morris, 1975).

While the present findings do not prove the existence of a Type C constellation, nor do they present a clear-cut case for a connection between components of Type C with prognosis or progression of malignant melanoma, they do suggest that the construct is a worthwhile one to pursue through further methodological refinements and research.

The National Cancer Institute Study[2]

The material below describes second- and third-year follow-up data to the first-year results of a study initiated in 1975 (Rogentine et al., 1979). The follow-up data are presented here for the first time.

Patient Sample and Study Design

The study was an adjunct to a randomized prospective clinical trial of adjuvant chemo- and immunotherapy being conducted at the National Cancer Institute. All measures were taken on 67 melanoma patients. Of the 67, 55 were in clinical Stage II (regional lymph node metastases) and 12 were in unfavorable prognostic categories of Stage I (local, or primary lesion only). Criteria for classifying unfavorable Stage I prognosis were the following: (a) Clark level IV with tumor thickness greater than 2.25 mm; (b) Clark level V; or (c) local recurrence (within 5 cm of the primary). All patients had undergone wide excision of the primary lesion as well as regional lymph node dissection, and thus were apparently disease free. At the time of the cut-off date for collection of data, there had not yet elapsed a year since surgery for 3 of the 67 patients, so the final analysis group consisted of 64 patients.

About two-thirds of the patients were studied in the hospital during evaluation for treatment protocol inclusion. The other third were studied in the immunotherapy outpatient clinic. Each patient was assigned randomly to one of four treatment groups: (1) observation (standard medical practice); (2) methyl CCNU (chlorethyl methyl cyclohexylnitrosourea); (3) vaccination with BCG; and (4) vaccination with a mixture of BCG and allogeneic melanoma tissue culture cells.

All patients knew they had cancer and had elected to accept referral to the National Cancer Institute for consideration of adjuvant cancer therapy. They ranged in age from 16 to 67 years. Fifty were male, 17 were female. Eighty percent of the 84 patients approached consented to participate in the psychological evaluation, yielding the 67 patients tested.

---

[2] We are grateful to Susan Fisher, R.N. (Clinical Center, National Cancer Institute [NCI]), through whose efforts the follow-up data in this study were made available for analysis. Our appreciation also goes to Dr. Charles Brown for statistical advice and analysis, and to Herman Heise and Josephine Smith for help in organizing the follow-up data (Biometry Branch, Field Studies and Statistics Program, NCI).

Psychological Testing and Clinical Variables

Rogentine et al. (1979) elected to examine psychological test results with respect to the clinical status (relapsed or disease free) at one year after lymph node dissection. Relapse was documented histologically or radiologically in all cases. Two consecutive groups of Caucasian patients were studied. In the first half of our patient population (N = 31), as they appeared chronologically, an attempt was made to find promising predictive relationships with relapse status at one year so that they could be applied prospectively to the chronological second half of the patient population (N turned out to be 33). They are called, respectively, Group I and Group II.

The psychological tests administered were the RCLQ (Recent Life Changes Questionnaire) (Rahe, 1974); the SCL-90R (a symptom check list) (Derogatis, Lipman, & Covi, 1973); the Locus of Control Questionnaire (Rotter, 1966); and a number of scales from the Minnesota Multiphasic Personality Inventory (MMPI) (Dahlstrom, Walsh & Dahlstrom, 1972, 1975). In the RCLQ, an instrument designed to measure the occurrence and subjective effects of stressful events, the first question asks whether or not subjects have experienced an illness which kept them in bed a week or more or took them to the hospital. All replied that this did happen, and on later questioning, established that the reference was to melanoma surgery. Patients were asked to rate on a scale of 1 to 100 the amount of personal adjustment needed to handle or cope with this event. A high score indicated much adjustment. Rogentine et al. (1979) called this score "MAS" (melanoma adjustment score) rather than the name applied to all such scores by Rahe, "SLCU" (subjective life change unit score), to identify its unique characterization in their study. We shall follow the same convention here.

In addition, the following clinical variables, previously found to be associated with survival in melanoma patients, were measured: clinical stage, number of positive lymph nodes, clinical enlargement of nodes, histology of the primary tumor, Clark level of invasion in the skin, location of primary tumor, age, sex, and time from first symptom to diagnosis.

Mortality and Second and Third Year Relapse

During the first year after nodal surgery only two patients died in Group I, so that mortality did not enter the analysis of Rogentine et al. (1979) for that Group, nor was a prediction made for Group II. Since 1975–1976, however, not only have more patients relapsed, but enough additional ones have died in the second and third years after surgery to permit an analysis of mortality. The present analysis, therefore, addresses the predictive power for two- and three-year relapse in both groups, as well as their mortality. As will be shown, however, prediction for Group I in those years is quite biased, both for relapse and mortality, and will be made merely to demonstrate that fact. Analysis of second and third year outcomes, considering those variables found to be nonpredictive for Group I during the first year, will be dealt with elsewhere.

Results

To recapitulate the findings of Rogentine et al. (1979), none of the following variables discriminated first year relapsers in Group I from nonrelapsers: the SCL-90R (when sex was controlled); the Locus of Control Questionnaire; and all of the clinical variables. In a separate analysis, Fox et al. (1978) found that while some MMPI scales discriminated at the $p < 0.20$ level in Group I, none was cross-validated in Group II at the $p < 0.20$ level and none of the scales discriminated at $p < 0.10$ in Groups I and II combined.

The analytic methods used by Rogentine et al. (1979) will be followed here. They derived a predictive algorithm from Group I as follows: If number of melanotic nodes was >7, relapse was predicted irrespective of MAS. If number of nodes was <7, an MAS score <65 was a predictor of relapse and a score >65 predicted nonrelapse. This algorithm was applied to Group II. In addition, discriminant analysis was used to derive coefficients for best prediction of relapsers in Group I; these coefficients were then applied to test for their efficacy in a presumably random other sample from the melanoma population as defined here, Group II. Finally, discriminant function jackknife technique (Gray & Schacany, 1972) was used on all 64 patients in an attempt to eliminate the bias of testing the same sample for discrimination from which the discriminating coefficients were derived. While the jackknife technique accomplished this for all practical purposes, it will be seen that a more worrisome potential bias exists, which will be discussed later. The jackknife technique will not be applied here because of that bias.

To permit greater insight into the implications of the second and third year relapse results, all three years' results will be presented in two tables, one for the algorithm (Table I) and one for the discriminant analysis (Table II).

Table I. Prediction of Relapse or Death by Use of the Algorithm of Rogentine et al. (1979)

Group I (N = 31)

Relapse (Actual)

< 1 Year Predicted (a*)

Actual \ Predicted	Yes	No	
Yes	16	1	17
No	2	12	14
	18	13	31

< 2 Years Predicted (b*)

Actual \ Predicted	Yes	No	
Yes	17	3	20
No	1	10	11
	18	13	31

< 3 Years Predicted (c)

Actual \ Predicted	Yes	No	
Yes	17	4	21
No	1	9	10
	18	13	31

Death (Actual)

< 1 Year (d)

Actual \ Predicted	Yes	No	
Yes	2	0	2
No	16	13	29
	18	13	31

< 2 Years "Predicted" (e)

Actual \ Predicted	Yes	No	
Yes	13	2	15
No	5	11	16
	18	13	31

< 3 Years "Predicted" (f)

Actual \ Predicted	Yes	No	
Yes	14	3	17
No	4	10	14
	18	13	31

Group II (N = 33)

Relapse (Actual)

< 1 Year Predicted (g)

Actual \ Predicted	Yes	No	
Yes	9	2	11
No	6	16	22
	15	18	33

< 2 Years Predicted (h)

Actual \ Predicted	Yes	No	
Yes	10	5	15
No	5	13	18
	15	18	33

< 3 Years Predicted (i)

Actual \ Predicted	Yes	No	
Yes	10	8	18
No	5	10	15
	15	18	33

Death (Actual)

< 1 Year "Predicted" (j)

Actual \ Predicted	Yes	No	
Yes	4	0	4
No	11	18	29
	15	18	33

< 2 Years "Predicted" (k)

Actual \ Predicted	Yes	No	
Yes	7	5	12
No	8	13	21
	15	18	33

< 3 Years "Predicted" (l)

Actual \ Predicted	Yes	No	
Yes	8	6	14
No	7	12	19
	15	18	33

* a, b, etc, are designations for the matrices referred to in the text.

Algorithm Analysis

It will be seen from Table I that the bulk of the relapses took place in the first year after nodal operation. Part of the reason for this is that, while all patients showed no disease symptoms or signs after nodal dissection, the interval from removal of the primary lesion to nodal dissection involved times ranging from zero to many months. Hence, we cannot use the large-sample survival times of the National Cancer Institute (Axtell et al., 1976) as a guide to expected survival, let alone relapse times, which the Institute does not collect and publish. The results for the first year's relapse experience are seen in the first column of Table I; these data were published by Rogentine et al. (1979). Data for matrix *b*, designated < 2 years, reflect the cumulated experience of years 1 and 2, and data for < 3 years (matrix *c*) reflect the experience of the cumulated first three years, both in Group I. In that Group, during the second year an additional three patients relapsed, and during the third, one further patient relapsed. Of the first three new ones, two were incorrectly predicted: in matrix *b*, actual–yes, predicted–no = 3, whereas in matrix *a* that figure was 1. The fourth new relapse case, seen in the same location in matrix *c*, was also incorrectly predicted. The correctly predicted new relapser is found in matrix *b*, actual–yes, predicted–yes, showing an increase in the number of correctly predicted yeses from 16 in the first year to 17 during the first two years. It will be recalled that the algorithm was derived from Group I's relapse experience during the first year.

As for mortality, none of the patients in either group died of causes other than melanoma during the first three years. One patient died later, but is included as "not relapsed", and "not dead" as of the end of the third year. All analyzed deaths, therefore, were those of relapsers. It is of interest to ask how well both the algorithm and the discriminant analysis coefficients predicted death, as well as relapse, even though the determinations by Rogentine et al. (1979) and Fox et al. (1978) addressed only the question of relapse during the first year. Because these authors dealt only with relapse, the word "prediction" as applied to mortality in Table I is entered in quotes.

The data are straightforward. In Group I two relapsers died during the first year (matrix *d*). An additional 13 relapsers died during the second year – see matrix *e* – and two others during the third, for a total of 17. When the algorithm was applied for the cumulated first two years in Group I, 13 out of 15 were correctly predicted to die in those years, and one of the two third-year fatalities was correctly predicted.

For Group II, the presumably random group on whom the algorithm was tested, matrix *g* shows the data from Rogentine et al. (1979). During the second year four new relapses occurred, as shown by the change from 11 in matrix g to 15 in matrix h in the row for actual "yes" counts. Of these, three were incorrectly predicted. In year 3, as seen in matrix i, an additional three relapses occurred, increasing the total relapses from 15 at the end of year 2 to 18 at the end of year 3. Of those three new relapses, none was correctly predicted. Thus in Group II, out of seven new relapses in the second and third years, six out of seven were incorrectly predicted by the algorithm.

Mortality in Group II during the first two years was a little lower than in Group I: 12/33 as opposed to 15/31. In Group II, as in Group I, an additional two people died in year 3, for a total of 14 indicated in matrix l, an increase from the 12 shown in matrix k. As in group I, one of these two deaths was correctly predicted.

Note that in matrix a 17 out of 31 patients (55%) relapsed in Group I, but in Group II, only 11 out of 33 patients (33%) relapsed, as seen in matrix g. By the end of year 3, the respective proportions were more similar: 21/31 (68%) and 17/33 (52%).

Discriminant Function Analysis

Using the same two predictors, number of melanotic nodes and MAS, a discriminant analysis was done on Group I in year 1 and the coefficients derived were applied to Group II, year 1. The success of this prediction appeared in Rogentine et al. (1979). In the present analysis the same coefficients were applied to Groups I and II at the end of years 2 and 3 for relapse and mortality. These data are seen in Table II, matrices m through x.

As with the algorithm, relapse prediction was quite good through the third year in Group I, as was mortality prediction. Since only two people died the first year in Group I, that set of data is not indicated as a prediction (see matrix p). Of the four new relapses (matrices n and o) three were incorrectly predicted. Of the two new deaths in matrix n, one was successful, the other not.

In Group II, after the first year, four relapsers were added to the 11 of matrix s, of whom 3 were incorrectly predicted, and of the three additional relapses seen in matrix u, all were incorrectly predicted. Out of seven new relapsers in the last two years, six out of seven were incorrectly predicted. In the third year the proportion of actual relapsers correctly predicted is only slightly better than chance. A similar picture is seen in regard to Group II mortality. Of the eight new deaths in year 2 (matrix w), only three were correctly predicted. In year 3 the two new deaths were correctly predicted, with a total proportion of eight out of

Table II. Prediction of Relapse or Death by Use of Discriminant Analysis, Using Year 1 Coefficients

Group I (N = 31)

Relapse

		< 1 Year			< 2 Years Predicted			< 3 Years Predicted	
		Yes	No	m*		Yes	No	n*	
Actual	Yes	14	3	17		15	5	20	
	No	4	10	14		3	8	11	
		18	13	31		18	13	31	

		< 3 Years Predicted		
		Yes	No	o
Actual	Yes	15	6	21
	No	3	7	10
		18	13	31

Death

		< 1 Year			< 2 Years "Predicted"			< 3 Years "Predicted"	
		Yes	No	p		Yes	No	q	
Actual	Yes	2	0	2		13	2	15	
	No	16	13	29		5	11	16	
		18	13	31		18	13	31	

		< 3 Years "Predicted"		
		Yes	No	r
Actual	Yes	14	3	17
	No	4	10	14
		18	13	31

Group II (N = 33)

Relapse

		< 1 Year			< 2 Years Predicted			< 3 Years Predicted	
		Yes	No	s		Yes	No	t	
Actual	Yes	7	4	11		8	7	15	
	No	4	18	22		3	15	18	
		11	22	33		11	22	33	

		< 3 Years Predicted		
		Yes	No	u
Actual	Yes	8	10	18
	No	3	12	15
		11	22	33

Death

		< 1 Year			< 2 Years "Predicted"			< 3 Years "Predicted"	
		Yes	No	v		Yes	No	w	
Actual	Yes	3	1	4		6	6	12	
	No	8	21	29		5	16	21	
		11	22	33		11	22	33	

		< 3 Years "Predicted"		
		Yes	No	x
Actual	Yes	8	6	14
	No	3	16	19
		11	22	33

* m, n, etc. are designations for the matrices referred to in the text.

14 deaths correctly predicted. This, like the finding for relapse in Group II, was also not far from chance (matrix x).

Discussion: Statistical Issues

The Jackknife Technique. A basic flaw in the use of the jackknife technique was mentioned above. Considered only as a statistical approach, the technique cannot be particularly faulted; however, its application to the combined group I and II is problematic. The flaw is that since both the algorithm and the discriminant function coefficients were derived from Group I, and since the choice of variables was derived from the identification in a "semifishing expedition" among all the tests given, the possibility of chance significance among a number of tests or test items must be very seriously considered. For that reason, and to decrease the probability that this in fact happened, a second group was chosen to test the hypothesis that the two significant variables did indeed predict beyond chance expectation, namely, Group II. But it was precisely because the success rate in the fishing expedition was high for the two variables that they were selected. Hence, degree of success when using the combined groups for any test of predictive capability, including the jackknife technique, is artificially inflated by the inclusion of Group I as part of the test group. For that reason, the results of that method for the 64 cases are not used here to predict success in years 2 and 3. On the other hand, if a test of the combined groups were indeed to be done and turned out to be *not* significant, one would be somewhat more confident than in other circumstances that the null hypothesis was not disconfirmed, and that the variables in question predicted relapse or death with no more than chance success. Such a test (using a different statistic) was done, such a result was found, and such a conclusion was drawn, in fact, by Fox et al. (1978) in regard to MMPI data for year 1. We do not address here differences already observed that had no significant relationship to relapse and nonrelapse.

The Algorithm. Many of the results reported above are to be expected. For example, 16 out of 17 actual relapsers were correctly identified in Group I as part of the algorithm development process. If only four more relapses occurred in three years, the process of testing the algorithm should properly be addressed only to them, as a new sample analogous to the testing of a different sample called Group II (ignoring the time difference for the moment). If these four are grouped with the first 17 relapsers, at least 16 of the 21 must be correct. Thus, the proportion of relapsers correctly identified in year 3 cannot be lower than 16/21, or 72 percent. One cannot, however, draw a valid conclusion from only four relapsers. Moreover, because only the Group I first year data can be used as the source of the algorithm, and the prediction was made at the time the first year data were collected, the proportion predicted to relapse must remain the same throughout the three years: 18 predicted to relapse, 13 not to relapse. Thus, the maximum possible success is 18 correct, and all additional relapsers beyond 18 *must* be incorrectly identified. Since most patients who die have previously relapsed, then, as time goes on, the proportion correct is forced to decline once all 18 are predicted correctly and additional relapses occur. This has not happened here yet, but it is pointed out as a limitation of using an algorithm based on a test group such as Group I for predicting later relapse.

A similar argument could be raised for mortality, but the number correct was not too close to the maximum possible correct (14 out of 18, matrix *f*). A more important issue is troublesome here, however. Since death is almost always preceded by relapse, a high success rate for relapse will increase the chance of a high success rate for mortality. Such is the case with the present set of data. In matrix *c* we see that 21 people relapsed; in matrix *f* we see that 17 people died. Even if all four people who were predicted in matrix *c* not to relapse, not only relapsed, but actually died, the least success achievable in matrix *f* is 13 out of 17 deaths correctly predicted, a respectable proportion. As more deaths occur, the number who relapse and the number who die come closer together, and the success rate of mortality prediction will more closely resemble the success rate of relapse prediction. The correlation between relapse and death in the years after the first is too high to separate the two as independent variables.

Group II data are subject to the same caveats. It happens, however, that the number of additional relapses (7) is not too far from the original number relapsing in year 1 (11), so the effect of successful prediction in year 1 does not carry so much weight as in Group I. In fact, the poor record in predicting the relapse of the additional seven relapsers led to an almost chance division of correct and incorrect prediction of the cumulative three year relapses: 10/18 (see matrix *i*). The results for mortality in Group II show a similar picture (matrix *l*). If success had been higher in this group, it would have been even closer to the ceiling of possible success, based on the fact that the algorithm predicted only 15 relapsers, rather than 18, as in Group I.

The Discriminant Function. In this case the number predicted to relapse in Group I (matrix *m*) was 18, as in the case of the algorithm. Since the prediction does not change as more people relapse, precisely the same arguments can be advanced here as in the case of the algorithm. With only four more relapses in years 2 and 3, no severe change in the success rate is expected; nor does it happen. The arguments and the findings in regard to death are very similar to those advanced in the case of the algorithm (see matrices p, q and r). In Group II the number predicted to relapse, 11/33, was quite low (see matrix x). This imposed a severe lower limit of success, although it was not reached because of the poor success rate in predicting the seven new relapsers. It was so poor, in fact, and the first year success rate for relapsers was so low (7/11, or 64 per cent–see matrix s), that the additional relapsers actually dropped the predictive capability to a level lower than 50 percent correct: 8/18, or 44 per cent correct. A similar picture, although not quite so dismal, is reflected in matrices v, w and x.

Prediction. While it is clearly not possible to achieve greater confidence in the prediction of first year relapses based on the new data, it might seem possible do so for second and third year newly occurring relapses, since they were not included in the predicted relapse groups of the first year. But that possibility is illusory. While the new relapsers were not first-year relapsers, they were clearly *nonrelapsers* then, and hence the algorithm as well as the discriminant coefficients were based, in part, on their scores as nonrelapsers. Obviously, then, one expects the new relapse cases in Group I to tend toward incorrect prediction, since they would normally show a small number of nodes and a high MAS score, following their earlier status as nonrelapsers in the training group, Group I: as expected, three out of four new relapsers were incorrectly predicted. In the test group, Group II, however, no such dependence on prior selection exists–neither in the first year nor in later ones. Hence the rate of incorrect identification among new relapsers–a significant six out of seven–is important to note. It may mean that the first high success rate was chance, and that the total count tends toward a possible mean true rate of 50 percent successful prediction; or it may be that one harbors, incorrectly, an expectation that the discriminating formulas are correct and apply to years 2 and 3, when, in fact they are correct, but are restricted in their correctness to year 1. Another interpretation is that the formulas predict in one direction for year 1, but in the opposite direction for years 2 and 3. Whatever the case, this study, encompassing two more years of observation, has not added anything substantial to help answer with confidence the question of whether MAS successfully predicts relapse in a group of melanoma patients like this.

Conclusions

From the NCI study one can conclude that, starting with the initial induction from the results of Group I tests that led to the hypotheses tested on Group II, additional data from years 2 and 3 did not increase confidence in the tentative conclusion based on success in predicting prognosis in Group II; if anything, they decreased it. This was true both for further relapses and for the substantial number of deaths occurring in years 2 and 3.

Integration: Conclusions to be Drawn from Considering Delay Behavior in Both Studies

In the San Francisco study, delay was found to be strongly and significantly related to prognostic indicators, and correlated with but did not predict 18-month follow-up status. While unfavorable prognostic indicators would theoretically predict earlier relapse among patients with longer delays, it would be unwise to go beyond the data and predict relapse in subsequent years.

The NCI study examined delay with respect to whether early relapse could have been the result of longer delay, rather than the relationship of delay to histopathology, and found that delay did not predict relapse (Rogentine et al., 1979, p. 649).

Some of the reasons that people may delay cannot be educed from the NCI study, although valuable hypotheses can be derived from the results of the San Fancisco study. The dynamics of delay and psychosocial characteristics associated with cancer patients are not isolated psychological elements; their interrelation must be complex.

Other Psychosocial Variables

We are aware of the pitfalls in attempting to infer the nature of a premorbid or even of a stable post-diagnostic personality or coping style from variables derived from interviews and psychological tests administered to patients who already have malignant melanoma. We feel that any relationship proposed between unfavorable prognostic indicators and psychosocial variables in the San Francisco study depend, in part, upon the stability of characteristic coping styles or "traits" in the presence of (1) a profound stressor which has life-threatening implications, (2) the possible somatopsychic effects of melanoma, and (3) the well-known psychological effects of having cancer (Fox, 1978).

It is of interest to record the findings of a follow-up study on the Western Collaborative Group, from which Friedman and Rosenman (1959) derived their Type A and B concepts. Follow-up for cancer in their study has, to this time, not been done, but recently a beginning was made toward such an analysis on their cohort of 3154 men. Ragland et al. (1982) determined cause of death on about 80 percent of those who died through 1977. Cancer caused 97 of the 315 deaths ascertained. After correcting for the effect of age on the distribution of men with Type A and B, the relative odds (proportion with Type A ÷ proportion with Type B) among those dying of cancer were 1.32, $p < .22$. While one cannot conclude that Type A people are at greater risk of cancer mortality than Type B, if the same proportions hold when the study is extended through 1982, and when false negatives are reduced to 3–4 percent with intensive followup, Type A's would be at significantly greater risk than type B's. It is obvious that there is confounding here, since the Type B's of this group contain the Type C's posited above, as well as the type B's defined above as distinct from Type A's and C's. If it is found that 1) the follow-up to the study by Ragland et al. (1982) strengthens the tentatively observed excess risk of Type A's of dying of cancer, and 2) Type C's are not only at greater risk of poor prognosis if they have cancer, as suggested above, but are also at greater risk of getting cancer, then there may be greater risk of cancer death at both ends of the continuum: Type A's (Are extreme Type A's at even greater risk?) *and* Type C's.

The findings from both the San Francisco study and the NCI study relating *disease progression* to patients' self report of relatively little need for adjustment as a result of their surgery or hospitalization are another matter, however. In the San Francisco study, this melanoma adjustment variable was as predictive of nonrelapse status (but not of relapse or death) as were the three best medical prognostic indicators combined. The relationship between progression and this variable, which emerged as the strongest predictor of relapse after one year in the NCI study, unfortunately could not be clarified by waiting two years, as was noted in the discussion of the NCI study above.

A kind of denial could be attributed to patients who claim little need for adjustment to having a life-threatening disease. Rogentine derived a denial scale based on delay measures assessed in the NCI study (Rogentine et al., 1979), but found no relation between denial and relapse. As the authors of the 1979 study observed (p. 653), a low adjustment score may indicate acceptance of life's difficulties rather than denial. Alternatively, it may indicate low emotional reactivity or suppressed expression of emotion. This latter possibility is congruent with the findings of lower self-reports of dysphoric emotion among patients who relapsed or died by the 18-month follow-up to the San Francisco study, as well as with reports of other researchers who have related suppression of emotions to tumor malignancy (Greer and Morris, 1975) and to poor prognosis (Derogatis et al., 1979).

Whatever subsequent research reveals to be the explanation for these results, the two studies discussed here suggest that components or measurements of a denial-like construct may be related to prognosis and progression of malignant melanoma.

References

Ackerman, A. B., & Su, W. P. D. The histology of cutaneous malignant melanoma. In A. W. Kopf, R. S. Bart, R. S. Rodriguez-Sains, & A. B. Ackerman (Eds.), *Malignant melanoma*. New York: Masson, 1979.

Averill, J. Personal control over aversive stimuli and its relationship to stress. *Psychol. Bull.*, 1973, *80*, 286–303.

Axtell, L. M., Asire, A. T., & Myers, M. H. (Eds.). *Cancer patient survival*. Report Number 5. SEER Program, National Cancer Institute, U. S. Dept. of Health, Education and Welfare, Bethesda, MD, 1976.

Bahnson, C. B., & Bahnson, M. B. Denial and repression of primitive impulses and of disturbing emotions in patients with malignant neoplasms. In D. M. Kissen & L. LeShan (Eds.), *Psychosomatic aspects of neoplastic disease*. London: Pitman, 1964.

Bahnson, C. B., & Bahnson, M. B. Ego defenses in cancer patients. *Ann. N. Y. Acad. Sci.*, 1969, *164*, 546–559.

Bahnson, C. B., & Bahnson, M. B. Role of the ego defenses: Denial and repression in the etiology of malignant neoplasm. *Ann. N. Y. Acad. Sci.*, 1966, *125*, 335–343.

Beck, A. T., Ward, C. H., Mendelson, M., Mock, J., & Erbaugh, J. An inventory for measuring depression. *Arch. Gen. Psychiatry*, 1961, *4*, 561–571.

Bendig, A. W. The development of a short form of the Manifest Anxiety Scale. *J. Consult. Psychol.*, 1956, *5*, 384.

Berkman, L., & Syme, S. Social networks, host resistance, and mortality. A nine-year follow-up study of Alameda County residents. *Am. J. Epidemiol.*, 1979, *109*, 186–204.

Brand, R. J., Rosenman, R. H., Sholtz, R. I., & Friedman, M. Multivariate prediction of coronary heart disease in the Western Collaborative Group Study. *Circulation*, 1976, *53*, 348–355.

Breslow, A. Thickness, cross-sectional area, and depth of invasion in the prognosis of cutaneous melanoma. *Ann. Surg.*, 1970, *172*, 902–908.

Carey, R. Emotional adjustment in terminal patients: A quantitative approach. *J. Counseling Psychol.*, 1974, *21*, 433–439.

Cassel, J. The contribution of the social environment to host resistance. *Am. J. Epidemiol.*, 1976, *104*, 107–123.

Cassileth, B. R. Personal communication to first author, 1982. U. of Pennsylvania Cancer Center, 3400 Spruce St., Philadelphia, PA 19104.

Cassileth, B. R., Clark, W. H., Jr., Heiberger, R. M., March, V., & Tenaglia, A. Relationship between patients' early recognition of melanoma and depth of invasion. *Cancer,* 1982, *49,* 198–200.

Clark, W. H., From, L., Bernardino, E., & Mihm, M. C. The histogenesis and biologic behavior of primary human malignant melanoma of the skin. *Cancer Res.,* 1969, *29,* 705–726.

Cohen, J., & Cohen, P. *Applied multiple regression/correlation.* New York: Wiley, 1975.

Cox, T., & Mackay, C. Psychosocial factors and psychophysiological mechanisms in the aetiology and development of cancers. *Soc. Sci. Med.,* 1982, *16,* 381–396.

Crowne, J. P. & Marlowe, D. A new scale of social desirability independent of psychopathology. *J. Consult. Psychol.,* 1960, *24,* 349–354.

Dahlstrom, W. G., Welsh, G. S., & Dahlstrom, L. E. *An MMPI handbook, Vol. I. Clinical interpretation* (Revised). Minneapolis: University of Minnesota Press, 1972.

Dahlstrom, W. G., Welsh, G. S., & Dahlstrom, L. E. *An MMPI handbook, Vol. II. Research applications* (Revised). Minneapolis: University of Minnesota Press, 1975.

Derogatis, L., Abeloff, M., & Melisaratos, N. Psychological coping mechanism and survival time in metastatic breast cancer. *J. Am. Med. Assoc.,* 1979, *242,* 1504–1508.

Derogatis, L. R., Lipman, R. S., & Covi, L. SCL-90; An outpatient psychiatric rating scale – A preliminary report. *Psychopharmacol. Bull.,* 1973, *9,* 13–28.

Engel, G. L. The need for a new medical model: A challenge for biomedicine. *Science,* 1977, *196,* 129–136.

Fox, B. H. Premorbid psychological factors as related to cancer incidence. *J. Behav. Med.,* 1978, *1,* 45–133.

Fox, B. H., Boyd, S. C., Van Kammen, D. P., & Rogentine, G. N., Jr. *Further analysis of psychological variables in predicting relapse after Stage II melanoma surgery.* Presented at III International Symposium on Psychobiologic, Psychophysiologic, Psychosomatic and Sociosomatic Aspects of Neoplastic Disease. Bohinj, Yugoslavia, 1978.

Friedman, M., & Rosenman, R. Association of specific overt behavior patterns of blood and cardiovascular findings. *J. Am. Med. Assoc.,* 1959, *169,* 1289–1296.

Glaser, B., & Strauss, A. *Awareness of dying.* Chicago: Aldine, 1965.

Gray, H. L., & Schacany, W. R. *The generalized jackknife statistic.* New York: Marcel Dekker, Inc., 1972.

Greene, M. H., & Fraumeni, J. F. The hereditary variant of malignant melanoma. In W. H. Clark, L. I. Goldman, & M. J. Mastrangelo (Eds.), *Human malignant melanoma.* New York: Grune and Stratton, 1979.

Greer, S., & Morris, T. Psychological attributes of women who develop breast cancer: A controlled study. *J. Psychosom. Res.,* 1975, *19,* 147–153.

Greer, S., & Morris, T. Psychological response to breast cancer and survival: Eight-year follow-up. Presented at the American Psychological Association Meeting, Los Angeles, September, 1981.

Gumport, S. L., Harris, M. N., Roses, D. F., & Kopf, A. W. The diagnosis and management of common skin cancers. *CA-A Cancer J. for Clinicians,* 1980, *31,* 79–90.

Holman, C. D. J., Mulroney, C. D., & Armstrong, B. K. Epidemiology of preinvasive and invasive malignant melanoma in western Australia. *Int. J. Cancer,* 1980, *25,* 317–323.

Huggan, R. R. A critique and possible reinterpretation of the observed low neuroticism scores of male patients with lung cancer. *Brit. J. Soc. Clin. Psychol.,* 1968, *7,* 122–128.

Kissen, D. M. Psychosocial factors, personality and lung cancer in men aged 55–64. *Brit. J. Med. Psychol.,* 1967, *40,* 29–43.

Lazarus, R. *Psychological stress and the coping process.* New York: McGraw-Hill, 1966.

LeShan, L. An emotional life-history pattern associated with neoplastic disease. *Ann. N. Y. Acad. Sci.,* 1969, *164,* 546–557.

Levy, S. The expression of affect and its biological correlates: Mediating mechanisms of behavior and disease. In C. Van Dyke, L. Temoshok, and L. S. Zegans (Eds.), *Emotions in health and illnes: Applications to clinical practice.* New York: Grune and Stratton, Inc. (In press).

Levy, S. Remarks on a presentation by B. H. Fox at the National Cancer Institute: Ragland, D. R., Brand, R. J., Rosenman, R. H., Fox, B. H. & Moss, A. R. *Type A behavior and cancer: A preliminary report,* 1982.

MacKie, R. M. & Aitchison, T. Severe sunburn and subsequent risk of primary cutaneous melanoma in Scotland. *Br. J. Cancer,* 1982, *46,* 955–960.

Magarey, C. T., Todd, P. B., and Blizard, P. T. Psycho-social factors influencing delay and breast self-examination in women with symptoms of breast cancer. *J. Sci. Med.,* 1977, *11,* 299–232.

McLachan, J. F. A scale for the evaluation of psychological distress. *J. Clin. Psychol.,* 1977, *33,* 159–161.

McNair, D., Lorr, M., & Doppleman, L. F. EDITS *manual: Profile of mood states.* San Diego, CA: Educational and Industrial Testing Service, 1971.

Morris, T., & Greer, H. S. A 'Type C' for cancer? Low trait anxiety in the pathogenesis of breast cancer. *Cancer Detection Prev. 3,* 1980, Abstract No. 102.

Pettingale, K. W., Greer, S., and Tee, D. E. H. Serum IgA and emotional expression in breast cancer patients. *J. Psychosom. Res.,* 1977, *21,* 395–399.

Rahe, R. H. The pathway between subjects' recent life changes and their near-future illness reports: Representative results and methodological issues. In B. S. Dohrenwend & B. P. Dohrenwend (Eds.), *Stressful life events: Their nature and effects.* New York: Wiley, 1974.

Rogentine, G. N., Jr., Van Kammen, D. P., Fox, B. H., Docherty, J. P., Rosenblatt, J. E., Boyd, S. C., & Bunney, W. E. Psychological factors in the prognosis of malignant melanoma: A prospective study. *Psychosom. Med.,* 1979, *41,* 647–655.

Rosenman, R. H., Brand, R. B., Jenkins, C. D., Friedman, M., Strauss, R., & Wurm, M. Coronary heart disease in the Western Collaborative Group Study: Final follow-up experience of 8 $^1/_2$ years. *J. Am. Med. Assoc.,* 1975, *233,* 872–877.

Rotter, J. B. Generalized expectancies for internal versus external control of reinforcement. *Psychol. Monogr.,* 1966, *80,* 1–28.

Shiloh, A. *Type C. The cancer-prone personality.* Unpublished paper. Dept. of Anthropology, U. of South Florida, Tampa, FL, 1982.

Stavraky, K. M., Buch, C. W., Lott, S. S., & Wanklin, J. M. Psychological factors in the outcome of human cancer. *J. Psychosom. Res.,* 1968, *12,* 251–259.

Temoshok, L., DiClemente, R. J., Sweet, D. M., Blois, M. S., & Sagebiel, R. W. Factors related to patient delay in seeking medical attention for cutaneous malignant melanoma. Manuscript under review, 1983.

Temoshok, L., & Grand, S. Reliability and validity of an inventory to assess character style. Manuscript submitted for publication, 1983.

Temoshok, L., & Heller, B. W. Introducing a "Type C" constellation into psychosocial research on cancer: Evidence for validity. Manuscript submitted for publication, 1983.

Temoshok, L., Sweet, D. M., Sagebiel, R. W., & Blois, M. S. Biological and psychosocial factors in melanoma progression at 18-month follow-up. Manuscript under review, 1983a.

Temoshok, L., Sweet, D. M., Sagebiel, R. W., Blois, M. S., Heller, B. W., DiClemente, R. J., & Gold, M. L. The relationship of psychological factors to prognostic indicators in cutaneous malignant melanoma. Manuscript under review, 1983b.

Whiting, D. A. Some thoughts on moles and melanomas. *Int. J. Dermatol.,* 1978, *17,* 485–487.

Worden, T. W., & Weisman, A. D. Psychosocial components of lagtime in cancer diagnosis. *J. Psychosom. Res.,* 1975, *19,* 69–79.

Author Index

Author Index   289

Baxter, J.D. 22, 31, *36, 52,*
Baylin, S.B. 130, *141*
Beaudet, A. 16, *50*
Bechtol, K.B. 7, *45,*
Beck, A.T. 266, *284*
Becker, F.F. 96, *134*
Beering, S.C. 61, *81*
Belenky, M.A. 16, *36*
Belovova, R.A. 180, 185, *203*
Benacerraf, B. 7, 8, 9, *36,* 213, *273*
Bendig, A.W. 266, *284*
Benfenati, F. 23, *35*
Bengtsson, M. 128, *134*
Benike, C.J. 9, *40*
Benjannet, S. 18, *38*
Ben-Jonathan, N. 20, *50*
Benner, R. 200, *203*
Bennett, A. 98, *134*
Bennett, J.M. 153, 154, *177*
Bennett, M.V.L. 20, *36*
Benson, H. 167, 173, *177*
Berczi, I. 111, *134*
Berebitsky, G.L. 71, *83*
Berger, D. 95, *145*
Berger, P. 68, *85*
Berghoffer, B. 128, 130, *136*
Bergland, R.M. 21, 22, *36, 49*
Bergmann, K. 2, *36*
Bernardino, E. 260, 264, *285*
Bernardis, L.L. 180. *206*
Bernstein, D.A. 160, *175*
Bernstein, I.L. 152, *175*
Berstein, I.M. 70, 74, 76, *82, 85*
Besedovsky, H.O. 10, 33, *36, 37,* 78, *81,* 95, 134, 180, 186, 189, 202, *204, 206*
Bezin, G.I. 180, 181, *204, 206*
Bhattacharyya, A.K. 77, *81,* 97, *135*
Bieliauskas, L.A. 101, 104, 106, 107, *135, 145*
Bielski, M. 96, *139*
Biozzi, G. 213, *223*
Birnbaumer, L. 31, *44*
Biryukov, V.D. 185, *206*

Bishop, J.M. 95, *135*
Bisset, G.W. 17, *37*
Biswas, C. 98, 128, *138*
Björklund, A. 15, 16, 23, *37, 46*
Black, P.H. 113, *135*
Blagosklonnaya, Y.V. 70, *82*
Blalock, J.E. 23, 25, 26, 33, 37, *54,* 247, *252, 254*
Blanchard, E.G. 153, 154, 155, *176*
Bleier, R. 20, *37*
Blichert-Toft, M. 64, *81*
Bliss, E.L. 67, *81*
Blizzard, P.T. 271, *286*
Block, B. 18, *38*
Blois, M.S. 263, 266, 267, 268, 269, *286, 287*
Blomgren, H. 192, 199, *203*
Bloom, F.E. 16, 19, 23, 25, 28, *37, 41, 48, 52,* 93, *138,* 227, 236, 247, *253, 255*
Bloor, F. 236, *254*
Blume, H. 22, *37*
Blume, H.W. 11, 14, 17, 18, 20, *50, 51*
Blumenfield, M. 61, *81*
Bobrov, Y.F. 70, *82*
Boccuzzi, G. 61, *81*
Bodner, W.F. 8, *48*
Bodwin, J.S. 128, 130, *136*
Bogerd, H. 96, *139*
Bohn, W.H. 94, 100, *145*
Bohus, B. 21, 22, 24, *37, 45,* 93, *137*
Bolles, R.C. 245, *253*
Booth, G. 208, *223*
Boraschi, P. 124, *135*
Borison, H.L. 167, *175*
Borkovec, T.D. 160, 167, *175*
Boros, L. 153, 154, *177*
Borysenko, J.(Z.) 101, 107, 108, 109, 127, *135,* 173, *177*
Borysenko, M. 109, *135*
Bottazzi, B. 124, *135*
Botticelli, L.J. 250, *253*
Bourne, H.R. 31, *37,* 67, *84*
Bovbjerg, D. 13, 34, *37, 38*
Bower, G.H. 244, 251, *252*

Boyd, M.R. 128, *135*
Boyd, S.C. 108, 125, *135, 144,* 259, 270, 272, 273, 274, 276, 277, 279, 282, 283, *285, 286*
Boyle, D.A. 117, 118, 119, 123, 126, *142*
Boyse, E.A. 218, *224*
Bozzone, J.M. 27, *48,* 227, 247, *255*
Brack, C. 8, *37*
Brady, J.V. 91, 93, *135*
Branceni, D. 110, *135*
Brand, K.G. 95, *135*
Brand, R.J. 262, *284, 286*
Braun, W. 31, *37*
Brawer, J.R. 16, 20, *37*
Breslow, A. 260, 264, *284*
Bresnick, E. 92, *135*
Brightman, M.W. 20, 29, *37, 38*
Briles, R.W. 92, *135*
Briles, W.E. 92, *135*
Briziarelli, G. 97, *139*
Broder, S. 26, *56*
Brooks, F. 127, *146*
Brooks, W.H. 3, 10, 11, *38, 39, 52*
Brown, D.M. 71, *82,*
Brown, G.M. 22, 44, 109, *137*
Brown, G.W. 105, *135*
Brown, M.L. 244, *254*
Brown, R. 106, 107, *140*
Brownstein, M.J. 16, 17, 18, 19, 22, *38, 40, 47*
Bruni, J.F. 23, *38,* 93, *146*
Brunner, K.T. 71, *82*
Bruno, S. 148, 157, *178*
Bruns, R.R. 98, 128, *138*
Bruto, V. 116, 121, *145*
Buch, C.W. 258, *286*
Buckingham, J.C. 67, *81*
Bugnon, C. 18, *38*
Bulbrook, R.D. 64, *81*
Bull, J.M.C. 92, 129, *135*
Bullock, K. 27, 33, *38*
Bunney, W.E. 67, *84,* 108, *144,* 259, 270, 272, 273, 274, 276, 277, 282, 283, *286*
Burchfield, S.R. 121, *135*

294 Author Index

Subject Index

in negative feedback, 22
and opioid peptides, 25–26
recognition sites on, 10
thymosin sensitivity of, 180
Lysosomes, 70, 71

Macrophage, 8, 26, 80, 227, 248
chemotaxis in, 32, 124
in humoral immunity, 179, 201
and metabolism, 70, 71, 73
in non-specific immunity, 114–115
stress effect on, 209, 21–218, 223
Major histocompatibility complex, 8–9
Malignancy. See Cancer; Neoplastic
processes; Tumor(s)
Mammary tumors, 96–98. See also Breast
cancer hormones in, 97–98
stress in, 222
Mast cells, 10, 11, 223
Medial forebrain bundle, 15, 16
Median eminence, 15–18, 20–21, 27, 34
α-Melanocyte-stimulating hormone
(MSH), 18, 23, 93
Melanoma, prognostic factors in, 259–284
Melanoma adjustment score, 270, 273,
283
Membranes, 5, 6, 28–32
degradation of, 125
plasma cell, 32, 74
receptor, 30
Memory
consolidation, 24
cyclic necleotides in, 31
immunologic, 5
short- and long-term, 3
Metabolic immunodepression, 59, 70–76,
79
Metabolism, 4, 91
glucocorticoid effect on, 179
in median eminence, 20
in various conditions, 59
Metastases, 98–100, 125
to brain, 95, 151
and decreased hormone sensitivity, 124
internal loop effects on, 129
in malignant melanoma, 260
specific immunity in, 115
Methionine-enkephalin
([Met]enkephalin), 18, 24, 25, 247
Methylcholanthrene, 96, 124, 125
Metyrapone (Metopirone), 11, 103, 246
Midbrain, 14, 16, 97

Migration ability, 180, 181
Mineralocorticoids, 111, 185, 188
Mitogen, See Concanavalin A;
Phytohemagglutinin
Monoamine, 19, 23, 67, 69. See also
Dopamine; Epinephrine;
Norepinephrine; Serotonin
Monocyte, 32, 73, 114, 115
glucocorticoids and, 195, 199, 201
Mood, 7, 69, 77, 259
Morphine, 244–245, 247, 250
Mortality, 274–281
Motivation, 7, 95, 243
MSH. See α-Melanocyte-stimulating
hormone
Muscle relaxation. See Relaxation
training
Mutations, 88, 95

Naloxone, 236, 237, 245, 247
Naltrexone, 236–237, 239, 247, 251
Natural killer cells, 110, 114–115, 248
in natural resistance, 227–228, 246–250
and readjustment, 12, 109
suppression of, 227
Natural resistance, 227–228
augmentation of, 237–242, 248–250
conditioning in, 252
effect of inescapable shock on,
229–232, 251
as internal loop effect, 86, 92, 97, 103,
114
natural killer cells in, 227–228, 248, 250
opiate antagonists in, 229, 236–237, 239
opponent processes in, 246–250
suppression of, 235–237, 248–250
Nausea, 148, 149
anticipatory, 150, 153
behavioral interventions for, 159–165
pharmacological interventions for,
157–158
Neo-endorphin, 19
Neoplastic processes, 6, 86–87, 88–89,
94–99. See also Cancer; Melanoma;
Tumor(s)
effect on host of, 94–95
and psychosocial factors, 132–133
Neostriatum, 16
Nervous system, 6–7, 28–30. See also
Central nervous system
autonomic, 7, 33, 217, 223
and glucocorticoid level, 186